Governing for Resilience in Vulnerable Places

Governing for Resilience in Vulnerable Places provides an overview and a critical analysis of the ways in which the concept 'resilience' has been addressed in social sciences research. In doing so, this edited book draws together state-of-the-art research from a variety of disciplines (i.e. spatial planning, economic and cultural geography, environmental and political sciences, sociology and architecture) as well as cases and examples across different spatial and geographical contexts (e.g. urban slums in India; flood-prone communities in the UK; coastal Japan). The cases present and explore challenges and potentials of resilience-thinking for practitioners and academics. As such, *Governing for Resilience in Vulnerable Places* aims to provide a scientifically robust overview and to generate some conceptual clarity for researchers, students and practitioners interested in the potential of resilience thinking as well as the application of resilience in practice.

Elen-Maarja Trell is Assistant Professor of Spatial Planning and Environment at the Faculty of Spatial Sciences, University of Groningen, The Netherlands. In 2014, she was the lead organizer of the international workshop 'Resilience: Just do it?! Governing for Resilience in Vulnerable Places' (with Britta Restemeyer, Melanie M. Bakema and Gwenda van der Vaart). She is interested in the role of local-level initiatives and public participation in creating more resilient and sustainable places. The themes she explores within this context include: community resilience in declining (rural) areas, flood resilience, urban food systems and gardening, and governance of renewable energy initiatives. In her previous projects, she has explored young people's place attachment and influential aspects for the well-being of rural youths in their everyday context.

Britta Restemeyer, MSc, is a lecturer and PhD researcher at the Faculty of Spatial Sciences, University of Groningen, The Netherlands. Her research focuses on resilience, adaptive governance and flood risk in urban areas. By studying the cases of Hamburg, London and Rotterdam, she explores how policy-makers deal with the tension between accepting uncertainties and providing security for people and businesses on a strategic as well as local level. Overall, she aims at informing policy strategies for creating more flood resilient cities, by improving the linkage between flood risk management and urban planning. In the past, she has participated in various German, as well as European, research projects (RIMAX, Climate Proof Areas, KLIFF, MARE) on climate change adaptation and flood risk.

Melanie M. Bakema, MSc, is a PhD researcher at the Faculty of Spatial Sciences, University of Groningen, The Netherlands and the Department of Earth and Environmental Sciences, University of Leuven, Belgium. In her PhD research, she focuses on resilience in the context of disasters. Her interest lies in disaster governance as a multi-level approach to overcome the social vacuum in disaster studies. Cases that she is investigating for her PhD research include Christchurch, New Zealand, Chiloé, Chile and the North of the Netherlands. By exploring the dynamic interactions between nature and societies in these cases, she aims at fostering transitions towards improved governance structures for creating more resilient social-ecological systems in the face of disasters.

Bettina van Hoven is Associate Professor of Cultural Geography at the Faculty of Spatial Sciences, University of Groningen, The Netherlands. Her recent research has concentrated on the feelings of belonging, the attachment of various population groups to the place where they live. In addition, she is researching community resilience and the role of arts practice and expression in building resilient communities in coastal areas. In the past, she has worked on projects involving: women in Eastern Europe, diaspora and migration, institutions, ethnicity, sexuality, disabilities, youth and nature. She is a member of the editorial board for 'Emotion, Space and Society' and has co-edited various publications in the past (e.g. den Toonder and van Hoven, 2012; van Hoven and Hoerschelmann, 2005).

Urban planning and environment
Series Editors: Donald Miller and Nicole Gurran

Maintaining and enhancing living conditions in cities through a combination of physical planning and environmental management is a newly emerging focus of governments around the world. For example, local governments seek to insulate sensitive land uses such as residential areas from environmentally intrusive activities such as major transport facilities and manufacturing. Regional governments protect water quality and natural habitat by enforcing pollution controls and regulating the location of growth. Some national governments fund acquisition of strategically important sites, facilitate the renewal of brownfields, and even develop integrated environmental quality plans. The aim of this series is to share information on experiments and best practices of governments at several levels. These empirically-based studies present and critically assess a variety of initiatives to improve environmental quality. Although institutional and cultural contexts vary, lessons from one commonly can provide useful ideas to other communities. Each of the contributions is independently peer reviewed, and are intended to be helpful to professional planners and environmental managers, elected officials, representatives of NGOs, and researchers seeking improved ways to resolve environmental problems in urban areas and to foster sustainable urban development.

Titles in the series:

Urban sprawl in Western-Europe and the United States
Chang-Hee Christine Bae and Harry W. Richardson

Integrating city planning and environmental improvement
Practicable Strategies for Sustainable Urban Development, 2nd Edition
Gert de Roo
Edited by Donald Miller

Nordic experiences of sustainable planning
Policy and Practice
Edited by Sigríður Kristjánsdóttir

Governing for Resilience in Vulnerable Places

Edited by Elen-Maarja Trell, Britta Restemeyer, Melanie M. Bakema and Bettina van Hoven

Routledge
Taylor & Francis Group
LONDON AND NEW YORK

First published 2018
by Routledge
2 Park Square, Milton Park, Abingdon, Oxon OX14 4RN

and by Routledge
711 Third Avenue, New York, NY 10017

Routledge is an imprint of the Taylor & Francis Group, an informa business

British Library Cataloguing-in-Publication Data
A catalogue record for this book is available from the British Library

Library of Congress Cataloguing-in-Publication Data
A catalog record for this book has been requested

ISBN: 978-1-138-21649-5 (hbk)
ISBN: 978-1-315-10376-1 (ebk)

Typeset in Sabon
by codeMantra

Contents

Figures and tables

Figures

Tables

Information on contributing authors

Dr Deepika Andavarapu received her PhD in Regional Development Planning program at University of Cincinnati. Her doctoral dissertation is based on an ethnographic research on a slum in Visakhapatnam, India. Prior to starting her academic career, Deepika worked as an urban planner in public and private sectors for over six years. She is currently exploring gender issues in the use of public spaces in the context of an urban slum in India.

Prof Mahyar Arefi is affiliated with the University of Cincinnati and received his PhD in planning from the University of Southern California. He is the recipient of different awards and scholarships including the U.S. HUD doctoral dissertation award (1999), Goody Clancy's Summer Faculty Fellowship (2005) in Boston, and the Fulbright fellowship in Turkey (2006) where he explored the concept of placemaking. His publications have appeared in edited volumes including the Companion to Urban Design (Routledge, 2011), the Routledge Handbook of Planning Research Methods (2015), and journals including Journal of Planning Education and Research, Cities, Town Planning Review, Built Environment, and Planning Practice and Research. His latest book Deconstructing Placemaking: Needs, Opportunities and Assets was published by Routledge in 2014.

Melanie M. Bakema, MSc, is a PhD researcher at the Faculty of Spatial Sciences, University of Groningen. In her PhD research, she focuses on resilience in the context of disasters. Her interest lies in disaster governance as a multi-level approach to overcome the social vacuum in disaster studies. Cases that she is investigating for her PhD research include Christchurch, New Zealand, Chiloé, Chile and the North of the Netherlands. By exploring the dynamic interactions between nature and societies in these cases, she aims at fostering transitions towards improved governance structures for creating more resilient social-ecological systems in the face of disasters.

Jessica de Boer, MA, is a PhD researcher at the Faculty of Spatial Sciences, University of Groningen. With a background in public administration (University of Twente) and artscience (Royal Academy of Arts), De Boer is interested in the practical application of theoretical concepts and ideas. For her PhD research, she developed an area-based approach to study the transition towards a sustainable energy system. Her approach combines insights from research on multilevel governance, complex systems and area-based planning. By analysing the interaction of local energy initiatives with the landscape in physical, socio-economic and institutional senses, she explores the interdependence of the energy system with the landscape. She participated in projects on decentralised energy systems (MACREDES) and decentralised energy landscapes (DELaND).

Sage Brice, MSc, entwines a lively contemporary art practice with doctoral studies in Cultural Geography at the University of Bristol. Previous academic experience includes Environmental Art (BA *hons*, Glasgow School of Art, 2006) and Human Geography (MSc with distinction, University of Bristol, 2015). Her practice-led doctoral research is on the intersection of human and nonhuman animal cultures, as mobilised in the figure of the common crane (*Grus grus*) at two wetland sites. Recent exhibitions include *The Power of the Sea* (Royal West of England Academy) and *The Water Knows All My Secrets* (Pratt Manhattan Gallery). She is currently working with Seila Fernández Arconada on *Some:when*, a socially-engaged project in Somerset, UK, supported by a grant from the Somerset Community Foundation.

Prof Simin Davoudi is Director of Global Urban Research Unit (GURU) at School of Architecture, Planning and Landscape and Associate Director of Newcastle University Institute for Sustainability. She is past President of the Association of the European Schools of Planning (AESOP); Fellow of the Academy of Social Sciences and Fellow of the Royal Society of Arts. She led the UK Office of Deputy Prime Minister's Planning Research Network; was a member of expert panels for: 3 UK government departments (DCLG, DECC and DEFRA), 2 EU Directorate Generals (Environment and Regional Policy), the ESRC Grant Assessment Panel, Research Excellence Framework (REF), and several European research councils; held visiting professorships at the universities of: Amsterdam and Nijmegen (Netherlands), Karlskrona (Sweden), Tampere (Finland), Virginia Tech (USA) and RMIT (Australia) and served on several advisory councils (including Hong Kong University); is co-Editor of the *Journal of Environmental Planning and Management*. Her research on urban planning, environmental governance, climate change and resilience is published widely. Selected books include: *Justice and Fairness in the City* (2016, Policy Press), *Town and Country Planning in the UK* (2015, Routledge), *Reconsidering Localism* (2015, Routledge), *Climate*

Change and Sustainable Cities (Routledge, 2014), *Conceptions of Space and Place in Strategic Spatial Planning* (Routledge, 2009), *Planning for Climate Change* (Earthscan, 2009), *Planning Governance and Spatial Strategy in Britain* (Macmillan, 2000).

Seila Fernández Arconada is an independent artist-researcher currently working on a number of projects including *The Land of the Summer People* (with the Water Engineering Department, Bristol University, funded by EPSRC) and *Some:when*, a socially-engaged project in collaboration with the artist Sage Brice. Her academic experience includes BA-MA Fine Art (with distinction, University of the Basque Country, 2009) and MA Fine Art (with distinction, UWE, 2012). Seila has delivered numerous cross-disciplinary workshops and interventions including *Transnational Dialogues*, *AGU Fall Meeting*, *On Earth* and *UkraineLab: Communities Development in (Post-) Crisis Regions*. She has exhibited internationally, recently at *Imagined Landscapes* at the Royal West of England Academy. Her work focuses on exploring artistic methodology, its boundaries and new approaches.

Steven Forrest, MA, is a PhD researcher at the Faculty of Spatial Sciences, University of Groningen. His PhD research focuses on flood resilience at the local level in the UK and the Netherlands. Steven is particularly interested in the role that communities play in flood resilience and their associated influences on local governance arrangements. The distribution of flood risk and resources, power relations between actors, and justice appear prominently in his research. Understanding the local level in this way can benefit attempts to improve flood resilience in the face of predicted climate change-induced increases in flooding. Prior to his PhD, Steven worked as a consultant at Collingwood Environmental Planning (London) where he focused on flood resilience, climate change and energy projects.

Kevin Gooley, MSc, is an urban sustainability advocate based out of Portland, Oregon. Through his educational and professional background, he has become engaged in grassroots efforts to ecologically balanced living, environmental protection, social justice and community-built resilience. He is currently a writer for the urban planning and design website The Global Grid (www.theglobalgrid.org) focusing on stories based out of the Portland, Oregon area.

Dr Kevin Grecksch is a postdoctoral researcher at the Centre for Socio-Legal Studies (CSLS), University of Oxford. He is a social scientist who specialises in water governance and climate change adaptation. His research interests include water governance, climate change adaptation, governance of societal transformation, property rights and natural resources and ecological economics. His current work focusses on drought and water scarcity in the UK, where he is reviewing and analysing drought management options. His previous projects focussed on climate change adaptation, sustainable bioenergy supply chains and marine energy potentials. Kevin's case study experience includes Germany, South Africa, the UK and the Netherlands. Kevin is also a Research Fellow of the Earth System Governance Project.

Dr Thomas Hartmann is Assistant Professor of Human Geography and Spatial Planning at Utrecht University; he is also affiliated with the Czech UJEP University in Ústí nad Labem. His special expertise is on land and water governance, with a specific focus on land policy for flood risk management. Beyond this field, he is an expert in land policies and planning instruments as well as in planning theory. Thomas Hartmann is one of the initiators of the network FLOODLAND (www.floodland.org), vice-president of the International Academic Association on Planning, Law, and Property Rights (www.plpr-association.org), speaker of the board of the German Flood Competence Centre (www.hkc-online.de) and member of the OECD water governance initiative. He speaks English, German, and Dutch.

Dr Bettina van Hoven is Associate Professor of Cultural Geography at the Faculty of Spatial Sciences, University of Groningen. Her recent research has concentrated on the feelings of belonging, the attachment of various population groups to the place where they live. In addition, she is researching community resilience and the role of arts practice and expression in building resilient communities in coastal areas. In the past, she has worked on projects on: women in Eastern Europe, diaspora and migration, institutions, ethnicity, sexuality, disabilities, youth and nature. She is a member of the editorial board for 'Emotion, Space and Society' and has co-edited various publications in the past (e.g. den Toonder and van Hoven, 2012; van Hoven and Hoerschelmann, 2005).

Prof Paulus P. P. Huigen is Professor of Cultural Geography at the Faculty of Spatial Sciences, University of Groningen, the Netherlands.

Prof Catherine Leyshon is Associate Professor of Human Geography in the Centre for Geography, Environment and Society at the University of Exeter's Penryn Campus. Her background is as a cultural geographer with an interest in sense of place, identity, and landscape. Catherine has written widely on the importance of local and familiar landscapes in understanding climate and environmental change, place as inspiration, sense of place, individual and community resilience, wellbeing, and environmental volunteering. Catherine's work is characterised by a strong commitment to co-production within a range of research networks and knowledge exchange partnerships with, *inter alia*; Natural England, the National Trust, Cornwall's Area of Outstanding Natural Beauty, the NHS, Cornwall Council, Age UK, and Volunteer Cornwall.

Malka Older is a PhD candidate at the Centre de Sociologie des Organisations of Institut d'Études Politiques (Sciences Po). Named Senior Fellow for Technology and Risk at the Carnegie Council for Ethics in International Affairs for 2015, she has more than a decade of experience in humanitarian aid and development. Her doctoral work explores the dynamics of multi-level governance and disaster response using the cases of Hurricane Katrina and the Japan tsunami of 2011. Her other research interests include the paradox of well-funded disaster responses and the effects of competition among actors in humanitarian aid. She has also conducted research for the Institut de Radioprotection et de Sûreté Nucléaire (IRSN) on human and organizational factors of the Fukushima Daiichi crisis.

Henk Ovink is a special envoy for International Water Affairs of the Kingdom of the Netherlands. Henk Ovink was appointed by the Dutch Cabinet as the first Special Envoy for International Water Affairs (2015). As the Ambassador for Water, he is responsible for advocating water awareness around the world, focusing on building institutional capacity and coalitions among governments, multilateral organizations, private sector and NGO's to address the world's urgent needs with regards to water and help initiate transformative interventions. Ovink is also Sherpa to the High-Level Panel on Water, installed by UNSG Ban Ki-Moon and President of the World Bank Jim Kim and including ten Heads of State / Government to catalyse change in water awareness and implementation. Henk is Principal for Rebuild by Design, the resilience innovation competition he developed and led for President Obama's Hurricane Sandy Rebuilding Task Force where he was Senior Advisor to the Chair. He has been Director General for Planning and Water Affairs and Director for National Spatial Planning in The Netherlands. Ovink teaches at the London School of Economics and at Harvard GSD and is member of the International Advisory Board for the City of Rotterdam. He was Curator for the 5th International Architecture Biennale Rotterdam 2012 'Making City', and curated the debate series 'Design and Politics: the next phase' for Aedes network Campus Berlin. He initiated the research program and is chief editor of the series of publications with nai010 Publishers on Design and Politics.

Dr Stephen Platt is a director of Cambridge Architectural Research and was its Chairman from 2001 to 2016. He is a social anthologist with higher degrees in engineering and architecture. His main research interest is in developing indicators and modelling disaster resilience and recovery. Over the past eight years, he has been studying socio-economic, planning and governance issues in post-disaster recovery following disasters in the USA, Pakistan, Thailand, Chile, Italy, New Zealand, Japan, China, Turkey and Iran. His other research interests include managing urban growth and change, and stakeholder and community involvement in strategic decision-making. He is currently working on tropical cyclone preparedness and recovery in the tourist sector in South-East Asia.

Britta Restemeyer, MSc, is a lecturer and PhD researcher at the Faculty of Spatial Sciences, University of Groningen. Her research focuses on resilience, adaptive governance and flood risk in urban areas. By studying the cases of Hamburg, London and Rotterdam, she explores how policy-makers deal with the tension between accepting uncertainties and providing security for people and businesses on a strategic as well as local level. Overall, she aims at informing policy strategies for creating more flood resilient cities, by improving the linkage between flood risk management and urban planning. In the past, she has participated in various German as well as European research projects (RIMAX, Climate Proof Areas, KLIFF, MARE) on climate change adaptation and flood risk.

Tom Scholten, MSc, works at Ministry for Infrastructure and the Environment and at the regional water board Vallei and Veluwe (Waterschap Vallei en Veluwe) as water trainee, where he is involved in water practice but also publications on water issues. In addition, he is an external PhD researcher at the Faculty of Geosciences, Utrecht University. His research focuses on the governance on frontiers of water and land. By studying cases in the Netherlands, he explores possibilities of governance arrangements for differentiation of integrative governance approaches of water and land. His interest lies in both water management and spatial planning.

Dr Elen-Maarja Trell is Assistant Professor of Spatial Planning and Environment at the Faculty of Spatial Sciences, University of Groningen. In 2014, she was the lead organizer of the international workshop 'Resilience: Just do it?! Governing for Resilience in Vulnerable Places' (with Britta Restemeyer, Melanie Bakema, Gwenda van der Vaart). She is interested in the role of local level initiatives and public participation in creating more resilient and sustainable places. The themes she explores within this context include: community resilience in declining (rural) areas, flood resilience, urban food systems and gardening, and governance of renewable energy initiatives. In her previous projects, she has explored young people's place attachment and influential aspects for the well-being of rural youths in their everyday context.

Gwenda van der Vaart, MSc, is a PhD researcher at the Faculty of Spatial Sciences, University of Groningen. In her PhD, Gwenda focuses on the role of the arts in community resilience. Her PhD research consists of a case study in the Dutch Wadden area, in which a participatory approach relying on art-based methods is adopted. In 2014, she was co-organizer of the international workshop 'Resilience: Just do it?! Governing for Resilience in Vulnerable Places' (with Elen-Maarja Trell, Britta Restemeyer, Melanie Bakema). During the workshop, she chaired the track 'the social side of resilience'.

Dr Tim Walker is a research associate in the Centre for Geography, Environment and Society at the University of Exeter's Penryn Campus. His PhD research focused on the process of catchment management; specifically, the seemingly intractable problem of managing diffuse water pollution risk in Cornwall. By thinking through risk relationally this research provided new insights into the practice of catchment management and the socio-cultural geographies around the water-environment. Methodologically Tim's work is underpinned by the principles and practice of Participatory Action Research. As such Tim works closely with local agencies such as Natural England, Environment Agency, National Trust, and Cornwall Wildlife Trust *inter alia*.

Dr Maik Winges currently works for the Deutsche Gesellschaft für Internationale Zusammenarbeit (GIZ) GmbH as adviser to the Eastern Cape Department of Economic Development, Environmental Affairs and Tourism. His work aims at improving resource-efficiency in the manufacturing sector in South Africa's Eastern Cape via easily applicable environmental management approaches. Before joining GIZ, Maik was a PhD candidate and post-doctoral researcher at the Carl von Ossietzky Universität Oldenburg and his research focused on social aspects of climate change adaptation, regional planning, (multi-level) governance, corporate environmental policy, sustainability, and development studies. Maik studied political science, economics, and modern history (MA) at the Friedrich-Schiller-Universität Jena and the Matej Bel University Banská Bystrica (Slovakia).

Prof Johan Woltjer is Professor of Urban Infrastructures and Head of Department at the University of Westminster, UK. He also is an Honorary Professor at the University of Groningen and a Visiting Professor at the University of Reading. Johan Woltjer focuses on water and infrastructure development and urban planning. He contributes an internationally comparative view to policy design for urban planning, particularly focusing on the UK, Europe and Asia. The impact of his work is visible through funded projects and publications on urban governance, regional development, infrastructure development, water management, policy evaluation, and capacity building, appearing in high-impact journals. Recent books are 'Place-Based Evaluation for Infrastructure and Spatial Projects (Ashgate)', and 'Evaluation for Participation and Sustainability in Planning' (Routledge).

Dr Christian Zuidema is Assistant Professor in Spatial Planning at the Department of Spatial Planning and Environment, Faculty of Spatial Sciences, University of Groningen. Zuidema has a background in environmental planning and has done extensive research on topics such as sustainable urban management, energy landscapes and governance renewal in environmental planning. His studies have focused on developments in the Netherlands and the EU. His teaching addresses courses on themes such as environmental planning and sustainable development. Following his research, he has published various books, such as Stimulating Local Environmental Policy (2011), Decentralization in Environmental Governance (2016) and, as co-author, Smart Methods for Environmental Externalities (2012). Furthermore, he is board-member of the International Urban Planning and Environment Association.

Acknowledgements

This edited collection is inspired by and draws on the international workshop *'Resilience: Just do it?! Governing for resilience in vulnerable places'* organized by the *Groningen Resilience Research Group* in Groningen, the Netherlands in October 2014. The editors would like to thank the workshop participants, the researchers as well as practitioners, for inspiring discussions about the potential of resilience thinking for both theory and practice. The editors would also like to thank the Netherlands Graduate School of Urban and Regional Research (NETHUR); the RGS Planning and Environment Research Group (PERG); Sustainable Society (University of Groningen); and the Department of Spatial Planning and Environment (University of Groningen) for the financial support for organizing the international workshop. The editors are grateful to Natasja Nienhuis for providing the photo for the cover and to Madison for agreeing to be our cover-girl. We would also like to acknowledge all our authors for their hard work on each individual chapter and for sticking with us throughout the process. The editors are extremely grateful to professor Simin Davoudi for kindly agreeing to write a critical reflection about resilience based on her extensive research and engagement with the concept as well as to Henk Ovink for sharing his international experiences and insights for the ways resilience could be used in practice.

Finally, we would like to thank the external reviewers of each chapter who, with their critical and constructive insights, helped to increase the quality of this edited collection:

Prof Angie Hart
Anna Martini, MSc
Prof Arjan van Timmeren
Dr Arjan Wardekker
Dr Becky Heaver
Dr Caroline McDonald-Harker
Claudiu Forgaci, MSc
Dr Constanza Parra
Dr Daniela Perrotti

Dr Elizabeth Maly
Dr Emmanuel Raju
Dr Erick Mas
Dr Hannah MacPherson
Prof Iain White
Prof Johan Woltjer
Prof John Handmer
Dr Margo van den Brink
Dr Martin Zebracki
Prof Philip McCann
Dr Richard Sliuzas
Dr Sander Meijerink
Dr Tim Haney

1 Self-reliant resiliency and neoliberal mentality

A critical reflection

Simin Davoudi

Forget sustainability. It's about resilience

—(Zolli, 2012)

The above headline in a *New York Times* article is an indication of the extent to which resilience has side-lined sustainability in political agendas, popular imaginations and academic writings. The academic literature on resilience, which has shown a steep rise in the last decade, ranges from engineering and ecology to economics, socio-technical studies, public policy theories, disaster management, climate change adaptation and urban planning. Seeking resilience has become a global agenda involving international institutions and public and private organisations. These have developed a growing array of evaluation frameworks and indicators to assess the resilience of cities and communities in the face of a multitude of uncertainties from financial crises, to extreme weather events and terrorist attacks. For example, the United Nations Office for Disaster Risk Reduction launched a campaign in 2012 on *How to Make Cities More Resilient.* In the same year, the World Bank published guidance on *Building Urban Resilience in East Asia.* Building on its 2008 *Asian Cities Climate Change Resilience Network*, the Rockefeller Foundation launched its much-publicised campaign for *100 Resilient Cities* in 2013 to help "cities around the world become more resilient to the physical, social and economic challenges that are a growing part of the 21st-century" (Rockefeller Foundation, 2014, no page number). Working with major consultancy firms such as Arup, the Foundation has also developed a toolkit for making cities more resilient.

Multiple meanings of resilience

Despite this rising popularity, resilience remains a contested concept with multiple meanings. It has been framed as persistence, adaptation and transformation. Persistence is one of the oldest definitions of resilience used by physical scientists and engineers to denote the capacity of systems to withstand external shocks and to 'bounce-back' to the original stable equilibrium. According to this *engineering resilience*, "the resistance to disturbance and the speed by which the system" snaps back are "the measures of resilience," (Davoudi, 2012, p. 300). Defining resilience as adaptation was pioneered by the work of Buzz Holling in the field of ecology. He suggested that "Resilience ... is a measure of the ability of these systems to absorb changes [...] and still persist" (Holling, 1973, p. 17). He later called this *ecological resilience* and defined it as "the *magnitude* of the disturbance that can be absorbed before the system changes its structure" (Holling, 1996, p. 33). In this perspective, the measure of resilience is "not just *how long* it takes for the system to bounce back, but also *how much* disturbance it can take and stays within critical thresholds" (Davoudi, 2012, p. 300). These two understandings of resilience share a common view based on the existence of a stable equilibrium in complex systems, "be it a pre-existing one to which a resilient system *bounces back* (engineering) or a new one to which it *bounces forth* (ecological)" (Davoudi, 2012, p. 301).

The idea of a stable equilibrium is rooted in Newtonian mechanical understanding of how the world works. This has been challenged by the complexity theory that considers systems as "complex, non-linear, and self-organising, permeated by uncertainty and discontinuities" (Berkes and Folke, 1998, p. 12). New approaches to resilience including the more recent work by Holling and his fellow ecologists in the Resilience Alliance use the term socio-ecological resilience to "advocate that the very nature of systems may change over time with or without an external disturbance" (Davoudi, 2012, p. 302). Some scholars have used the term 'evolutionary resilience' (Simmie and Martin, 2010; Davoudi, 2012; Davoudi *et al.*, 2013) suggesting that evolutionary resilience is not about a return to normality, but about "the ability of complex socio-ecological systems to change, adapt, and crucially, transform in response to stresses and strains" (Davoudi, 2012, p. 302, drawing on Carpenter *et al.*, 2005). Here, the emphasis is on transformation, and on breaking away from undesirable 'normal'.

From ecology to society

The evolutionary conceptualisation of resilience is now advocated by the Resilience Alliance as a *general* systems theory which can integrate society, economy and ecology. Hence, the notion of resilience has been extended beyond its engineering and ecological roots into the realm of society. This 'total complex system' is often dubbed as 'Panarchy' and defined as:

> the structure in which systems, including those of nature (e.g. forests) and of humans (e.g. capitalism), as well as combined human-natural systems (e.g. institutions that govern natural resources use such as the Forest Service), are interlinked in continual adaptive cycles of growth, accumulation, restructuring, and renewal.
>
> (Gunderson and Holling, 2002, cover text)

In this Panarchy model, systems function in a series of nested adaptive cycles that interact at multiple scales, speeds and timeframes. This means that, "small-scale changes [...] can amplify and cascade into major shifts (reflecting Edward Lorenz's idea of 'the butterfly effect') while large interventions may have little or no effects" (Davoudi, 2012, p. 303). Therefore, "past behaviour of the system is no longer a reliable predictor of future behaviour even when circumstances are similar" (Duit *et al.*, 2010, p. 367).

As I have suggested elsewhere, "the significance of Holling's work lies in his departure from Newtonian and mechanistic assertions of equilibrium – typical of the post-war cybernetics and closed systems theory – and his adoption of complexity science in the field of ecology" (Davoudi, 2016, p. 156). Given the unknowability of contingent outcomes, it is argued that there is a need for "a qualitative capacity to devise systems that can absorb and accommodate future events in whatever unexpected form they may take" (Holling, 1973, p. 21). Evolutionary resilience is a great step forward in systems thinking but when it is applied to the social context it is conceptually problematic and normatively contested. Conceptually, it is problematic because it overlooks human agency which is manifested in our ability to displace the effects of a crisis in time and space; the unequal distribution of power which can disrupt channels of communications and feedbacks; our ability to imagine and perceive "changes at a larger scale and longer term than our sensory abilities and immediate experience allow" and put in place mitigating measures; and our capacity to undertake organised collective action (Davidson, 2010, p. 1114). It is normatively contested because it raises questions of justice, fairness and inclusion depending on how it is interpreted as discussed below.

Self-reliance and neoliberal mentalities

The overemphasis on self-reliance, which is a misguided translation of self-organisation in complex systems, resonates closely with the neoliberal mentality and its emphasis on individualisation of responsibility (Davoudi and Madanipour, 2015). Indeed, it is this ideological fit with neoliberal mentality which has made resilience a favourable concept in public policy (Davoudi, 2016). Self-reliance implies that people and places should "pull themselves up by their bootstraps and reinvent themselves in the face of external challenges" (Swanstrom, 2008, p. 10). This means that to build resilience, the public sector should leave people and places to their own devices and resist supporting them. Officials claim that "if the government takes greater responsibility for risks in the community, it may feel under pressure to take increasingly more responsibility, thereby eroding community resilience" (RRAC, 2009, p. 6). The principle of self-organization, extracted from the complexity theory, offers a convenient match with both liberal understanding of responsibility and the freedom from the state intervention as well as the conservative value of self-help. Furthermore, it creates a contingently shared platform with communitarian's advocacy of self-sufficiency as an alternative to global capitalism. Such an alignment makes resilience a powerful discourse in which self-reliance is cast as "a common sense, neutral and universal measure of the resilient self; one that a responsible citizen should aspire to in the face of radical uncertainties" (Davoudi, 2016, p. 162). The move from the welfare to neoliberal modes of government in the late 1970s has been coupled with the liberal advocacy of individual responsibility which above all is aimed at entrepreneurship.

The intuitive fit between this interpretation of resilience and neoliberal values is not coincidental. According to Walker and Cooper (2011), the ideas that influenced Holling's ecological resilience run in parallel with the birth of neoliberalism. In the 1970s, when Holling was working on his ecological resilience, Friedrich Hayek was developing his theory of "spontaneous order". Similar to the idea of self-organization, this theory asserts that social order emerges from the interaction of self-serving individuals who rationally utilize the price systems to adjust their plans (Hayek, 1976). Like Holling, Hayek drew on complex systems theory to criticise "the state-engineered equilibria of Keynesian demand management" and called for the reform of "all social institutions in accordance with the self-organizing dynamic of the market" (Walker and Cooper, 2011, p. 149) which, he believed, could better maintain social order.

The overemphasis on self-reliance overlaps with the liberal view of society and the place of the individual within it. As Norberto Bobbio (1990, p. 43) put it, 'liberal individualism' "amputates the individual from the organic body ... plunges him into the unknown and perilous world of the struggle for survival". He distinguishes this from 'democratic individualism' which "joins the individual together once more with others like himself, so that society can be built up again from their union, no longer as an organic whole but as an association of free individuals" (ibid). The appropriation of resilience by the neoliberal agenda has turned the concept into a measure of the fitness of people and places to survive in the turbulent world; reiterating "the Darwinian law of natural selection and its interpretation as the survival of the fittest" (Davoudi, 2016, p. 164). It is claimed that "resilience, seen as an innate capacity of the biological species will diminish if people are exposed too much to dependency-inducing state welfare" (Davoudi, 2016, p. 163). Self-reliance is prescribed as a primary measure of resilience and a key "existential yardstick" (Rorty, 1999). It reproduces the wider process of "*existential politics*" by which "selective meanings and understanding of human subjectivity" are identified and institutionalized (Raco, 2009, p. 437, original emphasis). Living with threat, insecurity and vulnerability and standing on our own two feet is what the neoliberal interpretation of resilience is advocating. People are, therefore, expected to "carry the weight of the world on their shoulders" and become "responsible for themselves as a way of being" (Sartre, 1957, p. 51). Such a view has major implications for social democratic values of social justice, solidarity and inclusion. There is a danger in accepting resilience as a universally 'good' idea to promote and to which everyone should subscribe.

To avoid the pitfalls of resilience building ideas and activities, we should question their intended outcomes and ask: resilience for whom, "resilience from what to what, and who gets to decide?" (Porter and Davoudi, 2012, p. 331). If resilience is a "buffer capacity for preserving what we have and recovering to where we were" (Folke *et al.*, 2010, p. 20), we need to ask: is what we have a desirable condition that is worth preserving and returning to? Or, should we seek an alternative, more desirable path to move towards. We also need to be mindful of how 'desirable' is defined and by whom? Democratic procedures and inclusive decision making are, therefore, critical for ensuring that the outcome of resilience building is not prescribed by a few and applied to all.

Evolutionary resilience reflects a paradigm shift in science where nothing is certain except uncertainty itself. However, contrary to its dominant interpretation, the existence of uncertainty does not justify the acceptance of the status quo or inaction, because complexity and uncertainty provide the opportunity for trying an untried beginning. The contributions to this book provide a rich array of case study examples that demonstrate the opportunities and pitfalls of resilience building. They highlight the transformative potentials of resilience thinking, while at the same time unearthing the challenges of operationalising a concept which carries multiple meanings and risks being co-opted into the dominant neoliberal agendas. I share both the editors' enthusiasm for the opportunities which might arise from the application of resilience thinking in vulnerable places and their cautions about its potential challenges.

References

Berkes, F. and Folke, C. (eds.) (1998) *Linking Social and Ecological Systems: Management Practices and Social Mechanisms for Building Resilience*, Cambridge: Cambridge University Press.

Bobbio, N. (1990) *Liberalism and Democracy*, London: Verso.

Carpenter, S. R., Westley, F. and Turner, G. (2005) Surrogates for resilience of social-ecological systems, *Ecosystems*, 8(8): 941–944.

Davidson, D. J. (2010) The applicability of the concept of resilience to social systems: Some sources of optimism and nagging doubts, *Society and Natural Resources*, 23(12): 1135–1149.

Davoudi, S. (2012) Resilience: "A bridging concept or a dead end?", *Planning Theory and Practice*, 13(2): 299–307.

Davoudi, S. (2016) Resilience and the governmentality of unknowns, in M. Bevir (ed.) *Governmentality after Neoliberalism*, New York: Routledge.

Davoudi, S., Brooks, E. and Mehmood, A. (2013) Evolutionary resilience and strategies for climate adaptation, *Planning Practice and Research*, 28(3): 307–322.

Davoudi, S. and Madanipour, A. (2015) Localism and post-social governmentality, in S. Davoudi and A. Madanipour (eds.) *Reconsidering Localism*, London: Routledge, 77–103.

Duit, A., Galaza, V., Eckerberga, K. and Ebbessona, J. (2010) Governance, complexity, and resilience, *Global Environmental Change*, 20(3): 363–368.

Folke, C., Carpenter, S., Walker, B., Scheffer, M., Chapin, T. and Rockstrom, J. (2010) Resilience thinking: Integrating resilience, adaptability and transformability, *Ecology and Society*, 15(4): 20–28.

Gunderson, L. H. and Holling, C. S. (2002) *Panarchy: Understanding Transformations in Human and Natural Systems*, Washington, DC: Island Press.

Hayek, F. A. (1976) *Law, Legislation and Liberty, The Mirage of Social Justice*, Vol. 2, London: Routledge and Kegan Paul.

Holling, C. S. (1973) Resilience and stability of ecological systems, *Annual Review of Ecological Systems*, 4: 1–23.

Holling, C. S. (1996) Engineering resileince versus ecological resilience, in Schulze, P.C. (ed.) *Engineering within Ecological Constraints*, Washington, DC: National Academy Press.

Porter, L. and Davoudi, S. (2012) The politics of resilience for planning: A cautionary note, *Planning Theory and Practice*, 13(2): 329–333.

Raco, M. (2009) From expectations to aspirations: State modernisation, urban policy and the existential politics of welfare in the UK, *Political Geography*, 28: 436–444.

The Rockefeller Foundation (2014) *The 2013 Annual Report*, New York: The Rockefeller Foundation.

Rorty, R. (1999) *Philosophy and Social Hope*, London: Penguin.

RRAC (Risk & Regulation Advisory Council) (2009) *Building Resilient Communities, from Ideas to Sustainable Action*, London: RRAC.

Sartre, J. P. (1957) *Existentialism and Human Emotions*, New York: Wisdom Library.

Simmie, J. and Martin, R. (2010) The economic resilience of regions: Towards an evolutionary approach, *Cambridge Journal of the Regions, Economy and Society*, 3(1): 27–43.

Swanstrom, T. (2008) *Regional Resilience: A Critical Examination of the Ecological Framework, IURD Working Paper Series*, Berkeley, CA: Institute of Urban and Regional Development, UC Berkeley.

Walker, J. and Cooper, M. (2011) Genealogies of resilience: From systems ecology to the political economy of crisis adaptation, *Security Dialogue*, 42(2): 143–160.

Zolli, A. (2012) Learning to Bounce Back, *The New York Times*, 2nd November, available at: www.nytimes.com/2012/11/03/opinion/forget-sustainability-its-about-resilience.html?_r=0 (Accessed on 16 January 2016).

2 Governing for resilience in vulnerable places

An introduction

Elen-Maarja Trell, Britta Restemeyer, Melanie M. Bakema and Bettina van Hoven

In the past decades, the term 'resilience' has quickly gained currency in academia (including social, political and spatial sciences) as well as in practice. Nowadays, it is widely promoted as a promising concept to deal with shocks and uncertainties in the face of environmental, social and economic crises (cf. Davoudi, 2012; White, 2010). Originating in ecology, resilience was referred to as the ability of a system to return to stability or equilibrium after a disturbance (Pickett et al., 2004). According to an early formulation by Holling (1973), resilience indicates the ability of ecosystems to absorb changes and still be able to function properly. In the past decade, a so-called 'resilience turn' (Evans & Reid, 2014) has taken place in the social, political and spatial sciences where social-ecological resilience has been explored and applied as a useful concept to describe and organize responses to change by communities, institutions and economies (Adger, 2000; Klein et al., 2004; White, 2010). In spatial planning, for example, resilience is now widely acknowledged as a new approach to incorporate uncertainty into governance strategies, particularly with respect to natural hazards such as flooding (Davoudi, 2012; White, 2010).

Translating and applying the concept of resilience from its ecological and engineering roots to social sciences, however, remains a challenge. It is not surprising then that, due to the ambiguity of the concept 'resilience', research has largely focused on exploring the meaning of the concept (cf. Alexander, 2013; Davoudi, 2012; Pendall et al., 2010). However, there remains 'an apparent gap between the advocacy of socio-ecological resilience in the scientific literature and its take-up as a policy discourse on the one hand, and the demonstrated capacity to govern for resilience in practice on the other' (Wilkinson, 2012, p. 319). Current practices show that resilience is often used as a panacea to different problems (O'Hare & White, 2013). In some cases, 'resilience' might simply be a means to redress a problem and to justify an outdated or inherently unjust policy. In other cases, resilience may be so vague and far removed from its meaning that a so-called 'resilience approach' may lead to less desirable, not nearly resilient, outcomes (van der Vaart et al., 2015). The term 'resilience' therefore runs the risk of becoming a heavily contested buzzword.

As a result, there is a need for a better understanding of the potential and the challenges connected to the use of the concept of resilience in social sciences today. While an increasing number of books on resilience has been published in the past decade, the bulk of the books has focused on rather specific topics such as disasters (Comfort et al., 2010; Hicks Masterson et al., 2014; Lansford et al., 2016; Tidball & Krasny,2014; Tierney, 2014), climate change (Pelling, 2003,2011), water (White, 2010), or on one distinct spatial context such as the city (Beatley, 2009; Beatley & Newman, 2008; Eraydin & Tasan-Kok, 2012; Pearson et al., 2014; Rogers, 2012; Wamsler, 2009) and to some extent the rural regions (Brown & Schafft, 2011; Tamásy & Diez, 2013)[1]. The edited book *'Governing for Resilience in Vulnerable Places'*, however, draws together state of the art research from across a variety of social science disciplines (i.e. spatial planning, economic and cultural geography, environmental and political sciences, sociology and architecture) and across different spatial and geographical contexts (from urban slums in India to flood-prone smaller communities in the UK to coastal Japan). By doing so, the book is able to provide an overview and a critical analysis of the ways in which the concept 'resilience' has been 'translated' into and used in social and spatial sciences today. Acknowledging that resilience is a new powerful lens through which researchers and practitioners assess, discuss and make plans for major matters, special attention is paid to ethical, social and political issues at stake when trying to operationalize and use the concept of resilience in practice. As such, '*Governing for Resilience in Vulnerable Places*' is aimed to provide a scientifically robust overview and generate some conceptual clarity for researchers, students as well as practitioners interested in the potential of resilience thinking as well as the application of resilience in practice.

Governing for resilience in vulnerable places: summary of key themes

As the discussion above suggests, contemporary understanding of the concept of 'resilience' differs across and within disciplines and the concept has evolved from its roots in ecology and engineering to become increasingly influential in the social and spatial sciences today. Folke (2006) identifies several specific shifts in the development, understanding and usage of 'resilience' and argues that each 'type' of resilience has its own distinct characteristics (Table 2.1).

The fact that resilience has evolved from engineering and ecological sciences is one of the few aspects of resilience which the different authors who use the concept in social and spatial sciences seem to agree upon. The other aspect is the socially constructed nature of resilience and hence the significant political dimension of the concept (e.g. Burkhard & Gee, 2012; Chapin et al., 2009; Folke, 2006; Lloyd et al., 2013; Stokols et al., 2013). As Davoudi and Porter (2012) state: 'In the social world, resilience has as much to do with shaping the challenges we face as responding to them' (p. 306).

Table 2.1 The shifts in conceptualizing resilience

Time	*Resilience concepts*	*Characteristics*
1960s/early 1970s	Engineering resilience	Linearity, stable equilibria, time needed to recover from shock
1980s	Ecological resilience (social resilience)	Multiple equilibria, robustness, capacity to withstand shocks while maintaining the essential function, adaptation to short term external disturbances
1990s–2000s	Social-ecological resilience (evolutionary resilience)	Non-linearity, cross-scale dynamic interactions, renewal and reorganization, capacity to sustain and transform, regime shifts as a result of external or internal disturbances and gradual change

Source: Based on Davoudi & Porter (2012), Folke (2006) and Lloyd et al. (2013).

The challenge of finding a suitable cover image for this edited volume captures the illusive, all-encompassing and fuzzy nature of the concept 'resilience' well. A simple internet search illustrates that typically, resilience is visually captured in an image of a fragile plant or a seedling, blossoming, despite growing on a dry, harsh surface. While such an image reflects some facets of the concept of resilience well, particularly, the more ecology and perseverance related ones, the editors of this volume considered it to be missing the active, social, and perhaps more dynamic, creative and transformative potential of social-ecological or evolutionary resilience. This transformative potential, however, is crucial for social-spatial sciences, especially when discussing current governance challenges and potential governance changes. As Simin Davoudi argues in the opening chapter of this volume, the social context and 'human agency which is manifested in: our ability to displace the effects of a crisis in time and space [...] and our capacity to undertake organised collective action' should not be overlooked when conceptualizing resilience. To communicate the different facets of resilience as well as visually summarize the key themes of this edited volume, the photo of the little girl holding an umbrella and looking up to try to make sure what actions she should take next and whether she is safe from the rain, was created. The photo addresses the first key theme for this edited volume 'water and disaster risk' in the form of the raindrops that relate to the chapters discussing resilience specifically in the context of water management and community resilience to flooding. The little girl herself symbolizes the community and the social aspects of resilience, the second key theme of this edited volume. The cover is a mix of a photography as well as a cartoon (note the cloud, the 'painted' raindrops and the resilience graffiti on the wall) which points to the element of 'art' and 'creative practices and capacities' which are strongly present in the chapters of this book which discuss community resilience. Third, the 'human agency' and 'governance' aspects of this book which are further represented in most chapters is reflected by the active role that the girl on the photo is taking in trying to make a well-informed choice of whether she needs the umbrella or not to protect herself at that particular moment. By choosing the little girl for the cover the editors further wish to emphasize that while aiming to operationalize resilience, a critical eye should be kept on the ethical and social issues at stake as well as carefully consider the vulnerable groups in the society. Finally, the umbrella itself symbolizes the tendency of academics to consider 'resilience' as an 'umbrella' concept for a range of system attributes deemed desirable. Several chapters of this edited volume emphasize that such system attributes should be made operational to support planning and management.

As indicated above, the cover photo was specifically 'composed' to illustrate the interconnected themes of this edited volume. While the central focus of this volume is on exploring ways in which resilience is conceptualized and used in social and spatial sciences today, the volume is divided according to three dominant sub-themes:

I Governing for resilience: opportunities and challenges
II Resilience and disasters
III Community resilience, arts and capacity building

As the title of the volume suggests, first, explicit attention is paid to *'governing for resilience,'* introducing dilemma's and opportunities that planners and policy-makers face when trying to apply the resilience approach in practice (e.g. Zuidema & de Boer; Walker & Leyshon); legitimacy issues that may arise when 'doing' resilience (e.g. Scholten & Hartmann) and challenges of communicating the concept to different stakeholders (e.g. Greksch & Winges). The variety of ways in which resilience is and could be operationalized across different political, cultural and geographical contexts is discussed throughout the chapters. The chapters that more explicitly focus on governing for resilience (e.g. Zuidema & de Boer; Scholten & Hartmann; Gooley & Bakema; Forrest et al.; Walker & Leyshon) make clear that when using resilience in (policy-making) practice, it is necessary to be sensitive towards issues of power and justice and the different capacities that individuals have for self-sufficiency and self-organization. In addition, these chapters draw attention to the necessity to critically reconsider the changing responsibilities and the grounds for the legitimacy of the decision-makers when governing for resilience.

The second connecting strand centres around *'community resilience and capacity building'*. The discussions with regards to this broader theme focus on the importance of local level participation, knowledge and learning when planning for resilience in vulnerable places. Previous research shows that, to develop and enhance community resilience, community members must be able to actively engage in building the capacity to thrive in an environment that is characterized by change (Skerratt & Steiner, 2013). According to van der Vaart et al. (2015) resilience is often imposed onto supposedly vulnerable communities 'from outside', usually without much reference to the community members' ideas and priorities or without making use of their lived experiences (cf. Van der Voort & Vanclay, 2015). Using as examples case studies from different social, cultural and political contexts, the chapters that more explicitly centre around the 'community resilience' (e.g. van der Vaart et al.; Brice & Arconada; Forrest et al.; Andavarapu & Arefi) emphasize the need for trust and exchange between professionals/policy makers (and their expert knowledge) and the members of the local communities (and their local (expert) knowledge) and point the readers' attention to the capacities present on the local level. In this light, several contributions (e.g. Brice & Arconada; van der Vaart et al.) explore the potential role of arts in translating/mediating these different types of knowledge and thereby contributing to the resilience of vulnerable places.

Third, in a number of chapters resilience is considered in the context of *'disasters'*. These chapters (e.g. Platt; Older; Forrest et al.; Gooley & Bakema) introduce research on vulnerable places that have been or are prone to be impacted by disasters (e.g. Japan; Chile; Bangladesh; UK) and show that such contexts can also become places for innovation, learning and transformation. Several chapters in relation to this theme explore the multi-actor context of governing for resilience in vulnerable places. Considering the shift away from central control towards multi-level governance systems and stakeholder networks, new questions concerning the division of responsibilities between different actors (as illustrated by Scholten & Hartmann; Forrest et al.; Andavarapu & Arefi) on different levels in creating resilience strategies arise (Tierney, 2012). In addition, when implementing and designing resilience strategies new vulnerabilities may be created (e.g. Platt; Older). Throughout this theme and the chapters discussing it, the importance of collaboration and learning across different levels of government and between the state, market and the civil society is emphasized. In the context of the multitude of stakeholders, a key point raised by several authors and echoed in the opening chapter by Simin Davoudi is to be aware of from whose perspective resilience is 'done'.

In the concluding chapter '*Resilience in practice – a transformative approach?*' two of the editors (Bakema & Restemeyer) talk to Henk Ovink, the first Dutch Special Envoy for International Water Affairs about his experiences in 'making' vulnerable places resilient (to disasters), to provide a future perspective and directions for 'doing' resilience in practice. Bakema and Restemeyer discuss with Henk Ovink his idea of implementing resilience, termed 'the transformative approach', which essentially is a policy process based on inclusive collaboration. Based on his experiences around the world, Ovink stresses that there is no blueprint for creating resilience in practice and resilience strategies should always be tailored to the specific context and culture of a place. According to Ovink, political leadership is an important precondition for building resilience, and design can be a powerful tool for bringing the different stakeholders together and facilitating dialogue for co-creating new (transformative) visions.

In the chapter '*Self-reliant resiliency and neoliberal mentality: a critical reflection*' Prof. Simin Davoudi rightfully points out that resilience is 'a concept which carries multiple meanings and risks being co-opted into the dominant neoliberal agendas.' Through the contributions within this edited volume, the editors hope to bring the discussion on the concept of resilience a step further by highlighting some of these risks while also acknowledging the potential of resilience thinking for practice.

Note

1 Exceptions include the book by Evans & Reid (2014) providing critique on the concept of resilience and exploring the political and philosophical stakes of the 'resilience turn', the work by Zolli & Healy (2012) discussing the concept of resilience and the bouncing back abilities of systems, people and places; exploration of spatial resilience by Cumming (2011) and the book by Walker & Salt (2006) offering a conceptual overview of resilience thinking.

References

Adger, W. N. 2000.Social and ecological resilience: are they related? *Progress in Human Geography, 24(3)*, 347–364.

Alexander, D. E. 2013. Resilience and disaster risk reduction: an etymological journey. *Natural Hazards and Earth Systems Sciences Discussions, 1*, 1257–1284.

Beatley, T. 2009. *Planning for Coastal Resilience: Best Practices for Calamitous Times*. Washington, DC: Island Press.

Beatley, T. & Newman, P. 2008. *Resilient Cities and Green Urbanism Down Under: Learning from Sustainable Australian Communities.* Washington, DC: Island Press.

Brown, D. L. & Schafft, K. A. 2011. *Rural People and Communities in the 21st Century: Resilience and Transformation.* Cambridge: Polity.

Burkhard, B. & Gee, K. 2012. Establishing the resilience of a coastal-marine social-ecological system to the installation of offshore wind farms. *Ecology and Society, 17(4)*, 32–46.

Chapin, F. S. III, Folke, C. & Kofinas, G. P. 2009. A framework for understanding change. In: Chapin, F. S. III, Kofinas, G. P. & Folke, C. (eds.) *Principles of Ecosystem Stewardship: Resilience-Based Natural Resource Management in a Changing World.* New York: Spring Science + Business Media.

Comfort, L. K., Boin, A. & Demchak, C. C. 2010. *Designing Resilience: Preparing for Extreme Events.* Pittsburgh: University of Pittsburgh Press.

Cumming, G. S. 2011. *Spatial Resilience in Social-Ecological Systems.* Dordrecht: Springer.

Davoudi, S. 2012. Resilience: a bridging concept or a dead end? *Planning Theory and Practice, 13*, 299–307.

Davoudi, S. & Porter, L. (eds.) 2012. Applying the resilience perspective to planning: critical thoughts from theory and practice. *Planning Theory & Practice, 13(2)*, 299–333.

Eraydin, A. & Tasan-Kok, T. 2012. *Resilience Thinking in Urban Planning.* Dordrecht: Springer.

Evans, B. & Reid, J. 2014. *Resilient Life: The Art of Living Dangerously*. Malden, MA: Polity Press.

Folke, C. 2006. Resilience: the emergence of a perspective for social-ecological systems analysis. *Global Environmental Change, 16*, 253–267.

Hicks Masterson, J. H., Peacock, W. G., Van Zandt, S. S., Grover, H., Schwarz, L. F. & Cooper, J. T. 2014. *Planning for Community Resilience. A Handbook for Reducing Vulnerability to Disasters.* Washington, DC: Island Press.

Holling, C. S. 1973. Resilience and stability of ecological systems. *Annual Review of Ecology and Systematics, 4*, 1–23.

Klein, R. J. T., Nicholls, R. J. & Thomalla, F. 2004. 'Resilience to natural hazards: how useful is this concept?' EVA working paper no. 9, DINAS-COAST working paper no. 14, Potsdam Institute for Climate Impact Research, Potsdam.

Lansford, T., Covarrubias, J., Carriere, B. & Miller, J. 2016. *Fostering Community Resilience.* London: Routledge.

Lloyd, M. G., Peel, D. & Duckm, R. W. 2013. Towards a social-ecological resilience framework for coastal planning. *Land Use Policy, 30*, 925–933.

O'Hare, P. and White, I. 2013. Deconstructing resilience: lessons from planning practice. *Planning Practice and Research (special issue), 28*, 275–279.

Pearson, L., Newton, P. & Roberts, P. 2014. *Resilient Sustainable Cities. A future.* London: Taylor & Francis.

Pelling, M. 2003. *The Vulnerability of Cities: Natural Disasters and Social Resilience.* London: Earthscan.

Pelling, M. 2011. *Adaptation to Climate Change: From Resilience to Transformation.* London and New York: Routledge.

Pendall, R., Foster, K. A. & Cowell, M. 2010. Resilience and regions: building understanding of the metaphor. *Cambridge Journal of Regions Economy and Society, 3*, 71–84.

Pickett, S. T. A., Cadenasso, M. L. & Grove, J. M. 2004. Resilient cities: meaning, models, and metaphors for integrating the ecological, socio-economic, and planning realms. *Landscape and Urban Planning, 69*, 369–384.

Rogers, P. 2012. *Resilience & the City: Change, (Dis)order and Disaster.* Surrey: Ashgate.

Skerratt, S., Steiner, A. 2013. Working with communities-of-place: Complexities of empowerment. *Local Economy, 28(3)*, 320–338.

Stokols, D., Lejano, R. P. & Hipp, J. 2013. Enhancing the resilience of human-environment systems: a social ecological perspective. *Ecology and Society, 18(1)*, 7–18.

Tamásy, C. & Diez, J. R. 2013. *Regional Resilience, Economy and Society.* Surrey: Ashgate.

Tidball, K. G. & Krasny, M. E. 2014. *Greening in the Red Zone. Disaster, Resilience and Community Greening.* Dordrecht: Springer.

Tierney, K. 2012. Disaster governance: social, political, and economic dimensions. *Annual Review of Environment and Resources, 37*, 341–363.

Tierney, K. 2014. *The Social Roots of Risk. Producing Disasters, Promoting Resilience.* Stanford, CA: Stanford University Press.

van der Vaart, G. Trell, E.-M., Restemeyer, B. & Bakema, M. M. 2015. Resilience: just do it?! Governing for resilience in vulnerable places, University of Groningen, 9–10 October 2014. *Resilience: International Policies, Practices and Discourses, 3(2)*, 160–171.

Walker, B. & Salt, D. 2006. *Resilience Thinking. Sustaining Ecosystems and People in a Changing World.* Washington, DC: Island Press.

Wamsler, C. 2009. *Urban Risk Reduction and Adaptation: How to Promote Resilient Communities and Adapt to Increasing Disasters and Changing Climactic Condition.* Saarbrücken: VDM Verlag.

White, I. 2010. *Water and the City: Risk, Resilience and Planning for a Sustainable Future.* London: Routledge.

Wilkinson, C. 2012. Urban resilience: what does it mean in planning practice? *Planning Theory and Practice, 13*, 319–324.

Zolli, A. & Healy, A.M. 2012. *Resilience: Why Things Bounce Back.* New York: Simon & Schuster.

3 Resilient energy landscapes

A spatial quest?[1]

Christian Zuidema and Jessica de Boer

Introduction

The past decade has seen a swift increase in societal and political commitment to shift towards a more sustainable energy system. This commitment is confirmed by European Union Climate and Energy targets (CEC, 2010). Among the prime means to accommodate such a shift is the increased use of renewables in the energy mix, which the European Union has set at a twenty percent share in 2020. The use of renewables will have vast spatial implications. Fossil fuels are often found below the surface and transported to centralised units to produce electricity or the distribution of fuels. Renewables such as wind, solar or hydropower are often above the surface, highly visible and require vast amounts of space. Hence, we will have to accept energy production becoming an increasingly prominent part of our landscapes.

The spatial dimension of a shift towards a more sustainable energy system is gradually becoming evident (e.g. de Boer and Zuidema, 2015; Nadaï and Van der Horst, 2010; Noorman and De Roo, 2011; Pasqualetti, 2012; Stoeglehner et al., 2011; Stremke and Koh, 2011). Some positive examples exist of towns and villages benefiting from renewable energy production (e.g. de Boer and Zuidema, 2015; Jenssen, 2010). Nevertheless, it is the societal resistance to larger installations such as biodigesters, wind farms and solar fields that are attracting the most societal attention (e.g. Cass et al., 2010; Jones and Eiser, 2010; Walker et al., 2010; Wüstenhagen et al., 2007). Although renewable energy enjoys strong societal support, such support easily fades once renewable energy becomes spatially manifest. In the meantime, it is also clear that renewable energy production in Europe remains 'modest'. The ambition of twenty percent renewables in 2020 is only a first step. A move towards a truly sustainable energy system will require a further doubling or quadrupling of this proportion in the decades to come. In Europe, only Sweden, Norway and Iceland are already reaching levels of fifty percent or more for renewable energy production. Most European countries hover around or below the fifteen percent mark. A tremendous increase in renewable energy production will, therefore, be required in most European regions. This is certainly true for the region this chapter discusses, which is the Northern Netherlands. The Netherlands is facing a serious challenge to increase renewable energy production as renewable sources contributed only a small proportion, just over five percent of overall renewable energy production in 2014. It is a challenge that will especially affect the Northern Netherlands as it is considered one of the prime areas where the energy shift is to become implemented spatially.

The spatial dimension of renewable energy urges the involvement of spatial planners in pursuing a more sustainable energy system. To date, such involvement has predominantly played a role only in finding appropriate locations for energy production and in streamlining project implementation. It is a role that is limited to addressing isolated projects. Hence, spatial planning has yet to fully grasp the challenges of a wider integration of energy production and distribution within our urban and rural fabrics. It is this integration of the energy system in its physical and socio-economic landscape that this chapter will discuss. This chapter draws from the notion of 'resilience' to explain why such integration is not only a societal *challenge* but might have important *benefits* too. The chapter will highlight how this integration can have important benefits for both regional resilience as well as the resilience of the energy system. This also leads to the central thesis of this chapter, which is that taking a spatial perspective can help us to make progress in addressing two tightly interrelated societal challenges: improving the resilience of the energy system and the resilience of the regions in which these energy systems will be embedded.

On the one hand, a spatial perspective can support the development of a more resilient energy system. Renewable energy production depends on local circumstances, ranging from climatic conditions, topography, economic investment opportunities and available social capital. Hence, taking a spatial perspective can assist in developing an energy system that, through adapting to diverse local circumstances, creates alternative development paths for regional energy systems. This will not only support the development and improvement of alternative technologies needed within the energy system but also allow for the exchange of energy between regions. For example, hydroelectricity or biomass can generate energy in one region to compensate for a lack of sun or wind due to weather conditions in another region.

On the other hand, adapting renewable energy systems to local circumstances helps renewable energy to become embedded within a regions' socio-economic fabric. The result is that renewable energy might well support existing economic activities such as agriculture, chemical industries, transportation or port activities. It can also create new economic pathways, generate jobs or support local liveability. The financial gains from energy production can be used for local investments in local services such as schools, mobility, housing or nature management. This could lead to renewable energy production becoming part of a strategy to improve a region's resilience.

The discussion below in section two focuses on how the shift towards a sustainable energy system urges us to discuss the relationship between the energy system and the physical and socio-economic landscape in which it is embedded. This discussion provides a background for the subsequent investigation. This investigation begins in section three with exploring the two interrelated challenges of the shift towards sustainable energy landscapes for spatial planning. In section four, the investigation continues by explaining how the notion of resilience can help us to better understand how spatial planners might respond to these challenges.

Sections five and six contain the results of an empirical investigation into how the shift towards a more sustainable energy system might assist in creating both more resilient regions and a more resilient energy system. Data was gathered within the 2012–2015 MACREDES ('MApping the Contextual conditions for Resilient Decentralised Energy Systems') project that the author participated in. Within this interdisciplinary project, the author was part of a team studying the spatial dimensions of the shift towards an energy system based on more renewables. The research involved a study of multiple cases of locally based renewable energy initiatives, of (regional and national) research reports, of supervising and guiding master theses, several workshop sessions and over ten semi-structured interviews with government representatives. Although MACREDES provides important empirical insights for this chapter, it is important to note that this overall chapter takes a more theory-led perspective to explicitly argue and illustrate the relevance and possible use of a resilience perspective in pursuing a transition towards a more sustainable energy system. Finally, in section seven, a reflection will follow and some concluding remarks are presented.

Changing energy landscapes

The energy system and the physical and socio-economic landscape were strongly interdependent until at least the late 19th-century. Noorman and de Roo (2011) describe such interdependence as the 'first generation' energy landscape. Energy harvesting and production often had a visible impact on the landscape, for example through deforestation, the extraction of peat from moorlands and of coal from localized sites. The limited possibilities in transporting energy over long distances resulted in energy production and consumption needing to be close together as energy needed to be produced where it was needed (Pasqualetti, 2012). Consequently, socio-economic activities often developed in close relation to the resources available. However, this close relationship between energy systems and the landscape changed during the industrial revolution due to the availability of high amounts of easily accessible fossil fuels. It created what Noorman and De Roo (2011) call the 'second generation' energy landscape.

Characteristic of the second-generation energy landscape is that the impact of the energy system on the landscape is relatively modest. Production units are often fairly limited in numbers and size while depending predominantly on underground resources. Furthermore, much of the fossil fuels come from relatively remote areas in the world (EIA, 2012). The result is that energy production has become less visible than before the 20th-century. In the meantime, energy consumption has also become spatially detached from energy production. The higher energy density of fossil fuels allowed for transport over large distances over rail, road, water and through pipelines. The invention of alternating current further enabled transport of energy, as electricity could now be transported over hundreds of kilometres (Jones, 2010). A network of electricity lines, gas pipes and petrol stations, emerged during the 20th-century that now connects almost every household, company and vehicle owner to non-stop power supply. The result is a 'footloose' energy system in which space is implicit (de Boer and Zuidema, 2015). A system where energy is no longer a real factor in deciding where certain functions are located. Hence, spatial planning of energy production and consumption has become marginal. Spatial planning continues to matter when planning pipelines, electricity lines and energy plants, but with only minimal attention paid to the relationship between the energy system and the physical and socio-economic landscape.

The shift towards a more sustainable energy system re-emphasizes the interdependence between the energy system and the physical and socio-economic landscape. It is what De Roo and Noorman (2011) describe as the 'third generation' energy landscape. The shift involves an increased share of renewable energy production and consumption over the next decades. Early 21st-century landscapes in Western Europe are already changing with the emergence of new forms of energy production, dominated by solar energy, wind farms, hydropower, geothermal heat and the utilisation of biomass (e.g. Jenssen et al., 2012; Langbroek and Vanclay, 2012; Nadaï and Van der Horst, 2010; Sijmons and van Dorst, 2012).

Many renewable energy sources (e.g. wind, solar and hydropower) are highly visible, while others (e.g. waste heat, geothermal and biomass) depend strongly on local linkages with both resource suppliers and consumers. Furthermore, renewable energy density is far lower than that of fossil fuels. Compensating the energy produced by one large coal-fired power plant will require up to 80–100 large wind turbines. This amount equals a wind park ranging from about $50km^2$ to maybe more than $100km^2$; an area similar in size to a city such as The Hague or Florence. The result is that generating enough energy for an industrialised society will require vast amounts of space, even with some additional technological advances. The shift towards a more sustainable energy system will partly be a return to the interrelatedness between energy systems and their landscapes as was common before the 20th-century. However, it is also different from the energy systems of the past in having to meet a far larger energy demand in an increasingly densely populated and intensely used landscape. This poses some significant challenges for spatial planning.

A spatial challenge

The first challenge facing spatial planners is to investigate the varying potentials of different landscapes to produce energy. Although some renewables seem rather generically applicable, specific local and regional circumstances often play a conditioning role in producing renewable energy (e.g. Noorman and De Roo, 2011; Pasqualetti, 2012; Stoeglehner et al., 2011; Stremke and Koh, 2011; van den Dobbelsteen et al., 2007). Variations in solar radiation, wind speed, the presence of mountainous areas, geothermal potentials and abundances of biomass all dictate alternative options on a larger spatial scale. For example, wood-fuelled power plants are common in Sweden, hydroelectricity is found in the Alps and energy from waste is more common in the Netherlands. On a smaller scale the presence of waste heat from industries, well-suited rooftops for solar energy or the availability of residual biomass also condition energy potentials. A spatial perspective becomes relevant for identifying the potentials that a specific urban or rural landscape offers for producing renewable energy (van den Dobbelsteen et al., 2007). But a spatial perspective implies much more than identifying potentials. After all, production of renewable energy will not take place on a 'tabula rasa'.

Secondly then, spatial planners today are urged to investigate how renewable energy might be integrated into the physical and socio-economic landscape (de Boer and Zuidema, 2015). Much of the European landscape is already used for alternative socio-economic functions. This is especially true in more urbanised areas where there is little space left unused. Instead, land uses such as housing, transport, industry, offices, nature protection, agriculture and recreation put large claims on the physical landscape. Sometimes these existing land uses offer great opportunities for renewable energy production, for example, for using residual biomass from agriculture or residual heat from industries. Sometimes only a few tensions exist, as seen with wind farms in areas of very low population density or solar panels on the roofs of warehouses. However, renewable energy production can *compete* with existing land uses and *infringe* upon existing landscape qualities.

Competition can occur when space is specifically used for renewable energy production instead of other land uses. The growing of bio crops is a good example as bio crops can easily compete with crops meant for food production. Another example is the development of wind farms that compete with ecological protection zones or locations for new urban development. In most cases, some form of mixed use is possible with renewable technologies being part of a multifunctional landscape; e.g. solar panels on roofs, wind farms on agricultural land or waste heat in industrialised areas. In the case of multifunctional use, it remains important to recognise that infringement might still be a constraint for development. Infringement can range from the smell produced by biodigesters or the noise caused by wind turbines to the visual impact of wind farms and solar panels. Competition and infringement can create conflicts, which are especially prone to occur in more densely populated areas. They are conflicts often associated with the so-called NIMBY (not in my back yard) phenomenon (Cass et al., 2010; Walker et al., 2010).

The integration of renewable energy in both the physical and socio-economic landscape remains a relatively novel practice for both spatial planners and practitioners in the energy sector. Some first attempts have been pursued for the physical integration of renewables in the landscape (e.g. Stremke and van den Dobbelsteen, 2012). These attempts show how landscape architects and spatial planners, sometimes with the participation of residents, can facilitate physical integration and potentially soothe conflicts (Sijmons and van Dorst, 2012). Some first examples of the socio-economic integration of renewable energy include examples of farms with biodigesters, households with solar panels and heat-cold storages, and municipalities using their own bio-waste to produce biogas (de Boer and Zuidema, 2016). Revenues are then distributed locally among companies and sometimes also citizens, showing how degrees of socio-economic integration of energy production can be achieved. Some novel tendencies where entire municipalities, villages or islands take charge of their energy production have also emerged, with examples including the Danish island of Samsø and city of Sønderborg and the German towns of Feldheim or Saerbeck. Nevertheless, deliberate attempts at the physical and socio-economic integration of energy systems in their landscapes are rare. Consequently, the large-scale production of renewable energy can take place in projects focussed on energy production isolated from the spatial context (e.g. Spijkerboer et al., 2014).

In the case of renewable energy, spatial planning is considered to go beyond having a role in only preventing or mediating societal resistance to the projects and smoothing project implementation. The vast number of renewables needed and their spatial impact call for a better understanding of how renewables are to be *integrated* into their physical and socio-economic landscapes. Such integration is an attempt at searching for how the vast amount of renewable energy needed can be combined and linked to the characteristics of the physical and the socio-economic landscape. This also applies vice versa with how spatial planning might help in coping with the required changes in the energy system. The underlying idea is the creation of what de Boer and Zuidema (2015) describe as an *integrated energy landscape*, i.e. a multifunctional physical and socio-economic landscape in which the energy system is an integrated part. If successful, integration can smooth the process of project implementation in allocating renewables in our landscape. More importantly, such integration might be beneficial from the perspective of both the regional or local society *and* the energy system. This chapter argues that by using the concept of resilience such benefits might be better understood.

Taking a resilience perspective

The concept of resilience has, within the realm of spatial and political sciences, rapidly gained in popularity and use over the past decades. To some extent, resilience seems to replace 'sustainability' as the 'buzzword' in academic debates on planning and political sciences in the early 21st-century (Porter and Davoudi, 2012). It is especially its use in relation to systems such as cities, regions, infrastructure or communities, for dealing with external shocks and conditions of continuous change that have fuelled the popularity of resilience within the realm of planning and political sciences. Following its introduction into the realm of ecological studies by Holling in the 1970s, resilience initially had only a limited impact on academic debates within spatial and political sciences. Nevertheless, it was the work of Holling together with Goldberg that set the stage for the introduction of resilience into the spatial sciences. Holling and Goldberg (1971) accommodated a translation of the ecological principle of resilience into that of policy and decision making. Their work allowed spatial planning academics to empirically investigate urban and regional systems based on ecological theory. It was an age of pioneering that set the stage for resilience being positioned outside of the realm of material systems, such as ecosystems, which were considered separate from human systems. Instead, Holling and Goldberg (1971) showed how human societies are directly interrelated with and embedded in ecological and physical systems (also Reed and Lister, 2014). Furthermore, they explained how resilience is a consequence of both human and natural forces in this interrelated system (Holling and Goldberg, 1971). Human behaviour is then not only a constituent part of a system but is also a force for the creation and destruction of resilience. It has allowed us, as spatial planners, to see resilience both as a lens for analysing and describing the world we interact with and as a framework for inspiring policy ambitions. This resonates with the ambitions of this chapter to consider resilience as a lens to investigate the actual and desired development of a renewable-based energy system in the context of both the physical and socio-economic landscape.

More recently, the rising importance of complexity sciences within spatial planning and political sciences has brought resilience to the forefront of the academic debate. Complexity sciences challenge conventional conceptions of predictable change and stable systems by showing the world that planners and policy makers aim to intervene in as being in a constant state of flux. In this understanding of the world, conceptions of stability and linearity are being replaced by those of dynamically interacting social and physical systems that are producing non-linear, emergent and co-evolutionary behaviour. As Davoudi (2012) explains, "among the prescribed remedies for dealing with [such] a state of flux, the one that is rapidly gaining currency is 'resilience'" (p. 299).

Although Holling (1973) already hinted towards the role of dynamics, unpredictability and nonlinearity, resilience was first adopted in relation to the capacity of ecological systems to withstand shocks and bounce back to their original state. This view on resilience focusses on systems in stable equilibria, on degrees of disturbance that systems can handle and on their return times, i.e. it is a view that "applies only to behaviour of a linear system, or of a non-linear system in the immediate vicinity of a stable equilibrium where a linear approximation is valid" (Folke, 2006, p. 256). Hence, it is also a view that fits in well with notions of control, certainty and traditional command and control policies. It is a view that has gradually been amended due to the growing acceptance of the complexity and non-linearity of many of the physical and societal processes that planners and policy makers face. The result is a more dynamic understanding of resilience that underlines its potential for planning and policy sciences in the past decade.

When taking a more dynamic perspective, resilience is linked to systems that use mechanisms of self-organisation to adapt and respond to both internal and external processes of change (e.g. Folke et al., 2010; Gunderson and Holling, 2002; Martin and Simmie, 2010). It is a view Davoudi (2012) calls 'evolutionary resilience' and that fits with the rise of complexity sciences and more specifically with studies on complex adaptive systems (e.g. Berkes and Folke, 1998; Holland, 1999; Kauffman, 1991). Resilience is, from such a perspective, not necessarily about a system's capacity to return to its original or 'normal' state of equilibrium. Instead, an evolutionary perspective on resilience "challenges the whole idea of equilibrium and advocates that the very nature of systems may change over time" (Davoudi, 2012, p. 302). Therefore, taking an 'evolutionary' perspective means that "resilience is not conceived of as return to normality, but rather as the ability of complex socio-ecological systems to change, adapt and crucially, transform in response to stresses and strains" (ibid., p. 302).

In trying to grasp the mechanisms by which a resilient system copes with change, reference is made to what Davoudi (2012, p. 306) summarises as the "dynamic interplay of persistence, adaptability and transformability across multiple scales and timeframes" (also see Folke et al., 2010; Gunderson and Holling, 2002; Walker et al., 2004). Persistence can be linked to the capacity of a system to absorb pressures and shocks without collapsing. Persistence, as seen from a dynamic perspective, need not be interpreted as a system's ability to maintain or move back to a fixed state or equilibrium. Rather, a system can also persist through processes of adaptation and transformation, allowing some of its key functions to remain (persist) while possibly undergoing some structural changes. Therefore, the notions of adaptability and transformability are also central to a dynamic understanding of resilience (also Folke et al., 2010).

While alternative interpretations exist, adaptability and transformability refer to two complementary capacities that give a system its ability to persist in the face of change and dynamics. As Folke et al. (2010, p. 2) summarise, adaptability refers to a system's capacity "to learn, combine experience and knowledge, adjust its responses to changing external drivers and internal processes, and continue developing within the current stability domain or basin of attraction" (also Berkes et al., 2003). Transformability goes one step further and is "the capacity to create a fundamentally new system when ecological, economic, or social structures make the existing system untenable" (Walker et al., 2004, p. 5). Arguably, transformability can be positioned outside of the realm of resilience. After all, if the system fundamentally changes, can we still consider it the same system and hence resilient, or did the original system collapse to be replaced by a new one? Alternatively, transformability might also be a critical element of resilience. This becomes especially clear once we understand a system as being nested across multiple scales. Resilience then stems from the dynamics within and between individual elements or subsystems. The subsystems' capacity to transform can then be considered to allow the wider system to adjust and be resilient. This can, for example, be the case when fuel stations transform from being stations selling gasoline to places for recharging electrical vehicles. It will transform the function of a fuel station towards that of a recharging station while facilitating the energy system and transport system to continue functioning.

Finally, a dynamic perspective of resilience tends to frame systems as constituting both societal elements and natural elements. A dynamic perspective can also be traced back to the work of Holling and Goldberg (1971) on seeing ecological and social systems to be interrelated. Often described as socio-ecological systems, social and ecological systems are seen to relate to each other in a dynamic fashion (e.g. Berkes and Folke, 1998). It is a holistic perspective that suggests that we need to understand how social systems, such as institutions, economies, cities or communities are intricately linked with the ecological contexts in which they reside, be it nature, waterways, air quality or the climate. Arguably related, the literature on so-called socio-technical transitions further adds to this holistic systems interpretation. It argues that, in addition to seeing social and ecological systems as closely interwoven, technologies should also be included (e.g. Foxon et al., 2008; Grin et al., 2009; Loorbach, 2010; Meadowcraft, 2009; Rip and Kemp, 1998; Rotmans et al., 2001). It is a relevant addition especially in the face of the significant changes in technologies designed to support the shift to a more sustainable energy system. Overall, resilience can be considered as encompassing material characteristics (ecological and technical) with institutional and cultural characteristics also being contributing to or constraining a system's resilience. It urges us to also consider elements such as social capital, identity and social learning as essential for the resilience of a system: be it cities, regions, infrastructure systems or communities (Olsson et al., 2006).

In this chapter, resilience is understood from a dynamic perspective. It is a choice not just informed by its wide usage within planning and policy sciences, but also by understanding that the emerging energy landscape highlights major changes that require adaptations and transformations (e.g. Loorbach, 2010). Section five below discusses these changes from the perspective of a specific region; the Northern Netherlands. In this context, resilience relates to the capacity of this region to adapt to the pressure of integrating renewable energy into the physical and socio-economic landscape. Section six turns the tables and discusses these changes from the perspective of the energy system. Resilience is related to the capacity of the system to continuously provide affordable and sufficient amounts of energy while having to integrate more volatile and unstable resources. These two perspectives are not isolated from each other. Instead, as will be discussed in section seven, important synergies become apparent when adopting the idea of an integrated energy landscape in pursuing regional resilience and the idea of a resilient energy system.

Energy and regional resilience

The Northern Netherlands is an area of about 9000km^2, it is home to 1.7 million inhabitants and is the most peripheral and rural region of the Netherlands. The region faces some of the typical problems that more peripheral and rural areas often face: population decline, unemployment, an aging population, decreased services and a stagnating economy (CBS, 2013; Provincie Groningen, Friesland, Drenthe, 2015). Located on the borders of the North Sea, and for a large part at about sea level, the area is also facing risks associated with climate change. Finally, part of the region faces earthquakes induced by natural gas extraction. This causes additional problems, especially in the province of Groningen, due to damaged property, societal unrest and the increased risks of flooding. Consequently, the Northern Netherlands seems to face a complex mix of challenges.

Some areas, most notably close to the urban agglomeration of Groningen-Assen and Leeuwarden, seem to escape some of the challenges faced and are even expecting additional growth. The rest of the North faces what can be called rural decline (Spijkerboer et al., 2014). Rural decline relates to issues such as (youth) out-migration, decline of human capital and relatively low-income levels (Measham and Fleming, 2014). The result is a decline in the region's vitality. As Koomen (2011) explains, vitality can be linked to a healthy demographic development, sufficient economic activity in the form of employment, the availability of service facilities, strong social cohesion and a strong community identity (Shucksmith et al., 2006). In the Northern Netherlands, the first two indicators of vitality are heavily under pressure, with service facilities increasingly undermined. The possible result is a loss of local liveability.

Liveability can be linked to vitality and relates to opportunities for people to develop a good quality of life in a specific location. Liveability is difficult to define, especially when accepting the highly diverse interpretations and values that different people use to express a place as being liveable.

Nevertheless, liveability, to a certain extent, relates to at least some commonly accepted conditions that spatial planning can influence. As Newton (2012) expresses, "the concept embraces measures of residential amenity, human capital, social capital, human health and the more qualitative elements of personal satisfaction and happiness" (p. 82). There is a wide range of conditions that can support liveability (e.g. Ley and Newton, 2010). In a material sense, these conditions can include infrastructure (internet, drinking water, roads, et cetera), good quality housing, a clean and healthy environment and the secure provision of sufficient amounts of affordable energy. In a social sense, both the availability of services such as education, health care, and employment are crucial as are opportunities for cultural self-expression, for being respected and treated fairly. In the meantime, as Newton (2006) explain, liveability should also be positioned in a wider resilience perspective. Doing so implies that conditions supporting liveability will change. Liveability can only be maintained if these conditions are based on sustainable practices and can resist or transform in the face of internal or external changes. The current reliance on fossil fuels is an example of an unsustainable practice that challenges the potential for future liveability. Transformation towards a renewable based system seems the only long-term option for regaining a stable and affordable flow of energy without further damaging the climate. The crucial realization is that such a transformation could also potentially offer new opportunities for regional development. Renewable energy might be among the strategies to enhance conditions supporting liveability, both in a material sense (e.g. clean environment, nature development, affordable energy) and a social sense (e.g. jobs, local identities, local services). Hence, this chapter argues that liveability can be considered as tightly linked to the transition of the energy system.

In the Northern Netherlands, the potential of renewable energy is directly connected to processes of rural decline and opportunities for enhancing liveability. The main government parties are aware that some of the conditions supporting liveability in the Northern Netherlands are under pressure. In response, several policy directions are elaborated for stimulating economic and social development. Key issues mentioned are the more abstract research and development and international accessibility, while more concrete examples include the development of tourism, agrifood and sustainable energy (Noordervisie, 2015). The choice for sustainable energy is not a surprising one. The Northern Netherlands has a long-standing link to the energy sector. The area is home to a large reserve of natural gas and related human capital and institutional networks. Furthermore, the area is a good place for the development of large-scale wind farms (Ministry of Infrastructure and Environment and Ministry of Economic Affairs, 2014). Energy, therefore, is part of both the region's history and future.

Renewable based energy might support the region's social and economic development. Renewable based energy has the potential to strengthen existing local and regional activities, such as farming (Muller, 2009) and local industries (Avelino et al., 2012), while effects on generating employment also seem positive (Lehr et al., 2012). Renewable based energy has additional benefits for the local society, for example in contributing to citizen commitment to energy projects and the creation of social capital supporting an energy transition (Seyfang and Haxeltine, 2012). These arguments are reinforced in the Northern Netherlands by the availability of relatively large amounts of biomass from nature management and agriculture, good wind potentials and a suitability for novel renewable technologies such as osmosis (Moskvitch, 2014).

Despite its potential, renewable based energy is contested in the Northern Netherlands as also became apparent in the research conducted by de Boer and Zuidema (2015) in the context of the MACREDES project. Part of this research was a focus on large-scale energy projects, which in the Northern Netherlands were only large-scale wind farms. A key example studied was the case of the Veenkoloniën ('Peat Colonies'). The Veenkoloniën are a peripheral area characterised by a low population density and a relatively high economic dependence on state subsidies and unemployment benefits (Commissie Structuurversterking Veenkoloniën, 2001). Wind farms with a total capacity of 700MW are planned in roughly 850km^2 (Ministry of Economic Affairs, 2011). Due to their size, the wind farms are managed by the state in a specific top-down programme to smooth implementation. Agreements were made between large energy companies and the state, while local landowners would gain some of the revenues (Sijmons and van Dorst, 2012). The wider civil society was largely isolated from these projects and linkages with local initiatives, stakeholder interests and economic functions were not explicitly considered. As a result, the local population and much of the existing economic fabric were overlooked in the plans. Part of the local population swiftly organised into pressure groups and started an anti-wind farm lobby. Interviews reveal that these pressure groups were not against wind energy per se. What seemed to cause most resistance was the sheer size of the projects; the fact people were not actively involved in decision making and felt they had to face only costs and no benefits.

The case of the Veenkoloniën is an example of large state-induced projects that are usually developed in high isolation from their physical and socio-economic context. Although state actors are trying to create an aesthetically responsible allocation there is little or no local spin-off created. Revenues would go to the large investors and energy companies, while a small set of local landowners (often farmers) also benefit. The generation of jobs, creation of local economic revenues that might support local investments, and synergies with local businesses are limited, if not absent. These projects hardly support regional economic or social development and have limited potential for enhancing regional resilience and liveability. Furthermore, they face low societal support and acceptance (Bijl, 2013). Although more recent projects show increased attention for creating financial compensation for residents, large wind farms remain highly contested in the Northern Netherlands.

In contrast, within the MACREDES project, many energy initiatives were studied that are locally embedded. They are often small scale initiatives based on neighbourhood or village communities. Citizens themselves develop renewable energy initiatives that focus on the local purchase of solar panels, use of biomass or improved isolation measures. The Windpark A7, close to the Frisian village of Pingjum (600 inhabitants), is a good example of such a locally embedded energy initiative. The local community owns about eight percent of the 28MW wind farm together with people from nearby villages (see Dorp Pingjum, 2016). The community invests financial revenues directly into the community. Consequently, a local school and community centre were subsidised and additional solar panels and heat pumps were bought. It is using these revenues that these small villages can gain more control over their destiny. Due to their small size and declining population, it is challenging to retain services such as schools and community centres. In such a context, renewable energy production can be of added value for liveability by generates resources and local pride.

Another example, which is currently on hold due to political reasons, was even more directly contributing to creating local spin-offs. The example is a public-private partnership in the municipality of Hoogeveen (de Boer and Zuidema, 2015). The partnership was established around a wood-fuelled bioenergy plant (1mw) supplied with local residual biomass. The initiative depended on local municipal and business interest and partners. The municipality's participation guarantees a basic amount of available biomass and allows the heat produced in the oven to be distributed to nearby municipality buildings. A local company collects and processes the biomass and benefits from a nearby stable consumption market, while its participation ensures biomass is available in the right quality. Finally, the participation of a local energy company allows for sufficient technological know-how and for creating the physical and institutional infrastructure to distribute the energy. In spreading the risks, combining different fields of expertise and using local potentials, the initiative became financially viable. At the same time, it also created new institutional linkages which fitted with local social and economic ambitions. Nevertheless, doubts about financial returns have put the project on hold at the time of writing.

Locally embedded initiatives often generate modest amounts of energy (e.g. Rijksoverheid, 2013). Their contribution to an energy transition, however, is also in showing that energy initiatives *can* create relevant local spin-offs. These projects help create local institutional capacity, commitments to energy targets and local identities (e.g. Dedden, 2016; Duisterwinkel, 2015; Sulman, 2014). Furthermore, some of these initiatives have the potential to be up-scaled by becoming larger themselves or by growing in impact through inspiring policies, politics or different initiatives. A key example of upscaling studied in MACREDES project is a community initiative around solar power in the municipality of Groningen: Grunneger Power. The initiative started by supporting its members with solar panel procurement and installation. Gradually, it grew into a green energy company selling electricity for fair prices to its customers as well (Grunneger Power, 2012). Within two years this community initiative grew to about 1,000 private members (Broere, 2013). The initiative has also inspired other institutional changes not necessarily related directly to Grunneger Power. For example, the initiative is strongly involved in developing municipal service points for citizens around renewables and energy saving (Natuur en Milieufederatie Groningen, 2015) and they helped develop the institutional position of energy cooperatives by co-founding an overarching cooperative for the Northern Netherlands (Coöperatieve vereniging NLD Energie U.A., 2013).

The examples illustrate a dynamic interplay between the material energy system and its societal embedding. It is not the isolated energy initiative that gives a region additional transformative power; it is the energy initiative embedded in its physical and socio-economic landscape that provides this additional transformative power. As a result, two key conclusions regarding the role of renewable energy in relation to regional resilience can be drawn from the above. First, renewable energy is not only challenging as it requires incorporation into our landscapes, but it is also a possible solution to local or regional socio-economic challenges. A resilience lens helps us to see why and how. When viewed from the perspective of a specific region, resilience relates to the capacity of this region to adapt to the pressure of integrating renewable energy into the physical and socio-economic landscape. It begs for transformative power where the region can hold on or revitalise its main functionalities, such as jobs, services and amenities in the face of larger global and regional trends. Renewable energy has the potential to give a region increased transformative power, i.e. it can create new jobs, support services and open new economic development models. The examples studied also provide evidence that renewable energy can indeed create economic, institutional or social spin-off. Certainly, this spin-off remains modest due to the small scale of the examples and even local initiatives might still be contested. But what is crucial is that at least the *potential* of creating this spin-off is clear.

Second, renewable energy appears to be highly contested due to its impact on the landscape. On the one hand, if renewable energy is to become part of a strategy to increase regional resilience, its impact will obviously become far larger than now. On the other hand, even without such intentions, current Dutch policies urge for a swift increase in renewable energy production, which will affect the Northern Netherlands. It is thus clear that this increase is unavoidable. It is also clear that this strategy will *also* require large-scale renewable energy initiatives and projects. But the potential of renewable energy to generate spin-offs is not only relevant when it comes to individual or small cases. This potential is also present in the case of larger projects; e.g. when a wind farm directly generates revenues for the region. As a result, upscaling might not necessarily imply initiatives grow themselves; it is also when larger initiatives copy the basic model of creating regional spin-off that upscaling might occur. If and how such larger projects can create the kind of local support and commitment remains to be explored and tested. However, the potential for spin-offs may well play a decisive role in increasing societal support for an increase in renewable energy production.

Regional integration and resilient energy systems

When viewed from the perspective of the energy system, resilience can be associated with the current need for the system to continuously provide affordable and sufficient amounts of energy while having to integrate more volatile and unstable resources. Volatility and instability relate to many renewables that depend on weather conditions such as wind and solar energy (e.g. Kleijn and Van der Voet, 2010). As a result, it can become difficult to balance the supply of energy with the demand for energy and to keep the energy system, especially the electricity grid, stable. Taking a spatial perspective might help support the development of resilient renewable based energy systems by pursuing combinations between spatial functions and a diversification in energy systems based on local conditions. The argument of combinations between spatial functions stays close to the debate in the previous section. Instead of seeing new energy initiatives and projects as isolated from their physical and socio-economic landscape, they are instead integrated with them. The argument in this section will focus on what such integration means for the energy system itself.

As a starting point, integrated initiatives are often based on overlapping interests, which gives the initiative a multifunctional purpose (de Boer and Zuidema, 2016). Energy initiatives that unite alternative local interests tend to be less vulnerable to economic changes and social pressure (ibid). Therefore, such multifunctional initiatives can help the development of a more resilient energy system. For example, farmers use biodigesters to reduce their need to export manure, generate heat, produce gas and produce humus (Muller, 2009). The other benefits help to continue with the project even if the profit from biogas or heat reduces. In an economic sense, this means that there is more capacity to adapt to market change. Furthermore, linkages with other interests provide more funding options for the initiative. For example, solar panels on the roof of a large distribution centre could be funded by the company itself, an energy company or even individual users. Moreover, the MACREDES findings suggest the embedding of the initiative in the local economy provides investors with more social trust and support. Local commitment may open possibilities for extra investments in innovations or for bridging difficult periods with regional support. Hence, a spreading of risks can be achieved, which might reduce the vulnerability of the energy system in the face of changed economic conditions or subsidy regimes. Furthermore, as findings from the MACREDES studies also illustrate, local involvement can also stimulate learning about the costs and benefits of local energy production by allowing for more public support for innovation of the energy system. The result is that integrated energy initiatives can become catalysts for the development of institutional networks, knowledge and support. Therefore, integrating energy initiatives might add transformative power to the current energy system from a social and institutional perspective.

A spatial perspective can also be relevant by stimulating local and regional diversification of the energy system. Local and regional diversification emerges from the fact that area-based energy initiatives draw on local or regional qualities for energy production. Initiatives make use of site-specific advantages that lead to local or regional specialisations in energy production. Some regions or localities will be specialised in solar energy, others in wind power or geothermal heat, and yet others in energy from biomass. Such diversification can also support the development of a more resilient energy system. First, spatial diversification creates improved opportunities for a stable energy supply. A more diversified system allows for the exchange of capacity between, for example, wind and solar on the one hand, and biogas and hydro energy on the other. Second, spatial diversification also helps avoid path-dependency (Martin and Simmie, 2008). After all, it creates possibilities to experiment and improve various technologies. Instead of relying on 'monocultures', the system creates alternative pathways, production opportunities, and diverse institutions. This all makes the overall system less vulnerable and more resilient.

A good international example is hydro energy from Norway, which is sought after to balance wind and solar fluctuations in Germany (Gullberg et al., 2014). Nevertheless, a truly diversified grid goes further than small scale initiatives or isolated large connections. Ideally, the harvesting of varied energy sources such as waste heat, geothermal, biomass, hydro, solar and wind are linked to each other in such a way that they can (partly) resolve the challenge of creating a more predictable supply of energy. A spatial perspective, therefore, is not just relevant in understanding how energy initiatives can be integrated with the local physical and socio-economic landscape. It is also relevant in assessing how the resilience of the (inter) national energy system can benefit from local and regional energy systems that specialise and complement each other.

During the MACREDES project, the researchers conducted a scan of fifty-five initiatives in the Northern Netherlands that feature on a national website (www.hieropgewekt.nl) functioning as a platform for local citizen based energy initiatives. Of fifty-five initiatives, forty-nine generated energy with two others in a start-up phase and four only focussing on efficiency measures. Two relevant conclusions could be drawn based on this scan. First, a strong diversity of resources was found, with initiatives using locally available potentials. Second, diversification also related to the location of the initiatives. The scan showed that solar energy is by far the dominant resource in urban areas, with only one out of the twelve urban cases also focussing on other resources (wind in Coevorden). The rural cases also mostly use solar energy (twenty-seven of the thirty-seven) but also rely on wind (fifteen of the thirty-seven), biomass (nine of the thirty-seven) and hydro energy (one case). Although these cases are mostly small scale initiatives, they are beginning to have an impact on the overall energy system especially by showing pathways for development and change.

In the meantime, other renewable energy related developments that occurred outside of the scope of the MACREDES project took place. The development of heat networks in Groningen and Hoogezand is very concrete examples of rather big projects that use the locally available residual heat and geothermal potentials (Gemeente Groningen, 2016; Provincie Groningen, 2015). Another example of a development crucial for the region is the development of large off-shore wind farms, which are benefiting from the high wind speeds on the North Sea. They are triggering specific transformations in the energy system on land, notably in the Eemshaven harbour (North Netherlands). The building and maintenance of wind farms attract economic activities, while the wind farms are also fuelling the development of large data centres (in Eemshaven) that use the wind energy. Furthermore, these wind farms are also triggering research into liquid natural gas for buffering and heat due to the expected highly differentiated amounts of energy generated in the face of varying weather conditions.

As is clear from these examples, the Northern Netherlands is exploring a variety of resources based on regional and site-specific potentials. Consequently, the developments traced in the Northern Netherlands both show the emergence of multifunctional initiatives and systems *and* of spatial diversification. Such diversification is relevant for reducing the dependency of initiatives on only energy and of the region on only a limited set of resources. It is too early to tell if the Northern Netherlands is indeed contributing towards the development of what can be considered a resilient energy system. But what is clear is that in drawing on local and regional potentials, the development of a renewable-based energy system in the Northern Netherlands does show signs of the kind of diversity required for a resilient energy system

A reflection

Although celebrated by widespread societal support, the shift towards a more sustainable energy system is contested when its large-scale spatial consequences manifest themselves. As a result, it is easy to consider this shift to be problematic for regions and localities, often simplistically summarised as the so-called NIMBY effect. While a sustainable energy system will have large and possibly undesirable spatial consequences, this chapter argued that spatial planners also need to look beyond these undesirable consequences. With the help of the notion of 'resilience', this chapter proposed a complementary set of arguments to do so.

First, a resilience lens helps to view renewable energy as a possible solution for local or regional socio-economic challenges. Renewable energy has the potential to give a region transformative power and increase its livability, i.e. it can create new jobs, support services and open new economic development models. As such, it can contribute to a region's resilience by supporting or revitalising its main functionalities in the face larger global and regional trends. For such a contribution to become manifest, however, a resilience perspective does refer to a dynamic interplay between the material energy system and its societal embedding. This perspective suggests that energy initiatives should be well-integrated within the physical and socio-economic landscape.

Second, the integration of the energy system in the physical and socio-economic landscape might also support the resilience of the energy system itself. A resilient energy system is both able to balance supply and demand (energy security) and to transform towards a completely different structure and resource basis without losing its main functionalities: a stable flow of affordable energy. Linking energy initiatives with a set of local socio-economic interests is a means of gaining resources, generating commitment and hence, spreading and decreasing risks. While this supports the vitality of individual initiatives, spatial diversification might further increase the energy system's resilience. Local and regional diversification follows energy initiatives drawing on local and regional qualities for energy production. The resulting specialisation creates improved opportunities for creating a stable energy supply by having complementary resources, while it also can help avoid path-dependency. Therefore, it holds opportunities for giving the energy system more vitality and transformative power.

Clearly, this chapter conveys and optimistic message. It is, however, not a message without nuances. Integration of energy initiatives in their physical and socio-economic landscapes is not always easy or widely supported. Therefore, the desired speed of implementing renewable energy projects might be incompatible with careful integration and embedding in these physical and socio-economic landscapes. Such integration might increase the resilience of regions and the energy system. But it remains difficult to establish whether such integration will achieve greater resilience. The purpose of this chapter is also not to convey any of these messages. Instead, the message is that understanding the relevance of integrating energy initiatives in their physical and socio-economic landscapes offers interesting opportunities, which the notion of resilience can help to demonstrate.

Note

1 This paper is based on research undertaken under Macredes, a 4-year research project funded by the European Delta Gas Research program (Edgar), and Deland a 3-year European research project of 'Groen Gas – Grünes Gas' funded by Interreg IV A, Germany, Netherlands programme of the European Union.

References

Avelino, F., Frantzeskaki, N. & Jhagroe, S. (2012). *Can citizens selforganise an energy transition? Analysing the political paradoxes of self-organisation.* Copenhagen: 3rd International Conference on Sustainability Transitions.

Berkes, F., Colding, J. & Folke, C. (eds.) (2003). *Navigating social-ecological systems: Building resilience for complexity and change.* Cambridge: Cambridge University Press.

Berkes, F. & Folke C. (eds.) (1998). *Linking social and ecological systems: Management practices and social mechanisms for building resilience.* New York: Cambridge University Press.

Bijl, B. (2013). *Gebiedsgerichte condities voor het ontwerpen van een windfonds case: Windpark N33.* Groningen: Rijksuniversiteit, Groningen, Department of Spatial Planning & Environment.

Broere, R. (2013). Lokale energie houdt het noorden leefbaar. *Kijk Op Het Noorden*, 385, 10–11.

Cass, N., Walker, G. & Devine-Wright, P. (2010). Good neighbours, public relations and bribes: The politics and perceptions of community benefit provision in renewable energy development in the UK. *Journal of Environmental Policy & Planning*, 12(3), 255–275.

CBS, Centraal Bureau voor de Statistiek [Dutch Central Bureau for Statistics] (2013). *Grote gemeenten goed voor driekwart van bevolkingsgroei tot 2025.* www.cbs.nl/nl-NL/menu/themas/bevolking/publicaties/artikelen/archief/2013/2013-062-pb.htm (Accessed on 17 June 2015).

CEC, Commission of the European Communities (2010). *EUROPE 2020: A European strategy for smart, sustainable and inclusive growth*, COM (2010) 2020. Brussels: Commission of the European Communities.

Commissie Structuurversterking Veenkoloniën (2001). *Van Afhankelijkheid naar Kracht.* Drachten: Commissie Structuurversterking Veenkoloniën.

Coöperatieve vereniging NLD Energie U.A. (2013). *NLD energie: Noordelijk lokaal duurzaam energie.* www.nldenergie.org/ (Accessed on 06 December 2013).

Davoudi, S. (2012). Resilience: A bridging concept or a dead end? *Panning Theory & Practice*, 13(2), 299–307.

de Boer, J. & Zuidema, C. (2015). Towards an integrated energy landscape. *Urban Design and Planning*, 168(5), 231–240.

de Boer, J. & Zuidema, C. (2016). Stimulating co-evolutionary behaviour of renewable energy systems; The integrated energy landscape as vehicle for the energy transition. In Boelens, L. & De Roo, G. (eds.) *Spatial planning in a complex unpredictable world of change – towards a proactive co-evolutionary planning* (pp. 170–184). Groningen: InPlanning.

Dedden, B. (2016). *De kracht van gezamenlijke energie*, Master Thesis, Department of Spatial Planning & Environment. Groningen: Rijksuniversiteit Groningen.

Dorp Pingjum (2016). *Een kwart eeuw dorpsmolen Pingjum [A quarter century Dorpsmolen Pignjum].* www.dorppingjum.nl/wp-content/uploads/2016/01/DM-25_jaar_wel_wee_van_dorpsmolen.docx (Accessed on 26 August 2016).

Duisterwinkel, M. (2015). *De meerwaarde van duurzame energieinitiatieven*, Master Thesis, Department of Spatial Planning & Environment. Groningen: Rijksuniversiteit Groningen.

Energy Information Administration (2012). *Annual energy outlook 2012*. US Energy Information Administration (EIA). www.eia.gov/forecasts/aeo/pdf/0383(2012).pdf (Accessed on 04 March 2016).

Folke, C. (2006). Resilience: The emergence of a perspective for social–ecological systems analyses. *Global Environmental Change*, 16, 253–267.

Folke, C., Carpenter, S. R., Walker, B., Scheffer, M., Chapin, T. & Rockström, J. (2010). Resilience thinking: Integrating resilience, adaptability and transformability. *Ecology and Society*, 15(4), 20.

Foxon, T. J., Stringer, L. C. & Reed, M. S. (2008). *Governing long-term social-ecological change: What can the resilience and transitions approaches learn from each other?*, Paper prepared for presentation at the 2008 Berlin Conference, 'Long-Term Policies: Governing Social-Ecological Change', Berlin, 22–23 February 2008.

Gemeente Groningen (2016). Ruim 1700 woningen aangesloten bij warmtenet noordwest. https://gemeente.groningen.nl/actueel/nieuws/ruim-1700-woningen-aangesloten-bij-warmtenet-noordwest (Accessed on 16 June 2016).

Grin, J., Rotmans, J. & Schot, J. (eds.) (2009). *Transitions to sustainable development: New directions in the study of long term transformative change*. London: Routledge.

Grunneger Power (2012). *Grunneger power: ons energiebedrijf*. http://www.grunnegerpower.nl/ (Accessed on 22 January 2013).

Gullberg, A. T., Ohlhorst, D. & Schreurs, M. (2014). Towards a low carbon energy future – Renewable energy cooperation between Germany and Norway. *Renewable Energy*, 68, 216–222.

Gunderson, L. H. & Holling, C. S. (2002). *Panarchy: Understanding transformations in human and natural systems*. Washington, DC: Island Press.

Holland, J. H. (1999). *Emergence: From chaos to order*. Reading, MA: Perseus Books.

Holling, C. S. 1973. Resilience and stability of ecological systems. *Annual Review of Ecology and Systematics*, 4, 1–23. doi: 10.1146/annurev.es.04.110173.000245.

Holling, C. S. & Goldberg, M. A. (1971). Ecology and planning. *Journal of the American Institute of Planners*, 37(2), 221–230.

Jenssen, T. (2010). The good, the bad, and the ugly: Acceptance and opposition as keys to bioenergy technologies. *Journal of Urban Technology*, 17(2), 99–115.

Jenssen, T., König, A. & Eltrop, L. (2012). Bioenergy villages in Germany: Bringing a low carbon energy supply for rural areas into practice. *Renewable Energy*, 61(1), 74–80.

Jones, C. F. (2010). A landscape of energy abundance: Anthracite coal canals and the roots of American fossil fuel dependence, 1820–1860. *Environmental History*, 15(3), 449–484.

Jones, C. R. & Eiser, J. R. (2010). Understanding 'local' opposition to wind development in the UK: How big is a backyard? *Energy Policy*, 38(6), 3106–3117.

Kauffman, S. A. (1991). Antichaos and adaptation. *Scientific American*, 265(2), 64–70.

Kleijn, R. & Van der Voet, E. (2010). Resource constraints in a hydrogen economy based on renewable energy sources: An exploration. *Renewable and Sustainable Energy Reviews*, 14(9), 2784–2795.

Koomen, E. (2011). *Indicators of rural vitality. A GIS-based analysis of socio-economic development of the rural Netherlands*. Research Memorandum

2011-50. http://degree.ubvu.vu.nl/RePEc/vua/wpaper/pdf/20110050.pdf (Accessed on 17 June 2015).

Langbroek, M. & Vanclay, F. (2012). Learning from the social impacts associated with initiating a wind farm near the former island of Urk, The Netherlands. *Impact Assessment and Project Appraisal*, 30(3), 167–178.

Lehr, U., Breitschopf, B., Diekmann, J., Horst, J., Klobasa, M., Sensfuß, M. & Steinbach, J. 2012. *Renewable energy deployment – do the benefits outweigh the costs?* Discussion paper. http://www.gws-os.com/discussionpapers/gws-paper12-5.pdf (Accessed on 22 May 2017).

Ley, A. & Newton, P. (2010). Creating and sustaining liveable cities. In Kallidaikurichi, S. & Yuen, B. (eds.) *Developing living cities: From analysis to action* (pp. 191–230). Singapore: World Scientific.

Loorbach, D. (2010). Transition management for sustainable development: A prescriptive, complexity-based governance framework. *Governance*, 23(1), 161–183.

Maesham, T. G. & Fleming, D. A. (2014). Impacts of unconventional gas development on rural community decline. *Journal of Rural Studies*, 36, 376–385.

Martin, R. & Simmie, J. (2008). Path dependence and local innovation systems in city-regions. *Innovation: Management. Policy & Practice*, 10(2–3), 183–196.

Meadowcraft, J. (2009). What about the politics? Sustainable development, transition management and long term energy transitions. *Policy Science*, 42, 323–340.

Ministry of Economic Affairs (2011). *Energierapport 2011*. Den Haag: Rijksoverheid.

Ministry of Infrastructure & Environment and Ministry of Economic Affairs (2014). *Structuurvisie Windenergie op land* [Structurevision Wind on Land]. www.rijksoverheid.nl/onderwerpen/duurzame-energie/documenten-en-publicaties/rapporten/2014/03/31/bijlage-1-structuurvisie-windenergie-op-land.html (Accessed on 19 May 2015).

Moskvitch, K. (2014). The white stuff; Salinity variation between different types of water could provide a valuable future source of renewable energy. *Journal of Professional Engineering*, 27(5), 59–69.

Muller, A. (2009). Sustainable agriculture and the production of biomass for energy use. *Climatic Change*, 94(3–4), 319–331.

Nadaï, A. & Van der Horst, D. (2010). Wind power planning, landscapes and publics. *Land use Policy*, 27(2), 181–184.

Natuur en Milieufederatie Groningen (2015). *Servicepunt Lokale Energie Voorwaarts*. www.lokaleenergievoorwaarts.nl/ (Accessed on 28 April 2015).

Newton, P. W. (2006) '*Human settlements*', *theme commentary prepared for the 2006 Australian State of the Environment Committee*. Canberra: Department of the Environment and Heritage.

Newton, P. W. (2012). Liveable and sustainable? Socio-technical challenges for twenty-first-century cities. *Journal of Urban Technology*, 19(1), 81–102.

Noordervisie 2040, Groningen Province, Friesland Province & Drenthe Province (2015). *Noorderzine: een co-creatieve verkenning van de toekomst van Noord-Nederland*. www.ikdrenthe.nl/pers/ontwerp-noordervisie-2040-gepresenteerd (Accessed on 06 May 2015).

Noorman, K. J. & De Roo, G. (eds.) (2011). *Energielandschappen-de 3de generatie. Over regionale kansen op het raakvlak van energie en ruimte*. Assen/Groningen: Provincie Drenthe & Rijksuniversiteit Groningen.

Pasqualetti, M. (2012). Reading the changing energy landscape. In Stremke, S. & Van den Dobbelsteen A. (eds.) *Sustainable energy landscapes: Designing, planning, and development* (pp. 11–44). Boca Raton, FL: CRC Press.

Porter, L. & Davoudi, S. (2012). The politics of resilience for planning: A cautionary note. *Planning Theory and Practice*, 13(2), 329–333.

Provincie Groningen (2015). *Hoogezand-Sappemeer krijgt nieuw duurzaam warmtenet.* www.provinciegroningen.nl/actueel/nieuws/nieuwsbericht/_nieuws/toon/Item/hoogezand-sappemeer-krijgt-nieuw-duurzaam-warmtenet/ (Accessed on 16 June 2016).

Reed, C. & Lister, N. M. (eds.) (2014). *Projective ecologies.* Cambridge, MA: Actar Harvard Graduate School of Design.

Rijksoverheid (2013). *Visie lokale energie*, Directoraat-generaal Energie, Telecom & Mededinging Directie Energie en Duurzaamheid, Den Haag.

Rip, A. & Kemp, R. (1998). Technological Change. In Rayner, S. & Malone, E. L. (eds.) *Human choice and climate change* (pp. 327–399). Columbus, OH: Battelle Press.

Rotmans, J., Kemp, R. & van Asselt, M. (2001). More evolution than revolution: Transition management in public policy. *Foresight*, 3(1), 15–31.

Seyfang, G. & Haxeltine, A. (2012). Growing grassroots innovations: Exploring the role of community-based initiatives in governing sustainable energy transitions. *Environment and Planning-Part C*, 30(3): 381–400.

Shucksmith, M., Cameron, S., Merridew, T. & Pichler, F. (2006). *First European Quality of Life Survey: Urban-rural difference.* Luxembourg: Office for official Publications of the European Communities.

Sijmons, D. & van Dorst, M. (2012). Strong feelings: Emotional landscape of wind turbines. In Stremke, S. & Van den Dobbelsteen, A. (eds.) *Sustainable energy landscapes: Designing, planning, and development* (pp. 45–68). Boca Raton, FL: CRC Press.

Simmie, J & Martin, R. 2010. The economic resilience of regions: towards an evolutionary approach. *Cambridge Journal of Regions, Economy and Society*, 3(1), 27–43. doi:10.1093/cjres/rsp029.

Spijkerboer, R., Trell, E. & Zuidema, C. (2014). *Rural resilience and renewable energy: In search of synergies.* Europäische Peripherien zwischen Stagantion und Aufbruch: Annual Conference of the German Rural Geographers Working Group. 13 November 2014.

Stoeglehner, G., Niemetz, N. & Kettl, K. H. (2011). Spatial dimensions of sustainable energy systems: New visions for integrated spatial and energy planning. *Energy, Sustainability and Society*, 1(1), 1–9.

Stremke, S. & Koh, J. (2011). Integration of ecological and thermodynamic concepts in the design of sustainable energy landscapes. *Landscape Journal*, 30(2), 194–213.

Stremke, S. & van den Dobbelsteen, A. (eds.) (2012). *Sustainable energy landscapes: Designing, planning, and development.* Boca Raton, FL: CRC Press.

Sulman, N. (2014). *Lokale duurzame energie-initiatieven: eigenheid, groeien en samenwerken*, unpublished Master Thesis, Department of Spatial Planning & Environment. Groningen: Rijksuniversiteit Groningen.

van den Dobbelsteen, A., Jansen, S., van Timmeren, A. & Roggema, R. (2007). Energy potential mapping: A systematic approach to sustainable regional planning based on climate change, local potentials and exergy. In Council for

Scientific and Industrial Research (ed.) *CIP world building conference proceedings* (pp. 2450–2460). Cape Town: Council for Scientific and Industrial Research.

Walker, B., Holling, C. S., Carpenter, S. R. & Kinzig, A. (2004). Resilience, adaptability and transformability in social–ecological systems. *Ecology and Society*, 9(2), 5.

Walker, G., Devine-Wright, P., Hunter, S., High, H. & Evans, B. (2010). Trust and community: Exploring the meanings, contexts and dynamics of community renewable energy. *Energy Policy*, 38(6), 2655–2663.

Wüstenhagen, R., Wolsink, M. & Bürer, M. J. (2007). Social acceptance of renewable energy innovation: An introduction to the concept. *Energy Policy*, 35(5), 2683–2691.

4 Resilience to what and for whom in landscape management

Timothy Walker and Catherine Leyshon

Introduction

It has long been recognised that global biodiversity is vulnerable to the conjoined effects of anthropogenic climate change, population growth and land use change, jeopardising the integrity of ecosystem services that support human life on earth (IPCC, 2014; Opdam and Wascher, 2004; Thomas et al., 2004; Thuiller, 2007) Land managers[1] are tasked with understanding the vulnerabilities in the natural systems they oversee and designing management strategies that promote resilience (Hannah et al., 2002; Hopkins and Britain, 2007).

Among the many possible approaches to managing for resilience the 'Ecological Network Approach' (Ecological Network Approach) has gained traction among land managers, conservation scientists and policy makers with its attractively straightforward principles: (1) improve existing habitats; and (2) increase structural connectivity between sites. Indeed, the Ecological Network Approach is endorsed by 'Biodiversity 2020' (DEFRA, 2011), which is England's strategy to ensure biodiversity is protected into the future, as well as being embedded within the Lawton Report (2010) 'Making Space for Nature' and the Natural Environment White Paper (2011) 'The Natural Choice: securing the value of nature' (Baker and Fuller, 2013).

This chapter traces through how the Ecological Network Approach was trialled at the landscape scale in Cornwall, UK. Exploring how the Ecological Network Approach was translated from a model to policy and then trialled in a localised management strategy tells us much about how resilience is achieved in practice. The dilemmas and opportunities that policy makers, landscape managers and ecologists face when trying to apply this resilience approach in practice at the landscape scale are critically explored. This chapter zooms in on two of the most significant challenges. The first is dealing with uncertainty, both in the epistemic and stochastic sense. The second is dealing with ambiguity in the presence of two or more equally valid frames or interpretations about the system of concern (Brugnach et al., 2007).

We begin with a closer look at the Ecological Network Approach as a form of resilience thinking. We then introduce our case study area – the Lizard Peninsula, Cornwall UK – and trace out how the application of the Ecological Network Approach was conditioned by the dilemmas faced by landscape managers. We conclude by arguing that understanding the dilemmas and opportunities faced by land managers reveals much about the problems of governing for resilience.

Rethinking ecological resilience

The traditional approach to reducing risks to biodiversity in Europe is through the designation and maintenance of nature reserves (Baker and Fuller, 2013). Despite the success of reserves, it is now accepted that alone they are insufficient to prevent biodiversity losses from the effects of climate change and land use pressures (Mora and Sale, 2011). Current approaches focus on the creation of resilient ecological networks, where resilience is understood as both the speed with which a system returns to equilibrium after perturbation and the magnitude of disturbance that can be absorbed before the system enters another regime of behaviour (Gunderson, 2000). Lawton et al. (2010: iv) define an ecological network as "a suite of high-quality sites which collectively contain the diversity and area of habitat that are needed to support species and which have ecological connections between them that enable species, or at least their genes, to move". The Ecological Network Approach is key to reducing the risk of biodiversity loss and enhancing resilience to climate change and other pressures (Emery and Franks, 2012). Ecologists have shown how fragmentation (often due to land use changes) multiplies the impact of climate change and thus the risk of biodiversity loss (Opdam and Wascher, 2004; Thomas et al., 2004). The principle behind the Ecological Network Approach is, therefore, to maintain and connect habitats to enable species to move (Hodgson, Thomas, Wintle, and Moilanen, 2009).

Opdam and Washer (2004) put forward a vision for conservation strategies based on the Ecological Network Approach which requires achieving three objectives. First, stabilisation of the key areas or 'nodes' which lower the risk of extinction during extreme weather perturbations and serve as sources of regional recovery; second, achieve heterogeneity by increasing spatial variation at the landscape scale and reducing the vulnerability of local populations to weather variability; third, create permeability by developing networks of narrow corridors in semi-natural landscapes enabling wildlife to pass infrastructural barriers such as roads. Implementation of the Ecological Network Approach therefore, demands landscape scale management to address habitat fragmentation (Emery and Franks, 2012) under the guiding principles of 'more', 'bigger', 'better' and 'joined' (Lawton et al., 2010). However, as Baker and Fuller (2013: 33) note "hidden within that simple phrase there are many unanswered questions and much complexity". It is through understanding this complexity, and how that is dealt with on the ground, that we gain insights into resilience as a practice as well as a philosophy – in management and governance.

Thinking through resilience as practice helps to position the Ecological Network Approach as a resilience *model* rather than a prescriptive *guide* to management or delivery of its underlying philosophy. Therefore, land managers face the significant challenge of translating this resilience model into practical interventions for realising resilience in practice. This is a significant challenge, as demonstrated through the case study, for two reasons.

The first challenge is that of uncertainty. The *sine qua non* of the Ecological Network Approach is vulnerability and lack of resilience. Füssel (2007) argues that vulnerability represents a "conceptual cluster" for integrative human-environment research, which despite considerable variety in its definition is usually understood as the outcome of four interacting factors: the system of analysis (such as a habitat), the attribute of concern that is threatened, the hazard or potentially damaging influence on the system; and the timescale over which this will happen. Vulnerability assessments[2] have become key instruments to localise climate change impacts and design management strategies (Dessai and van der Sluijs, 2008). In the Ecological Network Approach, vulnerability is visualised primarily through maps, which demonstrate spatially the extent of habitat fragmentation and those areas at risk to further habitat loss. But deploying vulnerability analysis at the landscape scale in the Ecological Network Approach inevitably entails working with uncertainty. In the original and technical sense, uncertainty refers to situations where not all possible outcomes are known in probabilistic or objective terms (Sigel Klauer and Pahl-Wostl, 2010). Subsequent work has shown how uncertainty can originate from incomplete knowledge, more often known as epistemic uncertainty, or/and from unpredictability, more often known as stochastic uncertainty (Figure 4.1) (Hoek, Brugnach, Mulder, and Hoekstra, 2014).

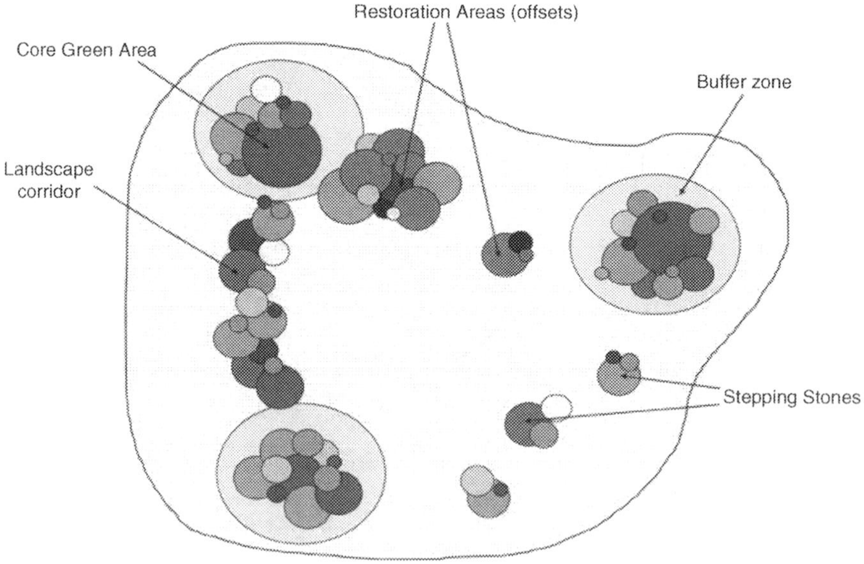

Figure 4.1 Components of an ecological network.
Source: adapted from Lawton, 2012.

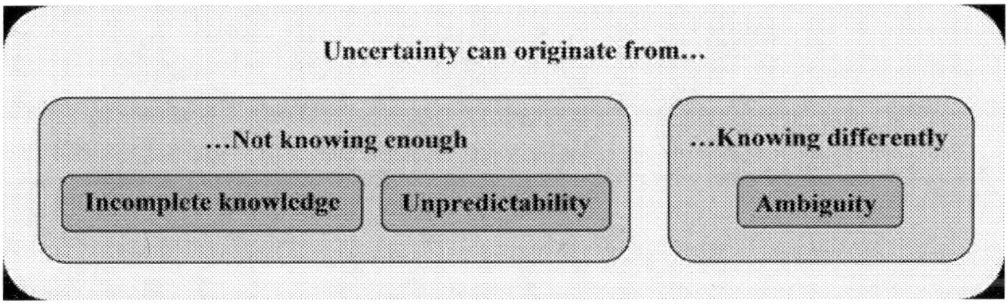

Figure 4.2 Diagram illustrating sources uncertainty in relation to ambiguity.
Source: adapted from Hoek et al., 2014.

Despite what is implied by the Ecological Network Approach model (Figure 4.2) landscapes are rarely comprehensively mapped – i.e. they exhibit epistemic uncertainty. Even where significant efforts have gone into detailed mapping, landscapes are never static – i.e. they exhibit stochastic uncertainty. Yet the implementation of the Ecological Network Approach is predicated on the existence of high-quality data on the current state of habitats to identify vulnerabilities and to target management interventions. Further, implementing the Ecological Network Approach also requires accounting for variabilities and the expected disturbances, for example, the extent to which climate change will affect different ecological components and in turn how those affected components will interact.

The second challenge is that of ambiguity. Contemporary research in multi-stakeholder environmental management has added a further layer of complexity to the problem of uncertainty. For example, Brugnach et al. (2007; 2011) assert that uncertainty has no meaning in itself but is a function of the relationship a decision maker establishes with the environment and other actors to make sense of a situation (Brugnach, Dewulf, Henriksen, and van der Keur, 2011; Brugnach et al., 2007). This situation is ambiguous in that there is "the simultaneous presence of multiple frames of reference about a certain phenomenon" Dewulf et al. (2005: 116). To clarify, frames or framing refers to how actors make sense of specific issues, connect them into a sensible whole, and delineate boundaries (Dewulf, Craps, and Dercon, 2004; Dewulf et al., 2009). How stakeholders frame issues is fundamentally important to how risks are managed, as Entman (1993: 52) explained, a framing will promote a "particular problem definition, causal interpretation and recommendation for treatment". Ambiguity is thus another dimension of uncertainty; it is not about the location, level or nature of uncertainty but is the presence of two or more equally valid frames or interpretations about the system of concern (Brugnach et al., 2007). This can also extend to many equally valid interpretations of what constitutes resilience in practice.

There are far more actors, human and non-human, in 'real' landscapes than suggested by the Ecological Network Approach model because landscape management cannot be done in isolation of the social, cultural and economic context. As such, one key problem with the Ecological Network Approach resilience model is the absence of humans, making it curiously out of step with the drive towards the greater understanding of conjoined human-environment relationships as socio-ecological systems. Further, there is an underlying assumption that if an ecological network was achieved it would satisfy all actors' agendas. But as decades of research on environmental governance have shown, conflicts always arise between different stakeholders around management strategies (Asah, Bengston, Wendt, and Nelson, 2012; Mazur and Asah, 2013). Therefore, land managers must work with ambiguity when trying to achieve resilience in practice.

FARM on the Lizard, UK

The empirical focus is an interdisciplinary project entitled Farm and Resilience Management (FARM) involving Natural England (NATURAL ENGLAND)[3], farmers on the Lizard Peninsula (Cornwall, UK) and academics from the Centre for Geography, Environment and Society (CGES) and the Centre for Conservation and Ecology (CEC) at the University of Exeter's Penryn Campus. It ran from 2013 to 2015. Natural England sought to apply the Ecological Network Approach to the Lizard landscape by spatially mapping the vulnerability of priority habitats to climate change, identifying appropriate management strategies, and then locating the barriers to their implementation.

As a peninsula jutting out into the Atlantic and surrounded on three sides by sea (Figure 4.3), Cornwall's weather and climate are dominated by maritime atmospheric and oceanic systems, including the Gulf Stream and the prevailing south-westerly winds which bring mild, but changeable weather and frequent winter storms. As in much of Great Britain, discernible changes to local weather, flora, fauna and landscapes are difficult to attribute directly to climate change and the scale at which regional models operate is too large to make accurate local predictions (for a critique of UKCP09 and the spatial and temporal scales at which it operates, see Brace and Geoghegan, 2011).

The Lizard landscape is characterized by small settlements, family farms of a few hundred acres (some operating under the soon-to-be-replaced Entry Level and Higher Level Stewardship schemes), the Goonhilly National Nature Reserve (covering 1600ha) and National Trust[4] properties. Parts of the Lizard are designated as part of Cornwall's Area of Outstanding Natural Beauty (ANOB). The Lizard includes some habitats and species which are unique to the peninsula and others which are extremely rare. Several land management organisations are active on the Lizard, namely Cornwall Wildlife Trust, the National Trust, Natural England, Cornwall AONB, and the National Farmers Union.

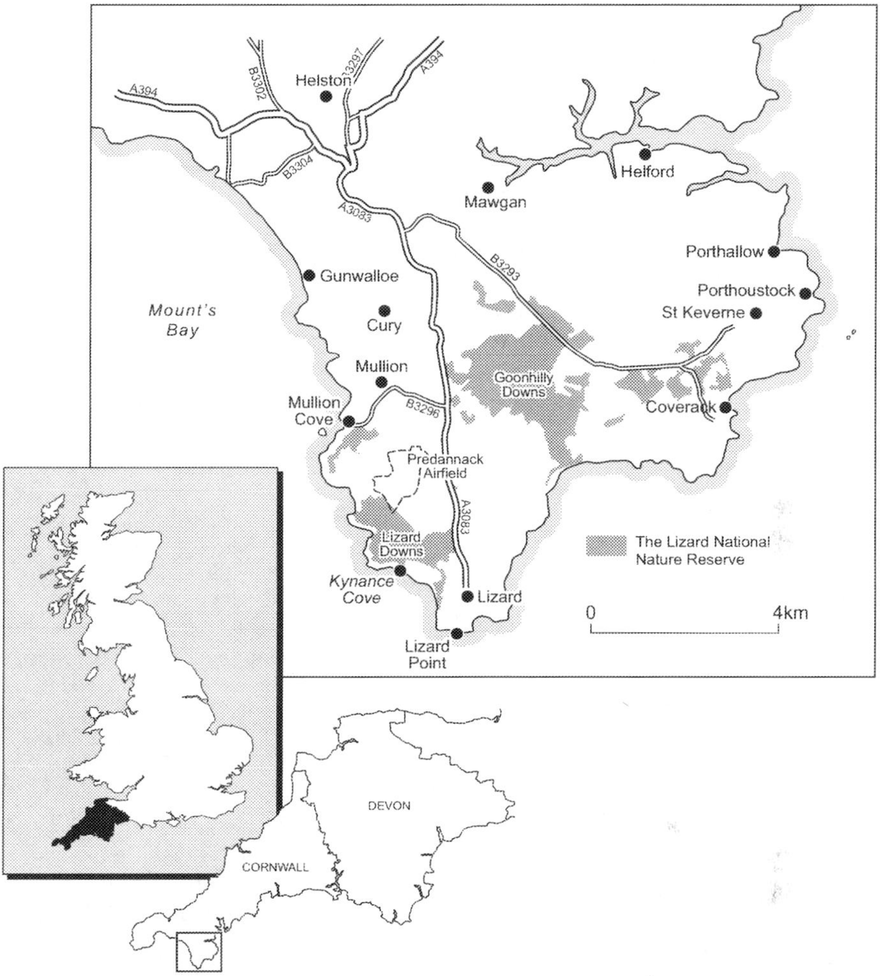

Figure 4.3 Map of Lizard Peninsula.
Source: University of Exeter Drawing Office.

However, in common with places worldwide (Brooks et al., 2002; Thomas et al., 2004), the unique and important biodiversity of the Lizard Peninsula – and the ecological and cultural benefits that it brings – are likely to be threatened by climate and other environmental changes. To help adapt to this threat, land managers are faced with building resilience to help natural systems absorb and respond to these changes (Hannah et al., 2002; Hopkins and Britain, 2007). The patchwork of designations and small family-run farms on the Lizard makes for particular challenges in respect of identifying, consolidating, and managing fragmented habitats.

The FARM project's intended aims were: first, understand where and how land management could be best targeted to safeguard the biodiversity of the Lizard Peninsula, Cornwall, UK, against future environmental changes; second, to understand the social, economic and practical constraints associated with implementing such land management; and, third, to ask how these findings could inform improved negotiations around land management elsewhere.

The original objective was for the CEC ecologists as part of the FARM project to take the findings of Natural England's National Biodiversity Climate Change Vulnerability Model (NBCCV) combine them with data from the ERICA database[5] to produce detailed biodiversity vulnerability maps for the Lizard in the context of climate change. They would evaluate the extent to which species persistence or local extinction is spatially correlated with environmental and habitat characteristics. These vulnerability maps would be used to determine management options needed to increase plant community resilience to climate change. These management suggestions would be based on *conservation.org* guidelines and advice from local specialists from Natural England. The ecologists intended to use existing microclimate models of the Lizard Peninsula (Maclean, Bennie, Scott, and Wilson, 2012;) to determine the types of management that would result in yearly variations in temperature and water conditions under future climate. Many of the species of highest conservation value on the Lizard Peninsula thrive because of the unique microclimatic conditions: relatively wet and mild conditions in winter, followed by drought-stressing in summer.

Management options were based on the Ecological Network Approach, intended to reduce habitat fragmentation and increase habitat connectivity to facilitate species range shifts, reduce species vulnerability and create coherent and resilient ecosystems in the face of climate change (Heller and Zavaleta, 2009). Examples of likely management solutions included extending the coastal strip further inland by altering field boundaries, reducing nutrient inputs to enable oligotrophic conditions, applying grazing regimes, and controlled burning.

The CGES geographers' role was then to take the maps to a select area of highest vulnerability on the Lizard (identified by the CEC ecologists in consultation with Natural England), and discuss the barriers and opportunities for farmers to take up proposed management options. This was considered necessary as the practical considerations and local opportunities that constrain and enable environmental management are not well understood. Nevertheless, it was assumed that the provision of detailed risk maps would reveal how farmers framed the issues.

The vulnerability mapping exercise revealed much about the process of science and knowledge production; specifically, that achieving land management objectives is not simply a linear process of identifying vulnerability and then overcoming barriers within the agricultural community. As we show below, the lack of an obvious course of action was primarily due to the uncertainties and ambiguities which plague the translation of the Ecological Network Approach resilience model into real world maps and downscaling for practical management strategies. In the following section, we examine the sources of these uncertainties and ambiguities along with the different stakeholders' conceptions of resilience. Through doing so the project raises questions about, first, the efficacy of traditional approaches to translating resilience models to practice; and second, the instrumentalist approach to identifying and operationalizing local land management decisions. Specifically, the process revealed a range of uncertainties and ambiguities which cannot necessarily be solved with better or more data. Instead of a purely scientist-led approach to resilience governance, the process points to the importance of local level participation, knowledge and learning.

Resilience – from policy to practice

Our approach to understanding how uncertainty and ambiguity condition management for resilience began by identifying the different actors involved and their usual frames, missions, interests, and roles. The actors in the FARM project were: local Natural England staff on the Lizard; CEC ecologists; CGES geographers; botanists with specialist knowledge of the Lizard; a sample of farmers on the Lizard. Their frames, missions, interests, and roles are summarised in Table 4.1.

Using a narrative-discursive approach, we then identified a series of six episodes (Table 4.2) in the data collection phase of the project as it evolved over the course of a year: (1) initiation; (2) ecologist-led risk mapping; (3) stakeholder focus group; (4) stakeholder-led risk mapping; (5) farmer consultations; (6) review and response.

These episodes saw the framings of key actors change, and interact, along with their use of risk analysis to arrive at management solutions. Each episode exposes knowledge traditions, the priorities of different stakeholders, and the configuration of different types of expertise and experience specific to the landscape in question.

Each of the episodes describes a particular shift in understandings of vulnerability, resilience, uncertainty, ambiguity. They describe, collectively, a shift from certainty (of approaches and outcomes), through uncertainty (especially in relation to the veracity of data) and finally ambiguity (in which several actors with different frames are seeking a resolution). We mapped evolution, or dissolution, of different actors' frames and their understanding of risk onto the six episodes. These are also associated with a shift from the macro-scale of national policy to the contingencies of local conditions. At the end of the project, the local delivery an Ecological Network Approach to management was complicated by uncertainty and ambiguity which had problematized the risk-logic underpinning the conservation strategy and the achievement of resilience in practice.

Table 4.1 Framings, mission, interests, and roles of key actors

Actor	*Epistemic frame*	*Mission*	*Specific interest*	*Role*
Natural England (National) A1	A positivist approach to knowledge wherein climate change models can be used to establish the condition and vulnerability of BAP[1] habitats nationally.	Produce a series of maps on the condition, conservation value, fragmentation, sensitivity, topographic variety and overall vulnerability of BAP habitats nationally using broad & consistent metrics to measure vulnerability.	Develop and adapt the maps to ensure their usefulness to local landscape managers.	Produce maps and take on feedback from regional land managers and users; overcome the problems of 'downscaling' climate models to produce locally relevant findings.
Natural England (Local) A2	Risks to biodiversity on the Lizard, under climate change, need to be mapped in order to provide the evidence base to underpin appropriate management options and strategic decision-making.	Qualify and validate the maps and use them to establish areas of heightened vulnerability and appropriate landscape management plans.	Engage ecologists to establish the specific characteristics of habitats and species present on the Lizard and their vulnerability. Engage the geographers to establish the cultural barriers that prevent farmers from managing their land for biodiversity and resilient habitats.	Oversee discussions between ecologists, botanical specialists, and geographers; receive the findings of the research; implement recommendations.
CEC Ecologists A3	Risk and vulnerability can be quantified using existing databases of species distribution.	Use existing databases (ERICA), Ellenberg indicators and RDB values to qualify the regional maps using data on monocots and diocots.	Demonstrate changes in plant communities between 1960 and 1985 and 1985 and 2013.	Utilise observational data to enhance the original maps and inform local land management decisions.

(*Continued*)

Actor	*Epistemic frame*	*Mission*	*Specific interest*	*Role*
CGES Geographers A4	A post-positivist approach in which risk is theorised as a social construction produced in particular contexts, and its effects are a matter of negotiation between different knowledge cultures.	To observe and participate in the negotiation between different knowledge cultures; to engage farmers in the validation of ecologists' risk maps; to explore the barriers to habitat-sensitive farming.	Gather qualitative data on the framings of different actors and the negotiations between them on risk, vulnerability, habitats and land management.	Facilitate knowledge exchange between different actors; participate in discussions about mapping risk.
Botanical specialists A5	An empiricist approach to risk based on local knowledge from detailed observations over a long time period provide the most robust information about local conditions. Rare species are most vulnerable.	Preserve rare species and natural habitats on the Lizard; developing their specialised, expert knowledge and championing the Lizard as a site of rare plants.	Ensure that botanical hotspots on the Lizard are adequately protected and preserved.	Contributed expert, local, observational knowledge to the mapping exercise, challenging the basis of risk mapping and the choice of management strategies.
Farmers A6	A practice-based approach to risk in which farming expertise, practical experience and daily observation form the basis of detailed local knowledge of their land.	Produce agricultural outputs such as beef, milk, brassicas, etc. Varying levels of commitment to farming for the environment & participation in agro-environmental schemes.	Maintain a livelihood while at the same time farming for the environment (with one exception).	Validate the risk maps against their local knowledge; explain the barriers to implementing further changes to their farming practice.

Source: Authors.

1 BAP habitats are priority environments which have been identified as being most threatened and requiring conservation action under the UK Biodiversity Action Plan (BAP).

2 The Ellenberg system describes the response of a species to edaphic and climatic parameters in comparison with other species. The Ellenberg's indicator values include a 9 point scale for each of six gradients: soil acidity, soil productivity or fertility, soil humidity, soil salinity, climatic continentality and light availability (Godefroid and Dana, 2007).

Table 4.2 Actions taken in different episodes in FARM

	Episode 1 – Initiation	*Episode 2 – ecologist-led risk mapping*	*Episode 3 – stakeholder focus group*	*Episode 4 – stakeholder-led risk mapping*	*Episode 5 – farmer consultations*	*Episode 6 – review and response*
Agency actors (A1 & A2)	Maps of condition of BAP habitat for Lizard National Character Area (A1, A2, A3)					
University (A3 & A4)		Maps produced based on local data (A2, A3).	Specialist consultation (A3, A5)	Specialist risk mapping (A3, A4, A5)	Farmer consultation (A4, A6)	Critical review and reflection (A3, A4)
Local actors (A5 & A6)						
	Time →					

Source: Authors.

Episode one

In February 2014, Natural England published their National Biodiversity Climate Change Vulnerability (NBCCV) model which undertook an analysis of current datasets to provide an assessment of the relative vulnerability of BAP habitats to climate change based on some simple metrics. In Episode one, the FARM team intended to use the NBCCV output maps of overall vulnerability to provide a guide for action within which local detail should define specific action based on the opportunities and constraints in the local ecology, the agricultural economy, and policy landscape. BAP habitats are priority environments which have been identified as being most threatened and requiring conservation action under the UK Biodiversity Action Plan (BAP) (Figure 4.4).

Recent policy shifts towards participatory decision making have disrupted, but not dissolved, the appeal to a coherent, robust, stable, objective evidence base for decision making. The vulnerability maps are an example of how the vulnerability of biodiversity can be framed as knowable and to some extent quantifiable through a series of rational data calculations. Initial anticipation from the FARM team was that the maps would straightforwardly point land managers towards the correct management strategies for resilience. This is what vulnerability scholars call the 'end point approach' where, at the end point in a series of analysis, a quantifiable

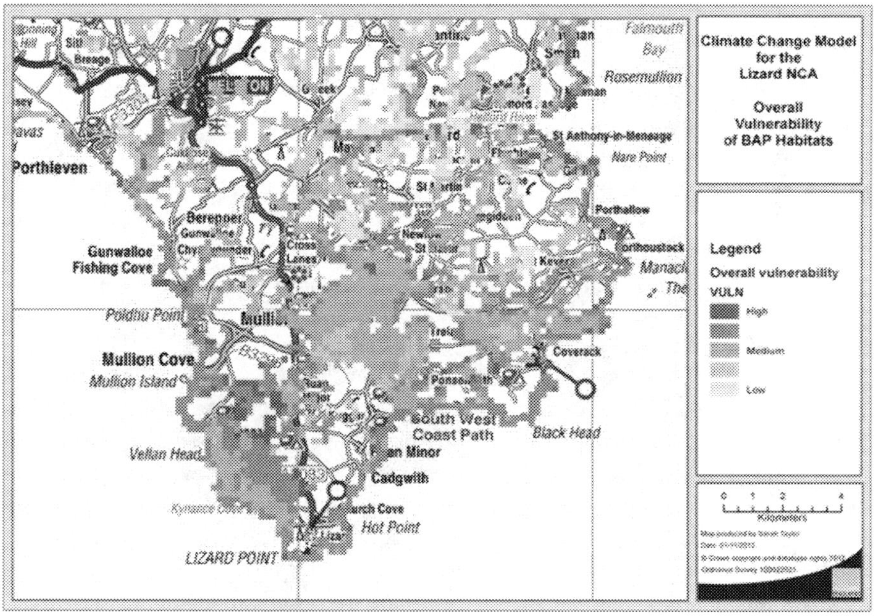

Figure 4.4 Overall vulnerability of BAP habitats.
Source: Taylor & Knight, 2012.

and static measure of vulnerability is produced (Kelly and Adger, 2000; Dessai et al., 2004). This approach is predicated on the instrumental conception of risk, which provides the evidence to underpin action. However, this is moderated by the policy imperative to support an adaptive management approach, defined as "a structured process of 'learning by doing' that involves much more than simply better ecological monitoring and response to unexpected management impacts" (Walters, 1997: 2). It should be noted that in Natural England's own climate change adaptation work, the NBCCVA is used alongside a range of resources and tools as well as expert judgement and local knowledge. For example, their National Character Area (NCA) Vulnerability Assessment methodology which is a feedback and user improvement process[6] (NE, 2013). Nevertheless, while the FARM team expected the vulnerability maps to be augmented with local knowledge they did not expect the results would be significantly challenged by the University ecologists or by local knowledge, as happened through the subsequent Episodes.

Episode two

The tidy linearity of this end point approach starts to break down in Episode two as other framings are brought into consideration, specifically those of the local Natural England representative (A2) and the CEC ecologists (A3). Amongst this group, there is still a strong commitment to risk as knowable and quantifiable, promising a clear and unequivocal view of management strategies from which resilience is the outcome. The ecologists' perspective was that the data underpinning the Natural England maps was inadequate for the Lizard because of epistemic uncertainty (i.e. lack of local data[7]). In response to this epistemic uncertainty, the ecologists took a different methodological approach. Rather than risk being assessed using a national scale model, the ecologists took a start point approach.

The ecologists started by attempting to model the existing state of the system – rather than a speculative projection of what might happen in the future – and focused on how the Lizard had already changed. Using local monitoring data (ERICA – Ecological Recording in Cornwall Automated, 2-million records, 25,000 species), recorded over the last 53-years which, along with RDB and the Ellenberg Values, the ecologists mapped the risks present at the local level. Ellenberg indicator values show whether that has been a change in mean reactivity, precipitation, moisture, nitrogen, light, RDB values, salinity, and temperature requirements of plants. Critically, the ecologist's position was that risk can still be quantified. But instead of risk being based on scenarios, their position was that any local risk map must be underpinned by empirics. This approach embodies resilience as practice, based as it is on a commitment to understanding change in the landscape.

Episode three

Scrutiny of the CEC ecologists' risk maps (Figure 4.5) through Episode three revealed three sources of uncertainty. First, potential epistemic uncertainty was identified in the data set by the ecologist. Second, it was acknowledged that this epistemic uncertainty might be interacting with the data's compilation, influenced by the specific interests of the botanical recorders. As Episode four confirmed, the interest of recorders is on the botanical hotspots and rare plants. Thus, the risk represented in the CEC ecologists' maps is more a reflection of the change in botanical hotspots than Lizard biodiversity as whole. The final, and most important, source of uncertainty was the issue of what these maps mean for a landscape management strategy based on the Ecological Network Approach. Because the maps show an overall change in plant composition, along the Ellenberg indicator values, it is difficult for land managers to interpret into specific action to assist one species.

Episode four

Through Episode four the different stakeholders' risk frames were explicitly exposed. The risk for the BSBI recorders was very much about the fate of the botanical hotspots, rather than biodiversity on the Lizard more generally. Resilience in practice lay in preserving these spaces. Yet the Ecological Network

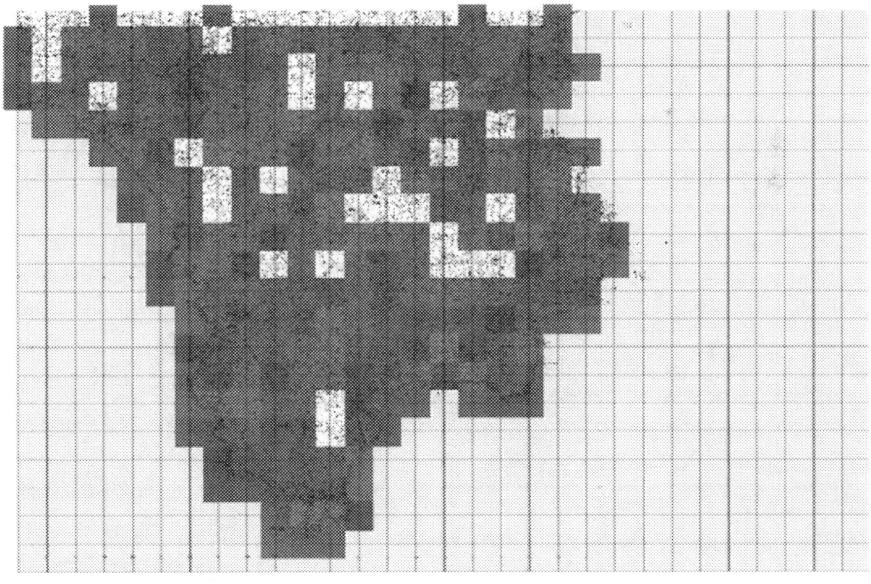

Figure 4.5 Example of ecologists risk map showing a reduction in precipitation across the Lizard.

Source: Owen Greenwood, unpublished.

Approach's emphasis on 'more, better, bigger, joined' promotes habitats which are, in the words of the scientific advisor (JH, 2014) "less 'unique' but none-the-less important". Episode four thus revealed ambiguity in landscape management and different conceptions of resilience in practice. Identifying where and how land management can be best targeted to safeguard biodiversity depends on a stakeholder's specialist interest and frames. In any landscape, the stakeholders involved and the data set drawn on in decision making will influence the resultant risks identified and the preferred management strategies.

The FARM project involved botanical specialist from the beginning and drew from their ERICA database. Arguably this influence drove the project away from the original aim to 'understand where and how land management could be best targeted to safeguard the biodiversity'. Instead, the FARM project produced maps which showed change, and potential risk, at botanical hotspots rather than risk at the 'less unique, but none-the-less important' sites; let alone identifying a strategy for delivering the Ecological Network Approach. This observation presents a fundamental challenge to the notion that environmental issues are 'out there' in the natural world to be managed through instrumental rationality and by the acquisition of more data. Instead, the argument here is that different actors will understand a landscape management decision differently, prioritize different problems, include or exclude different aspects, and favour different kinds of solutions (Dewulf et al., 2004; Brugnach et al., 2007). This has implications for how we understand resilience in theory and practice (Figure 4.6).

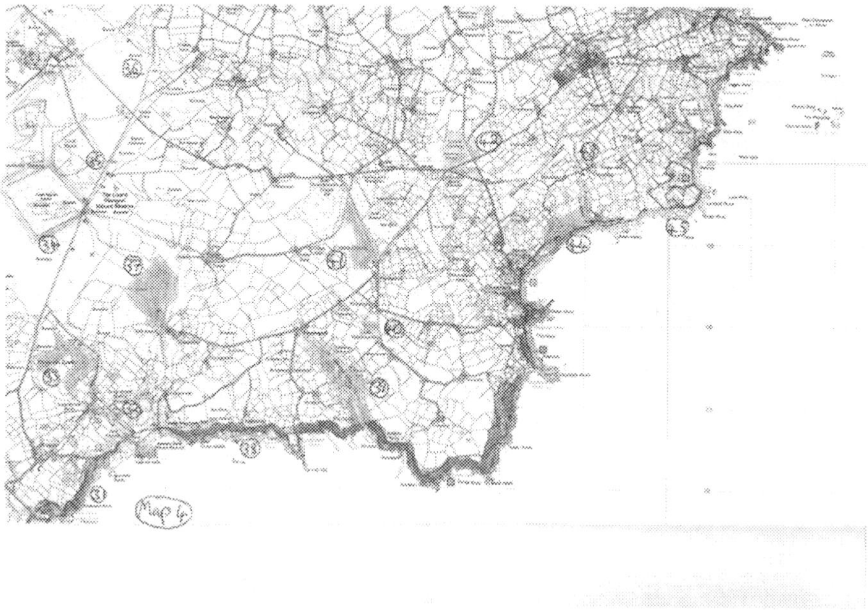

Figure 4.6 Risk Map of SE side of the Lizard annotated by project participants.
Source: Authors.

Episode five and six

In the final two Episodes, farmers emerge as arbiters between the inputs from different groups of experts. The farmers' critique of the validity of the ecological risk maps compelled the FARM team to review the original use of the ERICA database. The importance of this process, described in Episodes five and six, cannot be understated because without such process a landscape management strategy might have been predicated on contested data framed from a solely botanical perspective. In summary, the possible management solutions, underpinned by the Ecological Network Approach, are a matter of negotiation on the ground between actors with different and sometimes competing priorities who bring different frames to the discussion. Data and maps might be a starting point for this conversation but by no means define the scope of the issue or the viable solutions. Throughout each episode, scale became increasingly important as a modifier of the claims of each actor. The ecologists found the spatial scale of the NBCCV model was not detailed enough while the local expert stakeholders and farmers found the ecologist's risk maps to be temporally and spatially incomplete or inaccurate. At the scale of the farm, multiple frames of reference attempt to reconcile in a context in which ambiguity dominates. As the Natural England representative concluded; "in local contexts, the advantages of using broad and consistent metrics to measure vulnerability diminish and the specific characteristics of habitats and species present at that location become more important" (JC, 2014)

Conclusions and implications

Tracing through how the Ecological Network Approach was trialled at the landscape scale in Cornwall has exposed how resilience as a practice is conditioned by uncertainty and ambiguity. Resilience as a practice is revealed through the multiple, sometimes competing, framings on the Lizard of both the problem of and solutions for ecosystem fragmentation. Different experts – botanists, ecologists, farmers and others clearly held different ideas about what constituted resilience in that landscape (a similar finding to (Greksch and Winges, 2017). These framings become apparent through a series of episodes in which the interplay of uncertainty and ambiguity become apparent. This clearly shows that we need to be more attentive to what resilience as a practice means for different stakeholders working in a landscape where problem definition, approaches, solutions and possible outcomes are all a matter of negotiation. This also requires rethinking resilience in theory, especially its relationship to other concepts like risk and vulnerability.

Although resilience lies at the heart of much environmental management, it is frequently positioned as an *achievement* or *outcome* rather than a process or practice. Our research raises the question of how resilience as an achievement embedded within the Ecological Network Approach can be reconciled with resilience in practice in the multiple framings of the environment and its problems. While socio-ecological resilience is advocated in the scientific literature and policy discourse, as Wilkinson (2012) shows, it has not played out in a "demonstrated capacity to govern for resilience in practice". One possibility is that the post-hoc application of a frames analysis could be replaced with a priori process which would form part of grounded participatory governance for resilience. Such an approach would also include other actors – outside of agencies, land managers and farmers – who currently have little input into decision making.

Notes

1 The phrase 'land manager' is used here as an umbrella term for a wide range of individuals and statutory and non-statutory organisations involved in the conservation of landscape and biodiversity, the design and administration of agricultural stewardship schemes, management of designated areas, and the protection of the natural environment more broadly. In the UK, this includes Natural England, the National Trust, wildlife charities, and Defra, amongst others.
2 The term vulnerability assessment is used here in the broadest sense and means the process of identifying, evaluating and implementing actions to reduce risk to habitats.
3 Natural England is a statutory body responsible for looking after England's variety of wild plants and animals, its biodiversity and natural features www.gov.uk/government/organisations/natural-england.
4 The National Trust is a charity founded in 1895 to preserve built heritage and open spaces in England, Wales and Northern Ireland.
5 ERICA – Environmental Recording in Cornwall Automated. This is the largest and most comprehensive computerised natural history databank of any region in Britain with two million records covering 25,000 different species (www.cisfbr.org.uk/Documents/PRESS%20RELEASE.pdf).
6 There was not capacity to engage in this feedback process due to the scope of the project. But as set out in the conclusion, future research should take up opportunities in order to ensure that identified on the ground limitations are resolved.
7 The NBCCV assessment tool can use local data to amend analyses if required and time or the project remit permits.

References

Asah, S. T., Bengston, D. N., Wendt, K., & Nelson, K. C. (2012). Diagnostic reframing of intractable environmental problems: Case of a contested multiparty public land-use conflict. *Journal of Environmental Management, 108*, 108–119. doi:10.1016/j.jenvman.2012.04.041.

Baker, D. J., & Fuller, R. J. (2013). How can research help deliver a 'coherent & resilient ecological network'? *BTO Research Report*. online: British Trust for Ornithology.

Brace, C. & Geoghegan, H. 2010. Human geographies of climate change: Landscape, temporality, and lay knowledges. *Progress in Human Geography, 35*(3), 284–302.

Brooks, T. M., Mittermeier, R. A., Mittermeier, C. G., Da Fonseca, G. A. B., Rylands, A. B., Konstant, W. R., ... Hilton-Taylor, C. (2002). Habitat loss and extinction in the hotspots of biodiversity. *Conservation Biology*, *16*(4), 909–923.

Brugnach, M., Dewulf, A., Pahl-Wostl, C., & Tallieu, T. (2007). Towards a relational concept of uncertainty: About knowing too little, knowing too differently and accepting not to know. *Proceedings of the 14th International Conference on Multi-Organisational Partnerships, Alliances & Networks MOPAN*. Leuven, Belgium.

Brugnach, M., Dewulf, A., Henriksen, H. J., & van der Keur, P. (2011). More is not always better: Coping with ambiguity in natural resources management. *Journal of Environmental Management*, *92*(1), 78–84. doi:10.1016/j.jenvman.2010.08.029.

DEFRA. (2011). *Natural environment white paper*. London: HM Government: Stationary Office.

Dessai, S., Adger, W. N., Hulme, M., Turnpenny, J., Köhler, J. & Warren, R. 2004. Defining and experiencing dangerous climate change. *Climatic Change*, *64*(1), 11-25.

Dessai, S., & van der Sluijs, J. (2008). *Uncertainty and climate change adaptation—A scoping study*. The Netherlands: Utrecht University.

Dewulf, A., Craps, M., & Dercon, G. (2004). How issues get framed and reframed when different communities meet: Case study of a collaborative soil conservation initiative in the Ecuadorian Andes. *Journal of Community and Applied Social Psychology*, *14*, 177–192.

Dewulf, A., Craps, M., Bouwen, R., Taillieu, T., & Pahl-Wostl, C. (2005). Integrated management of natural resources: dealing with ambiguous issues, multiple actors and diverging frames. *Water Science & Technology*, *52*(6), 115–124.

Dewulf, A., Gray, L., Putnam, R., Lewicki, N., Aarts, R., Bouwen, C., & Woerkum, V. (2009). Disentangling approaches to framing in conflict and negotiation research: A meta-paradigmatic perspective. *Human Relations*, *62*, 155–193.

Emery, S. B., & Franks, J. R. (2012). The potential for collaborative agri-environment schemes in Engalnd: Can a well-designed collaborative approach address farmers' concerns with current schemes? *Journal of Rural Studies*, *28*(3), 218–231.

Entman, R. M. (1993). Framing: Toward clarification of a fractured paradigm. *Journal of Communication*, *43*(4), 51–58. doi:10.1111/j.1460–2466.1993.tb01304.x.

Füssel, H.-M. (2007). Vulnerability: A generally applicable conceptual framework for climate change research. *Global Environmental Change*, *17*(2), 155–167.

Greksch, K., & Winges, M. (2017). Resilience – A useful term for transdisciplinary projects? Experiences from the field. In E. Trell, B. Hoven, B. Restemeyer, & M. Bakema (Eds.), *Governing for resilience in vulnerable places* Groningen: University of Groningen.

Gunderson, L. H. (2000). Ecological resilience—In theory and application. *Annual Review of Ecology and Systematics*, *31*(1), 425–439.

Hannah, L., Midgley, G., Lovejoy, T., Bond, W., Bush, M., Lovett, J., ... Woodward, F. (2002). Conservation of biodiversity in a changing climate. *Conservation Biology*, *16*(1), 264–268.

Heller, N. E., & Zavaleta, E. S. (2009). Biodiversity management in the face of climate change: A review of 22 years of recommendations. *Biological Conservation*, *142*(1), 14–32.

Hodgson, J. A., Thomas, C. D., Wintle, B. A., & Moilanen, A. (2009). Climate change, connectivity and conservation decision making: Back to basics. *Journal of Applied Ecology, 46*(5), 964–969. doi:10.1111/j.1365-2664.2009.01695.x.

Hoek, V. D. R. E., Brugnach, M., Mulder, J. P. M., & Hoekstra, A. Y. (2014). Analysing the cascades of uncertainty in flood defence projects: How "not knowing enough" is related to "knowing differently". *Global Environmental Change, 24*, 373–388.

Hopkins, J., & Britain, G. (2007). *Conserving biodiversity in a changing climate: Guidance on building capacity to adapt.* Department for Environment, Food and Rural Affairs.

IPCC. (2014). Summary for policymakers. In C. B. Field et al. (Eds.), *Climate change 2014: Impacts, adaptation, and vulnerability. Part A: Global and sectoral aspects. Contribution of working group II to the fifth assessment report of the intergovernmental panel on climate change* (pp. 1–32). Cambridge and New York: Cambridge University Press.

Kelly, P. M. & Adger, W. N. 2000. Theory and practice in assessing vulnerability to climate change and facilitating adaptation. *Climatic Change 47*(4), 325–352.

Lawton, J. H., Brotherton, P. N. M., Brown, V. K., Elphick, C., Fitter, A. H., Forshaw, J., ... Wynne, G. R. (2010). *Making space for nature: A review of England's wildlife sites and ecological network.* London: DEFRA.

Maclean, I., Bennie, J. J., Scott, A. J., & Wilson, R. J. (2012). A high-resolution model of soil and surface water conditions. *Ecological Modelling, 237-238*, 109–119. https://doi.org/10.1016/j.ecolmodel.2012.03.029.

Mazur, K. E., & Asah, S. T. (2013). Clarifying standpoints in the gray wolf recovery conflict: Procuring management and policy forethought. *Biological Conservation, 167*, 79–89.

Mora, C., & Sale, P. F. (2011). Ongoing global biodiversity loss and the need to move beyond protected areas: A review of the technical and practical shortcomings of protected areas on land and sea. *Marine Ecology Progress Series, 434*, 251–266.

Opdam, P., & Wascher, D. (2004). Climate change meets habitat fragmentation: Linking landscape and biogeographical scale levels in research and conservation. *Biological Conservation, 117*, 285–297.

Sigel, K., Klauer, B., & Pahl-Wostl, C. (2010). Conceptualizing uncertainty in environmental decision-making: the example of the EU water framework directive. *Ecological Economics, 69*, 502–510.

Thomas, C. D., Cameron, A., Green, R. E., Bakkenes, M., Beaumont, L. J., Collingham, Y. C., & Hannah, L. (2004). Extinction risk from climate change. *Nature, 427*(6970), 145–148.

Thuiller, W. (2007). Biodiversity: Climate change and the ecologist. *Nature, 448*(7153), 550–552. doi:10.1038/448550a.

Walters, C. 1997. Challenges in adaptive management of riparian and coastal ecosystems. *Conservation Ecology, 1*(2), 1.

Wilkinson, C. (2012). Urban resilience: What does it mean in Planning Practice? *Planning Theory and Practice, 13*, 319–324.

5 Resilience thinking – is vagueness a blessing or a curse in transdisciplinary projects?

Experiences from a regional climate change adaptation project

Maik Winges and Kevin Grecksch

Introduction

Between 2008 and 2014 the German Federal Government supported climate change adaptation research in a large-scale funding initiative. Transdisciplinary research was a cornerstone of all seven funded projects across Germany (see Biebeler et al., 2014 for a summary of all projects) based on the following assumptions: The key to successful adaptation are regional and tailor-made solutions, measures and strategies that consider regional economic, ecological and social characteristics (Garrelts et al. 2013a,b; Grecksch, 2014; Winges, 2015). Researching climate change requires not only collaboration of different academic disciplines from environmental sciences to social sciences, but it also requires public participation to raise awareness and ensure legitimacy of mitigation and adaption measures. Therefore, climate change will not only be a challenge for disciplinary research but also contests the relationship between science and society. Research questions regarding climate change are characterised by high complexity, high pressure to react, and the necessity to produce solutions. Scientists have become advocates of mitigation and adaption leaving their (assumed) neutral position towards the research object. Therefore, the process of generating knowledge itself has been put into question by several discourses since the 1990s: post-normal science (Funtowicz and Ravetz, 1993), post-academic science (Ziman, 1996), triple-helix (Etzkowitz and Leydesdorff, 2000) or mode-II science (Gibbons, et al., 1994). This article discusses experiences from one of the seven funded projects, "nordwest2050-Prospects for Climate-Adapted Innovation Processes in the Model Region Bremen-Oldenburg in North Western Germany" (in the following "nordwest2050"). The project chose socio-ecological resilience as the theoretical framework (Folke et al., 2002, 2005), which is increasingly interesting for research projects (Van der Vaart et al., 2015). However, the assumption whether this is a good fit, especially when defined rather vaguely, has been discussed rarely so far. For this chapter, we assume that transdisciplinary research has special characteristics and procedural demands. The chapter focuses on the question whether resilience as boundary concept supports or hinders tackling these features. Resilience shares its vagueness with other boundary concepts, facing similar issues. In other contexts, such as the sustainable cities discourses, vagueness has been accused of impeding decision making (Tatham et al., 2014) and something that must be diminished (Seeliger and Turol, 2013). Therefore, our findings might provide insights beyond the resilience community.

To approach the question whether vagueness was a blessing or curse in transdisciplinary projects, in the following, we present experiences made during the above-mentioned research project. First, we briefly introduce transdisciplinary research, resilience and resilience thinking. This is followed by an introduction to the research project in order to understand the observations we made. Next is a discussion of our experiences against the design principles of transdisciplinary research outlined in Section two. The chapter closes with a conclusion summarising our findings.

Transdisciplinary research

Despite all differences between post-normal science, post-academic science, triple-helix science and mode-II science, all share the lowering of disciplinary barriers and the integration of non-scientific knowledge, i.e. transdisciplinarity (Hessels and Lente, 2008). Transdisciplinarity distinguishes itself from multidisciplinarity and interdisciplinarity, whereby the first means that different academic disciplines are cooperating and the latter means cooperation plus sharing methods and concepts. Transdisciplinarity aims at a common, open and reflexive learning process of science and society (Adomßent and Michelsen, 2011, p. 104) to solve societal problems. This includes forming connections between different knowledge bodies (between academic disciplines, between academic and non-academic knowledge), interests and communication practices and languages (Jahn et al., 2012). Transdisciplinary research ideally has a shared "knowledge body" of all actors, at least it has a "varied problem understanding" and therefore a broad spectrum of solutions (Adomßent and Michelsen, 2011). Hence, next to generating scientific effort in the sense of knowledge generation, the search for solutions to societal problems is at the heart of transdisciplinary research. This means an extended role for science though. Instead of just being purposeful, knowledge generation is also measured against its usefulness (Jahn et al., 2012). In a transdisciplinary context, science's purpose is not only to get closer to "truths", but also to contribute to a responsible transition towards a climate adapted lifestyle and economy (WBGU, 2011). The proposed research design for transdisciplinary knowledge generation is action research, a "process oriented and open search"

(Adomßent and Michelsen, 2011, p. 11) that focusses on the identification of problem-solving strategies and its barriers plus how to overcome the theory-practice and researcher-subject dualism (Adomßent and Michelsen, 2011).

Given the diverse disciplinary and professional backgrounds communication problems can arise though. Institutional logics can be different as well and transdisciplinary research projects fight against self-centredness too. Due to the focus on the problem-solving qualities, knowledge production that goes beyond the case studied is often pushed to the background (Adomßent and Michelsen, 2011). In addition, transdisciplinary action research lacks consistency of term definitions and approaches. A coherent research frame or standardised methods are yet to come (Brandt et al., 2013). Jahn et al. (2012) attest transdisciplinary approaches a marginal status and question whether it really is a new and genuine form of knowledge generation. Nonetheless, its importance with regards to urgent and complex issues such as environmental problems and climate change are widely acclaimed (Brandt et al. 2013; Deppisch and Hasibovic, 2013; Hagemeier-Klose et al., 2014; Scholz, 2013; Serrao-Neumann et al., 2015).

According to Lang et al. (2012, p. 28), transdisciplinary research processes consist of three phases: Phase A covers "Collaborative problem framing and building a collaborative research team". In phase B "Co-Creation and solution-orientated transferable knowledge and transferable knowledge through collaborative research are key issues. Phase C covers (Re-) integrating and applying the co-created knowledge. In phase C the results are applied and also reintegrated in scientific processes as well as societal practices (Lang et al., 2012). While a useful overall concept can help to successfully do so, it is not as essential as in phase A or phase B. The project did not cover phase C as nordwest2050's aim was to develop a strategy for making the study region climate adapted until 2050. It is now up to public authorities and stakeholders to implement the collaboratively developed adaptation steps since this process requires a democratically mandated authority. Hence, we concentrate on phases A and B in our analysis.

Lang et al. (2012) describe design principles for every phase. These are rather detailed process steps than general design principles. Still, without these steps, transdisciplinary processes are likely to create unsatisfying results. Based on these process steps we discuss the usefulness of resilience as a guiding principle in transdisciplinary research projects and clarify whether it supports or hinders the particular design principle.

Transdisciplinary research with a focus on climate change entails specific challenges: Many of the projected effects of climate change may only have an impact in the future, i.e. ten, twenty or thirty years from today. Hence, problem awareness and the incentive to act are low among stakeholders and decision makers (Garrelts et al., 2013a,b; Grothmann et al., 2013). In addition, research projects usually last several years, in the case of nordwest2050 five years, and this requires long-term commitment from stakeholders. They need to be appreciated and taken care of, especially if longer breaks between workshops occur. Generating interest and commitment is especially challenging for practitioners and the broader public since it brings about additional workload which often cannot be offset with day-to-day business. Hence, a benefit from participation must be visible during the whole process. Besides concrete results, this can be achieved through a desirable guiding concept like sustainability, which is, to many researchers, a rather fuzzy concept (Phillis and Andriantiatsaholiniaina, 2001). Large groups engage in the process of sustainable development, be it in their role as practitioners or as citizens and are willing to invest time and/or money. This commitment is often linked to specific projects.

Socio-ecological resilience and resilience thinking

Resilience is an increasingly popular term within the scientific debate, e.g. in psychology (Rutter, 1987), organisational theory (Vogus and Sutcliffe, 2007) or in the field of computer networks (Najjar and Gaudiot, 1990). Resilience, as we refer to it, has its roots in ecosystem theory as a counter-concept to the then prevalent perception of stable, single equilibrium ecological systems. Thus, the central goal is to focus on the maintenance of ecosystems and their functions. In this view, resilience has been defined as the ability of a system to withstand stress and still provide pivotal services (Brand, 2005; Carpenter et al., 2001; Folke et al., 2002). The concept was then transferred to socio-ecological systems (SES). SES are based on the idea that socio-economic and ecological systems are interconnected and mutually dependent (Adger, 2006). However, in contrast to ecological systems, social systems are purposeful and can be designed to a certain, even if limited extent (Walker et al., 2004; Folke et al., 2005; Davoudi et al., 2012).

Resilience is referred to as analytical tool as well as normative boundary concept (Brand, 2007). In the latter case, it is more precise to speak about "resilience thinking", which lies "on the vague end of the spectrum" when it comes to resilience concepts (Strunz 2012, p. 113). Resilience has been criticized for too often mixing these aspects, being ambiguous and therefore lacking clarity, blending descriptive and normative aspects, losing track of its core feature by diminishing ecological aspects and becoming a way of thinking rather than a well-defined concept (Brand and Jax, 2007). However, in this respect resilience has been praised as being a helpful "conceptional point of reference" (Deppisch and Hasibovic, 2013, p. 119; see also Brand and Jax, 2007) in interdisciplinary and transdisciplinary research.[1] In this regard, conceptual vagueness is useful in general and resilience thinking is considered a useful, but vague, term (Strunz, 2012). According to Strunz (2012), Vague terms: a) support creativity which relies on open, vague language; b) foster inter-and transdisciplinary communication (although precision should not hinder communication across disciplines; c) are more appropriate for problem-solving under high uncertainty and with a high need for action. In addition, Deppisch and Hasibovic (2013) see – among others – an advantage in the necessity of taking a close and critical look at the norms and values and the disclosure of feedback and dependencies between social and ecological systems. The advantages are countervailed by the disadvantages such as the lack of empirical testability, circumvention of scientific methods and the abandonment of the aim of establishing validity of concepts (Strunz, 2012).

The role and definition of resilience within the project "nordwest2050"

The project "nordwest2050-Prospects for Climate-Adapted Innovation Processes in the Model Region Bremen-Oldenburg in North Western Germany" (nordwest2050) was a five-year research project funded by the German Federal Ministry of Education and Research (BMBF). Nordwest2050 was driven by academic research but extensive stakeholder collaboration has been an essential and vital part from its onset. It was a practice-oriented research project aimed at increasing the ability of the Metropolitan Region Bremen-Oldenburg to deal with climate change in three selected policy fields – energy, agriculture and food production and ports and logistic – to implement measures into regional planning and development processes. Figure 5.1 shows the study region, a coastal region on Germany's North Sea coast.

After five years, the actors` awareness of climate change impacts should be increased and a common overall strategy to handle them on sectoral and regional level should be developed. The strategies were based on a vulnerability assessment of the current systems as well as possible future opportunities (innovation potential analysis) in a changing physical and normative environment, both for the sectors – previously mentioned – as well as the whole region. Furthermore, scenarios covered a range of other possible future developments apart from climate change. To address normative issues, the project also developed a "vision", the desired future all stakeholders would pursue. Within the project, we used an extensive set of stakeholder processes, which involved semi-structured expert interviews, workshops, a web-based participation tool, a project website, information material, regional conferences, a business competition, a project advisory board etc. The number and diversity of stakeholders were large and varied in the different subprojects (see also "Build a collaborative research team"). It ranged from small-scale farmers, small and medium-sized enterprises to public authorities and industry representatives as well as the media. Figure 5.2 illustrates the basic project structure and the stakeholder process.

The findings in this chapter are based on the authors' observations, and extensive minutes from project meetings, stakeholder meetings, one-to-one conversations with stakeholders and numerous project workshops. The authors were involved in the research project as social scientists analysing regional governance aspects and were, therefore, working on a cross-cutting issue. This enabled them to participate in most research and stakeholder processes within the project. The observations solely reflect the authors' views and experiences and are not representative for the project.

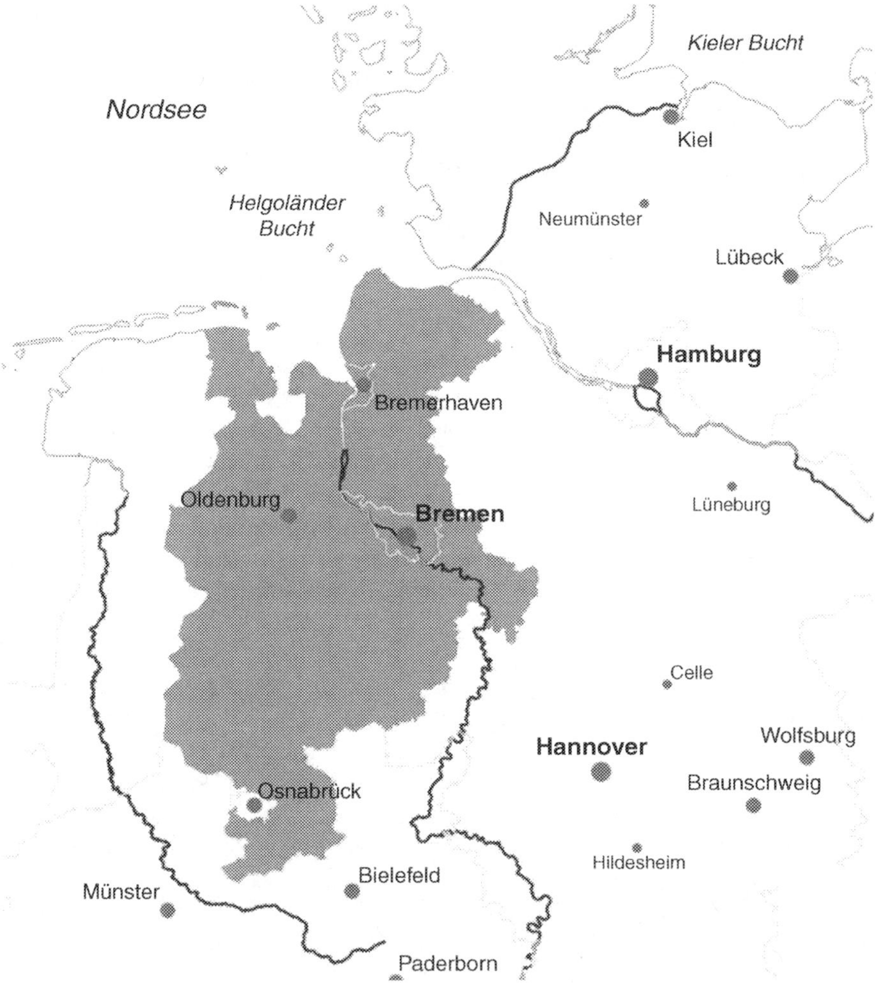

Figure 5.1 Map metropolitan region Bremen-Oldenburg.
Source: Data licence Germany – BBSR Bonn 2017 – Version 2.0.

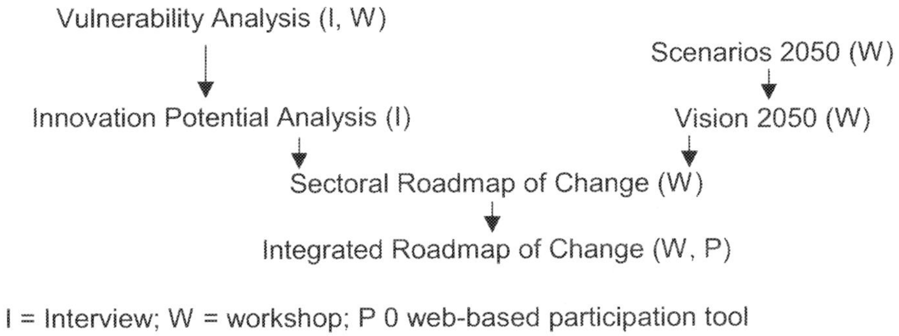

Figure 5.2 Stakeholder process "nordwest2050".
Source: Authors.

Resilience in the transdisciplinary research project "nordwest 2050"

In the project, resilience had a twofold function: It was used as an analytical tool as well as a normative boundary concept since the problem seemed complex and approaching it required involving a range of different stakeholders and scientists. The decision on a vague boundary concept was also driven by the attempt not to deter any actors and to be as inclusive as possible to provide the discussed broad spectrum of solutions.

In addition, there are indications that the term 'resilience' compared to 'adaptation' shifts the focus from individual to collective actions, although it is not clear yet whether this just discourages individual responses or indeed triggers community action (Wong-Parodi et al., 2015). Furthermore, resilience seemed to be a rather encouraging term in comparison to adaptation that harbours a more reactive connotation with a focus on preservation. In contrast, resilience has a strong focus on acquiring new capabilities (Wong-Parodi et al., 2015). As to resilience as the analytical tool, a definition was developed by an interdisciplinary working group. Discussing and agreeing on the concept took up almost the first project year.

Resilience was then a reference point for all project teams and their respective subprojects and work packages. The common definition of resilience in the project was as follows: "Resilience describes the capability of a system to maintain its services under stress and in turbulent environments (despite massive external disturbances and internal breakdowns)" (Gleich and Gößling-Reisemann, 2010, p. 25). In contrast to robustness, which refers to the ability of systems to maintain system characteristics when subjected to specific disturbances, the project's understanding of resilience emphasised the ability to cope with disturbances and its self-organisational capacity in a comprehensive way (Thissen et al., 2017). While robustness focusses on a partial challenge around a single metric, resilience approaches are qualitative in nature and suitable for multifaceted problems that are difficult to quantify (Thissen et al., 2017). Thus, resilience means a balanced relation between resistance, adaptive capacity, the ability to improvise and the ability to innovate. Resistance describes a systems' ability to withstand external stress factors, adaptive capacity refers to "the ability of a system to adjust to climate change (including climate variability and extremes) to moderate potential damages, to take advantage of opportunities, or to cope with the consequences" (Parry et al., 2007). The ability to improvise and the ability to innovate are concerned with actor's abilities and their access to material resources and social resources and they are also dependent on their willingness to learn, adapt and to take up opportunities (see also Gleich and Gößling-Reisemann, 2010). In nordwest2050 dimensions and design elements of resilient systems (system abilities, system resources, system structures) were identified (Gleich and Gößling-Reisemann, 2010). System abilities are for instance adaptiveness, the ability to learn or its self-healing ability. System resources refer to energy, materials and information among others. System structures describe aspects such as diversity, redundancy, positive and negative feedback loops as well as buffers. System resources and system structures are not only aimed at quantity and quality but are also directed towards their proliferation and diversification. The presence and diversity of redundancies of elementary structures, for example, increase the ability to maintain system functions even if external conditions dramatically change (Gleich and Gößling-Reisemann, 2010). We assumed that if actors learn to improve these elements they can work towards resilience of their reference system. While the terms were partially illustrated, the level of abstraction remained high.

The rather complex definition of the then barely known resilience concept seemed only little appealing to potential stakeholders when it came to its function as boundary concept. In addition, boundary concepts require an involvement of all involved parties. That is why stakeholders were given the opportunity to develop their own common resilience understanding based on a wide definition. For easier communication, the resulting boundary concept was called the project's guiding principle. Stakeholders did not reject the definition. However, despite encouragement they did not embrace it or alter it either: Their projects did not reflect elements of the definition let alone mentioned them. The differentiation between resilience as an analytical tool and as a guiding principle more often led to confusion among the participating researchers than adding value to the project.

Resilience in transdisciplinary research

This section is a discussion of our findings and experiences against the design principles of transdisciplinary research outlined in the section "Transdisciplinary research" above and according to Lang et al. (2012). The description follows Table 5.1.

Table 5.1 Design principles for transdisciplinary research

	Design principle	*Description*
	create interest and commitment	raise problem awareness and create incentives; demonstrate benefit for stakeholders to participate and to commit
Phase A	build a collaborative research team	identify scientists from relevant disciplines and stakeholders with experience and expertise; clarify competencies, decision rules and establish balanced structures between scientists and practice actors
	create joint understanding and definition of the (sustainability) problem to be addressed	define the problem as a societally relevant problem; involve all team members in the problem definition and establish a common reference point
	collaboratively define the boundary/research object, research objectives as well as specific research questions and success criteria	formulate the overall research object and objective; formulate it in a guiding question and sub-questions; specify in operationalised research questions
	design a methodological framework for collaborative knowledge production and integration	agree on methods and applied transdisciplinary settings; employ an evidence-based template for collaboration
Phase B	assign and support appropriate roles for practitioners and researchers	be as transparent as possible; balance societal relevance and scientific rigour; employ cognitive, structural and procedural leadership
	apply and adjust integrative research methods and transdisciplinary settings for knowledge generation and integration	make use and further develop methods; use tools to support teamwork and collaboration

Source: Authors, based on Lang et al. (2012).

Create interest and commitment

During the five years, the researchers involved in the project worked with numerous stakeholders. Some of them were already directly concerned with climate change issues, others knew they might be in the future. Furthermore, some stakeholders did not have a direct link to the topic, yet they agreed on exchanging on it (see Build a collaborative research team). However, the efforts to gain wide public interest were not as successful as hoped. For example, the project's communication team produced several short videos, which were published on the project website and on YouTube. However, the number of viewers remains low although we cannot attribute this directly to the resilience term. While resilience is not limited to either mitigation or adaptation the funding body's aim and stipulations were clear about the adaptation focus, which also manifests itself in the working definition and the available information material. At this point we might have taken some of the advantages of the vagueness of resilience thinking, by excluding mitigation aspects stakeholders would have associated with the term. Thus, we might have lost interested parties that focus on these issues. Mitigation would have given them a point of departure in the discussions. On the contrary, we had to draw the line and set some key pillars to assure the term is supporting the project to reach its goal. Vagueness and specificity are therefore binaries but form a spectrum.

Although the idea of climate change adaptation in a broader sense and resilience in particular gained acceptance during the process, the time and commitment spent on the project or at least the willingness to do so decreased. Stakeholders no matter whether they were from administration or private businesses were concerned with a wide range of issues and climate change adaptation was just one of them. In addition, climate change as – at least perceived – long term issue tends to be given a lower rank when it comes to prioritisation. The term did not create ideas of short-term goals that would have sparked off further motivation. The creativity in the sense of coupling short-term and long-term goals was rather low.

Build a collaborative research team

Nordwest2050 was conceptualised and developed as a research project involving researchers from different disciplines from the very beginning. Resilience (thinking) was chosen as guiding concept during the grant application phase and was, therefore, the central term from the very start. All researchers and practitioners were aware of that before joining the project. As 'bottom-up approach, which aims at strengthening the system,' (Thissen et al., 2017) it seemed to be the most appropriate concept to fulfil the funder's aim of holistic, inclusive transdisciplinary projects. Social scientists, economists, geographers, biologists, psychologists and industrial engineers were part of the team. As mentioned earlier, it took one year to agree on a common resilience definition. As it turned out, scientists from different fields knew the resilience term(s) in their research area but were partly unaware of the meaning in other research fields and the consequences it would pose on interdisciplinary communication. This came as a surprise since most of the scientists had worked in interdisciplinary contexts before. In addition, the project had an advisory board made up of regional representatives from administration, unions, chambers of commerce, business, religion, media and non-governmental organisations. As the project focussed on three economic sectors – agriculture and food production, energy and ports, and logistics, each sector team had a set of practice partners and stakeholders with whom they were collaborating over the project's course of time. Other subprojects, such as regional governance, formed problem-oriented alliances and collaborations with stakeholders.

Create joint understanding and definition of the problem to be addressed

The basic problem handled in the project were the inevitable climate change impacts from the past and ongoing man-made greenhouse gas emissions and the measures to adapt to them. Yet, this does not cover the question which impacts might occur and what qualifies them as problematic. The project was process-oriented. Both impacts and measures were supposed to be identified on the grounds of the resilience concept during the project. Hence, increasing resilience was set as both main objective and success criteria before any stakeholder consultation. During the project the overall vagueness of the concept fuelled the impression that every aspect is negotiable. Some stakeholders were not willing to deal with questions beyond their sphere of influence. Economic players were often not interested in talking about anything but their own business decisions. Politicians as well as high-level administrative personnel needed to reduce complexity to include results in their work, which could mean either transfer it in an indicator or into tangible (short-term) measures. In this regard, analytical and normative dimensions were mixed without reflecting on them.

Collaboratively define the boundary/research object, research objectives as well as specific research questions, and success criteria

At the beginning of the project, an interdisciplinary team with representatives from each subproject was given one year to define a common understanding of resilience and with that a common language (Groot et al., 2015). However, this group did not consist of stakeholders or representatives from the broader public. The practitioners were only involved after the researchers finalised their common definition. This is in part because stakeholders expect input. Still, it was astonishing how controversial the process had been, even without the challenge to integrate non-researchers into the debate about a complex academic term. The final definition (see section on Resilience) was a compromise in the best sense, meaning nobody got what they wished for. The debate lasted longer than the contemplated twelve-months and did not achieve a basic level of agreement. Conflicts about the normative aspects as well as the relation between resilience and sustainability remained unresolved.

In addition, not all the practitioners were happy with the term either. Within the administration, local actors did not know or embrace resilience as a term, higher-level public administration, on the other hand, supported it. The explanation seems simple. Discussing a conceptual term is easier and more fruitful for actors dealing with conceptual work in their everyday work than for actors doing 'groundwork'. Furthermore, business actors are often interested in solutions specific to their problems. From their point of view, conceptual discussions as well holistic problem solutions are often pointless.

Even agreeing on a broad definition did not lead to a joint understanding, since vagueness resulted in resilience to serve as "container". Some project partners simply relabelled their existing activities in many cases even mitigation measures such as usage of renewable energy sources – a widely known problem (O'Hare and White, 2013; Van der Vaart et al., 2015). We can only speculate to which end actors invested considerable time in the project if they did not intend to change their policies. One explanation might be the prospect of scientific legitimisation for their approaches. While these activities were not irrelevant in terms of resilience, they were not the result of a systematic resilience-oriented analysis either. This is not to say that all actors acted like this. Nevertheless, the resilience term bears the risk of such behaviour. A project definition might not even be the "lowest common denominator" since it might not be common.

The sectoral approach of the project further augmented the problem of apart drifting understandings of resilience. Just like in other fields, isolation (of the inner-sector discourses) led to incompatibility. The energy sector focussed on redundancies whereas the activities of the agriculture and food production sector centred on extending ranges of tolerance and diversity. Even though both elements play a crucial role in terms of resilience, it cannot be narrowed down to them alone. The regional dimension increased the diversity of problems, actors and interests. Urban and rural problems were often very different. Cities and rural districts in the study region have a long history of conflicts especially in terms of attracting businesses. The holistic approach of including big economic players and small, green companies underestimated not only the conflicts among them but also the difficulty in a common problem scoping.

On the plus side though, actor knowledge and interest in the term (and the overall topic) increased noticeable during the project, while the interest of the broader public was not overwhelming. Some actors even committed to the project via a formal contract. In those cases, subprojects with predetermined steps and co-funding have been realised. Other stakeholders participated in the wider transdisciplinary exchange process.

Design a methodological framework for collaborative knowledge production and integration

Even after defining the problem, research object, objectives, questions and success criteria, there are different choices available when it comes to methodology. Since resilience has been established as a term within multiple discourses, researchers from different academic disciplines might not be aware of the approaches of their colleagues and therefore choose established methods within their discipline, which can impede collaboration. In addition, we as researchers lost track differentiating between analytical tool and resilience thinking in different work streams. Actors are more likely to identify with resilience concepts close to their field of work. Farmers chose ecosystem science-based resilience understandings, whereas engineers were more attracted to technical approaches. The diverse range of actors in the project reflected this very well. It ranged from ecological forerunners willing to take up any opportunity to combine climate change adaptation and business success to companies unable to think beyond their traditional business model based on a stable physical environment. Resilience in their case was how to sustain this model against the projected effects of climate change. Unfortunately, we could not observe the advantage of disclosure of feedback and dependencies between social and ecological systems, at least not in all cases. Some stakeholders applied resilience aspects only to their technical systems. Not even social consequences were given a thought, let alone ecological ones. For that reason, choosing resilience as a guiding concept requires intensive dialogues at an early stage within the development of a methodological framework. The project involved different actors with different agendas, e.g. medium sized companies with a sustainability focus and established companies regarding this topic an imposition rather than an opportunity. It would have been a benefit if it had led to a knowledge exchange between them. Unfortunately, it did not and it rather led to separated and conflicting strategies.

Assign and support appropriate roles for practitioners and researchers

Roles have been assigned, however, practitioners alienated themselves from the project whenever they did not agree with the researchers' results. This is not a problem related to resilience rather than to transdisciplinary processes in general. Some actors understood resilience rather technical. The separation of resilience as analytical tool and resilience thinking as guiding principle proved easier said than done since it requires actors to be interested in doing so. If stakeholders suspect their business model might be questioned, they try to avoid the topic dealing with resilience as an analytical tool. If commitment in transdisciplinary research is based on gaining benefits, it comes with no surprise that commitment decreases once benefits were doubted.

This went as far as one actor trying to leave the process if certain assumptions of future economic development were altered in order to find out about the system's robustness towards such changes. "This scenario does not exist for us, not even hypothetically", one actor said. Without being able to reveal the identity of the actor, we can, however, say that the discussed scenario would have endangered his current business model. In another case, a suggested minor change in political responsibilities, which was co-developed by researchers and practitioners almost stalled the project. The affected political entities withdrew support without any substantive reason. Hence, resilience thinking failed to spark discussions that challenge actor positions as suggested by Strunz (2012) in this case, although over the course of the project many discussions about normative aspects did occur. Still, including economic or politically powerful actors might not always support discussions about normativity. In addition, these actors have negotiating power if they are indispensable in terms of project success. During the project, several actors threatened to leave the project when discussions did not go their way. Compromises overrepresented their interests and hence reproduced and reinforced the regional power balance. In the final stage of the project, a kind of memorandum of understanding was signed by important actors and stakeholders where they agreed and committed to basic principles regarding the project's results. Nonetheless, this document marked a very light version of results, which was agreeable by all actors yet controversially discussed among the project's researchers.

Apply and adjust integrative research methods and transdisciplinary settings for knowledge generation and integration

The above-described interpretation of resilience led to a lack of considering normative implications. Resilience was understood by some stakeholders as something, which can be described in simple construction rules like the n+1 rule for the electricity grid, which says that there should be at least one more unit of all critical features than necessary for operation under regular circumstances. This led to expectations that problems can be solved without altering societal rules and principles. In addition, it excludes issues of justice. Uneven distribution can decrease adaptive capacities at the level of disadvantaged individuals as well as at societal level (Adger et al., 2006; Paavola and Adger, 2006). Climate change itself as well as adaptation to it might have distribution effects. When it comes to climate change adaption measures, there are several modes of allocating resources. Since financial resources are scarce, cost-effectiveness is often used as a benchmark. It ensures that the money used results in the greatest possible effects. Nevertheless, it may be that the most vulnerable will not benefit from adaptation measures based on this criterion. Therefore, Paavola and Adger (2006, p. 607) argue for a "putting the most vulnerable first". However, debates within the project never reached this far. Resilience thinking with all the different connotations seemed to mask, if not increase the issue since its character as potential portmanteau has never been discussed. In addition, stakeholders seemed to appreciate this feature – it allowed them to avoid normative debates that might question their policies or business models. Hence, methodological problems of the research process design are amplified.

When it comes to production of generalizable, transferable knowledge, vague terms suffer from their disadvantages. Empirical testability requires clear and specific definitions and concepts. Without empirical testability, it is impossible to decide whether measures and assumptions have been successful and why (not). Therefore, even negative outcomes based on transdisciplinary approaches might not be detected.

Conclusion

Resilience had a twofold function in the project: It was used as analytical tool as well normative boundary concept for the interaction between researchers and practitioners. Regarding the latter, the project showed that a vague resilience thinking concept can lead to different understandings of resilience. This allows for a wide range of actors to identify themselves with the term and hence for several actors to be willing to cooperate and therefore support *building a collaborative research team*. On the contrary, broad definitions accessible to different stakeholders can easily lead to inconsistencies when it comes to *understanding and definition of the problem to be addressed* (Cook and Spray, 2012). Transdisciplinary research has been, among others, criticized for its inconsistency with regard to term definitions and approaches (Jahn et al., 2012). Using vague concepts such as resilience thinking bears the risk of intensifying or at least covering up such problems if they are not addressed properly and from the very beginning. If communication among different researchers and practitioners is only "improved" by masking differences and conflicts instead of mitigating them, the term failed to deliver. The different understandings and the reluctance to discuss normative issues became obvious when *research object, objectives, questions, and success criteria* should be defined and already resulted in subprojects to drift apart. Some actors were cherry-picking from the *methodological framework* using only those aspects they could identify with or worse, aspects they already addressed under different names thereby losing track of the holistic approach. Attempts to expatiate on normative aspects of resilience thinking led to practitioners threatening to give up their *assigned roles* and retreat *support for the roles* of dissenting practitioners and researchers. *Knowledge generation and integration* suffered from the issues of the preceding process steps. In addition, the difficulty to create transferable, generalizable, empirically testable knowledge is disadvantage of vague terms in general.

To sum up: In the case of nordwest2050 vagueness did not support creativity, communication and more effective problem solving, nor have normative questions been raised sufficiently. Due to the abundance of resilience definitions and concepts even within interdisciplinary discourses, clarity could not be achieved. This is not to say that resilience ultimately leads to this result. Nevertheless, it requires enhanced efforts to prevent vagueness, since it invites actors to avoid arduous conflicts. Especially business actors feel constrained to meet their (mostly short-term) business goals. Sectoral or in-company solutions may derive from a general strategy since they need to be tailor-made for specific problems. However, if the solution contradicts the solutions or approaches of other actors or aims of the overall system, resilience is not increased. Moreover, without a common understanding, a fragmented, incomplete and therefore counterproductive view on resilience of some actors is more likely.

Some of the aspects can be attenuated by thoroughly discussing normative goals from the very beginning. Normative discussions, in turn, most certainly lead to vivid discussions and the risk of losing some stakeholders who are not willing to or able to modify their positions. This leads to another important aspect that proved demanding but refers to handling normative aspects in transdisciplinary research in general (Lang et al., 2012). The selection of actors also determines the quality of results in transdisciplinary projects. Actors in nordwest2050 were quite diverse: they did have completely different "environments" that were supposed to be connected by resilience thinking. This was impeded by the different normative orientations, which were reflected in their understanding of resilience and led to both conflicts and hollowing out of the understanding of resilience. Thus, there seems to be a trade-off: The more diverse the set of actors, the vaguer resilience thinking needs to be to create interest and common commitment from stakeholders. However, this bears the risk of stressing resilience thinking or other vague terms to become an empty shell.

In a nutshell: Resilience thinking is a mixed blessing. It can, however, serve as a departure point. Existing activities might be viewed in a new light and hence expanded and supplemented. The creative contribution and the adaptability of the term itself are part of its merits. A diverse set of stakeholders can agree on the term resilience. However, that may be because they mean completely different things when using the term although especially parts of the broader public have not (yet) an image of the meaning of resilience whatsoever. This can lead to counterproductive results. A way to mitigate this problem is to expatiate on the normative aspects of the term from the very beginning. The question is: Will actors depart the moment you do so or rather how do you manage and motivate a broad actor spectrum to go along with that even if it questions some basic business principles? It is difficult to know their hidden agendas: Are they interested in the project goal or are they seeking for legitimisation of existing practices? In the case of nordwest2050 – despite considerable achievement in the sector projects – the deliberate use of a vague resilience concept fell short of its expectations. The lack of a common understanding could not be overcome by communication. The range of interests and problem perceptions seemed to be too wide. Hence, a relevant question for future transdisciplinary research projects is: How can boundary concepts be applied in a way that they are open and holistic without losing focus? Comparative studies of different projects might contribute to answering this question.

Note

1 In truly transdisciplinary projects the conceptual framework should not be predefined but developed commonly, although this might overstrain stakeholders who expect scientists to bring something to the table they can work with (Deppisch & Hasibovic, 2013).

References

Adger, W. N. (2006). Vulnerability. *Journal of Global Environmental Change*, 16(3), 268–81.

Adger, W. N., Paavola, J., Huq, S. & Mace, M. J. (eds.) (2006). *Fairness in Adaptation to Climate Change*. Cambridge, MA: MIT Press.

Adomßent, M. & Michelsen, G. (2011). Transdisziplinäre Nachhaltigkeits wissenschaften. In H. Heinrichs, K. Kuhn and J. Newig (eds.) *Nachhaltige Gesellschaft* (pp. 98–116). Wiesbaden: VS Verlag für Sozialwissenschaften.

Biebeler, H., Bardt, H., Chrischilles, E., Mahammadzadeh M. & Striebeck J. (eds.) (2014). *Wege zur Anpassung an den Klimawandel: Regionale Netzwerke, Strategien und Maßnahmen*. Köln: Institut der deutschen Wirtschaft Köln Medien GmbH.

Brand, F. S. (2005). *Ecological Resilience and Its Relevance within a Theory of Sustainable Development*. Leipzig: UFZ Centre for Environmental Research.

Brand, F. S. & Jax, K. (2007). Focusing the Meaning(s) of Resilience: Resilience as a Descriptive Concept and a Boundary Object. *Ecology and Society* 12(1): Art. 23.

Brandt, P., Ernst, A., Gralla, F., Luederitz, C., Lang, D. J., Newig, J., Reinert, F., Abson, D. J. & von Wehrden, H. (2013). A Review of Transdisciplinary Research in Sustainability Science. *Ecological Economics*, 92(0), 1–15.

Carpenter, S., Walker, B., Anderies, J. M. & Abel, N. (2001). From Metaphor to Measurement: Resilience of What to What? *Ecosystems*, 4(8), 765–81.

Cook, B. R. & Spray, C. J. (2012). Ecosystem Services and Integrated Water Resource Management. Different Paths to the Same End? *Journal of Environmental Management*, 109, 93–100.

Davoudi, S., Shaw, K., Haider, L., Quinlan J., Allyson E., Peterson, G. D., Wilkinson, C., Fünfgeld, H., McEvoy, D. & Porter, L. (2012). Resilience: A Bridging Concept or a Dead End? "Reframing" Resilience: Challenges for Planning Theory and Practice Interacting Traps: Resilience Assessment of a Pasture Management System in Northern Afghanistan Urban Resilience: What Does It Mean in Planning Practice? Resilience as a Useful Concept for Climate Change Adaptation? The Politics of Resilience for Planning: A Cautionary Note. *Planning Theory & Practice*, 13(2), 299–333.

Deppisch, S. & Hasibovic, S. (2013). Social-Ecological Resilience Thinking as a Bridging Concept in Transdisciplinary Research on Climate-Change Adaptation. *Natural Hazards*, 67(1), 117–27.

Etzkowitz, H. & Leydesdorff, L. (2000). The Dynamics of Innovation. From National Systems and "Mode 2" to a Triple Helix of University–Industry–Government Relations. *Research Policy*, 29, 109–23.

Folke, C., Carpenter, S., Elmqvist, T., Gunderson, L., Holling, C. S. & Walker, B. (2002). Resilience and Sustainable Development: Building Adaptive Capacity in a World of Transformations. *Ambio*, 31(5), 437–40.

Folke, C., Hahn, T., Olsson, P. & Norberg, J. (2005). Adaptive Governance of Social-Ecological Systems. *Annual Review of Environmental Resources*, 30, 441–73.

Funtowicz, S. & Ravetz, J. R. (1993). Science for the Post-Normal Age. *Futures*, 25(7), 739–55.

Garrelts, H., Grothmann, T., Grecksch, K., Winges, M., Siebenhüner, B. & Flitner, M. (eds.) (2013a). *Vulnerabilität und Klimaanpassung: Herausforderungen adaptiver Governance im Nordwesten Deutschlands*. Bremen/Oldenburg: nordwest2050 Projektkonsortium. www.nordwest2050.de/index_nw2050.php?obj=page&id=136&unid=a0a20e52fd43acfb68ea12e112905716 (Accessed on 28 March 2016).

Garrelts, H., Grecksch, K., Grothmann, T., Winges, M., Herbeck, J. & Siebenhüner, B. (2013b). *Sektorale Roadmap Regionale Governance. Handlungspfade und Handlungsempfehlungen auf dem Weg zu einer klimaangepassten regionalen Governance im Nordwesten*. Bremen/Oldenburg: nordwest2050 Projektkonsortium. www.nordwest2050.de/index_nw2050.php?obj=page&id=136&unid=a0a20e52fd43acfb68ea12e112905716 (Accessed on 28 March 2016).

Gibbons, M., Limoges, C., Nowotny, H., Schwartzman, S., Scott, P. & Trow, M. (1994). *The New Production of Knowledge: The Dynamics of Science and Research in Contemporary Societies*. London: Sage.

Gleich, A. von & Gößling-Reisemann, S. (2010). Resilienz als Leitkonzept. Vulnerabilität als analytische Kategorie. In K. Fichter, A. v. Gleich, R. Pfriem & B. Siebenhüner (eds.) *Theoretische Grundlagen für erfolgreiche Klimaanpassungsstrategien* (pp. 11–49). Oldenburg/Bremen: nordwest2050 www.nordwest2050.de/index_nw2050.php?obj=page&id=136&unid=a0a20e52fd43acfb68ea12e112905716 (Accessed on 28 March 2016).

Grecksch, K. (2014). *Adaptive Water Governance: Conclusions and Implications Regarding Adaptive Governance and Property Rights*. Oldenburg: University of Oldenburg.

Groot, A. M. E., Bosch, P. R., Buijs, S., Jacobs, C. M. J. & Moors, E. J. (2015). Integration in Urban Climate Adaptation: Lessons from Rotterdam on Integration between Scientific Disciplines and Integration between Scientific and Stakeholder Knowledge. *Building and Environment*, 83, 177–88.

Grothmann, T., Grecksch, K., Winges, M. & Siebenhüner, B. (2013). Assessing Institutional Capacities to Adapt to Climate Change: Integrating Psychological Dimensions in the Adaptive Capacity Wheel. *Natural Hazards and Earth System Sciences*, 13(12), 3369–84.

Hagemeier-Klose, M., Beichler, S. A., Davidse, B. J. & Deppisch, S. (2014). The Dynamic Knowledge Loop: Inter-and Transdisciplinary Cooperation and Adaptation of Climate Change Knowledge. *International Journal of Disaster Risk Science*, 5(1), 21–32.

Hessels, L. K. & Lente, H. v. (2008). Re-Thinking New Knowledge Production. A Literature Review and a Research Agenda. *Research Policy*, 37, 740–60.

Jahn, T., Bergmann, M. & Keil, F. (2012). Transdisciplinarity: Between Mainstreaming and Marginalization. *Ecological Economics*, 79(0), 1–10.

Lang, D., Wiek, A., Bergmann, M., Stauffacher, M., Martens, P., Moll, P., Swilling, M. & Thomas, C. (2012). Transdisciplinary Research in Sustainability Science: Practice, Principles, and Challenges. *Sustainability Science*, 7(1), 25–43.

Najjar, W. & Gaudiot, J. L. (1990). Network Resilience: A Measure of Network Fault Tolerance. *Computers, IEEE Transactions on*, 39(2), 174–81.

nordwest2050. (2014). Integrierte Roadmap of Change. Fahrplan für Klimaanpassung und Resilienz in der Metropolregion Bremen-Oldenburg im Nordwesten. www.nordwest2050.de/index_nw2050.php?obj=page&id=136&unid=a0a20e52fd43acfb68ea12e112905716 (Accessed on 28 March 2016).

nordwest2050. (2016). English Summary. www.nordwest2050.de/index_nw2050.php?obj=page&id=139&unid=a0a20e52fd43acfb68ea12e112905716 (Accessed on 28 March 2016).

O'Hare, P. & White, I. (2013). Deconstructing Resilience. Lessons from Planning Practice. *Planning Practice & Research*, 28(3), 275–79.

Paavola, J. & Adger, W. N. (2006). Fair Adaptation to Climate Change. *Ecological Economics*, 56, 594–609.

Parry, M. L., Canziani, O. F., Palutikof, J. P. & van der Linden P. J., Hanson. C. E. (2007). *Climate Change 2007: Impacts, Adaptation and Vulnerability. Contribution of Working Group II to the Fourth Assessment Report of the Intergovernmental Panel on Climate Change*. Cambridge: CUP.

Phillis, Y. A. & Andriantiatsaholiniaina, L. A. (2001). Sustainability. An Ill-Defined Concept and Its Assessment Using Fuzzy Logic. *Ecological Economics*, 37(3), 435–56.

Rutter, M., 1987. Psychological Resilience and Protective Mechanisms. *American Journal of Orthopsychiatry*, 57(3), 316–31.

Scholz, R. W. (2013). Transdisciplinarity: Theory and Visions on Global Transdisciplinary Processes for Adapting to Climate Change. In O.C. Ruppel, C. Roschmann, & K. Ruppel-Schlichting (eds.) *Climate Change: International Law and Global Governance: Volume II: Policy, Diplomacy and Governance in a Changing Environment* (pp. 327–56). Baden-Baden: Nomos Verlagsgesellschaft.

Seeliger, L. & Turok, I. (2013). Towards Sustainable Cities. Extending Resilience with Insights from Vulnerability and Transition Theory. *Sustainability*, 5(5), 2108–28.

Serrao-Neumann, S., Schuch, G., Harman, B., Crick, F., Sano, M., Sahin, O., von Staden, R., Baum, S. & Low Choy, D. (2015). One Human Settlement: A Transdisciplinary Approach to Climate Change Adaptation Research. *Futures*, 65, 97–109.

Strunz, S. (2012). Is Conceptual Vagueness an Asset? Arguments from Philosophy of Science Applied to the Concept of Resilience. *Ecological Economics*, 76, 112–18.

Tatham, E. K., Eisenberg, D. A. & Linkov, I. (2014). Sustainable Urban Systems: A Review of How Sustainability Indicators Inform Decisions. In I. Linkov (ed.) *Sustainable Cities and Military Installations* (pp. 3–20). Dordrecht: Springer Netherlands.

Thissen, W., Kwakkel, J., Mens, M., Sluijs, J., Stemberger, S., Wardekker, A. & Wildschut, D. (2017). Dealing with Uncertainties in Fresh Water Supply: Experiences in the Netherlands. *Water Resources Management*, 31, 703–725.

Van der Vaart, G., Trell, E.-M., Restemeyer, B. & Bakema, M. M. (2015). Resilience: Just Do It?! Governing for Resilience in Vulnerable Places, University of Groningen, 9–10 October 2014. *Resilience*, 3(2), 1–12.

Vogus, T. J. & Sutcliffe, K. M. (2007). Organizational Resilience: Towards a Theory and Research Agenda. *In Proceedings of the IEEE International Conference on Systems, Man and Cybernetics, 7–10 October 2007* (pp. 3418–22). Montreal, QC.

Walker, B., Holling, C. S., Carpenter, S. R. & Kinzig, A. (2004). Resilience, Adaptability and Transformability in Social–Ecological Systems. *Ecology and Society*, 9(2), 5.

WBGU (Wissenschaftlicher Beirat der Bundesregierung Globale Umweltveränderungen). (2011). *World in Transition – A Social Contract for Sustainability*. Berlin: WBGU.

Winges, M. (2015). *Klimaanpassungskapazität der Regionalplanung: Ein Bewertungsansatz für politisch-administrative Systeme*. Marburg: Metropolis.

Wong-Parodi, G., Fischhoff, B., & Strauss, B. (2015). Resilience vs. Adaptation: Framing and Action. *Climate Risk Management*, 10, 1–7.

Ziman, J. (1996). "Postacademic Science". Constructing Knowledge with Networks and Norms. *Science Studies*, 9, 67–80.

6 Flood resilience and legitimacy – an exploration of Dutch flood risk management

Tom Scholten and Thomas Hartmann

Introduction

Floods can be approached at a given location with two different concepts in mind: defending against floods or adapting to floods (Saurí-Pujol et al., 2001) (further, the option of mitigation exists, but this is a rather long-term and large-scale approach). First, resistance-based flood protection is the traditional approach to flood risk; second is resilience, which is linked with the concept of flood risk management. Flood protection usually requires dykes, technical flood protection measures, and strong water management institutions with technical skills; resilient flood risk management asks for comprehensive and integrative concepts, encompassing many stakeholders and asking for collaboration at various levels. The advantage of resistance-oriented flood protection is that it facilitates using protected land efficiently without the necessity of making compromises because of the flood risk. However, this approach has boundaries and constraints when flood risk increases, protection measures fail, or extreme floods occur. Thus, complementary resilient flood risk management is necessary, which comes with costs for adaptation and compromises for land use, but allows for coping much better with the management of increasing risk and extreme events because it reduces vulnerabilities.

In the past, resistance-based flood protection was the predominant approach (Moss and Monstadt, 2008; Saurí-Pujol et al., 2001). However, in acknowledging the statement by the International Decade of Natural Disaster Reduction (IDNDR) that it is neither technically feasible nor economically affordable to protect all properties from flooding (Plate, 2001; Vogt, 2005), a paradigm shift from the defence against floods to the more comprehensive and integrated management of flood risks (including vulnerabilities) has taken place during the last twenty-years (Grünewald, 2005; Schanze, 2006).

Particularly in the Netherlands, resilience becomes increasingly an imperative. The Netherlands is located downstream to large rivers and to a large extent below sea-level. Accordingly, flooding is an important issue for the country. In addition, with major settlements (e.g. Randstad) in the coastal region and along the rivers (e.g. cities of Maastricht, Nijmegen) it is highly vulnerable (Tempels and Hartmann, 2014). In an urbanized delta area like the Netherlands, floods are an imminent and urgent threat. Water virtually comes from all sides: the North Sea, through groundwater, through flash floods, and from rivers upstream to the Netherlands. The Intergovernmental Panel on Climate Change (IPCC) confidently states that damages by river floods will substantially increase in Europe, which will require action to reduce the impact of river floods (IPCC, 2014). Accordingly, flood risk management is needed that does not solely focus on defending against the water but also considers accommodating it (Hartmann and Spit, 2016; Stead, 2014). For the Netherlands, that means a shift towards increasing flood resilience.

The basic idea of flood-resilience is that cities and landscapes become capable of absorbing the negative consequences of flooding (Begum et al., 2007; de Bruijn, 2005; Petrow et al., 2006) – in other words, allowing them to be flooded with minimal damage (Holling, 1973). The present Dutch landscape is intensively used with many different land uses, such as housing, business or infrastructure. Therefore, the balancing of spatial activities has become an issue on its own. But cities and intensively used landscapes are not meant to be inundated. Making them resilient requires physical adjustments, such as using streets as discharge flumes or for retention, creating evacuation routes, and installing calamity polders (IKSR, 2002) or even constructing floating homes. Non-structural measures are also necessary, such as financial recovery capacity, insurance schemes (Berke and Campanella, 2006), information structures, or management mechanisms. Resilience comes with costs for adaptation and compromises for land uses, whereas resistance-oriented flood protection provides lines of defence. These lines are boundaries that separate wet and dry areas. Resilient flood risk management challenges clear boundaries between land and water. This has crucial consequences for the allocation of land uses and requires collaboration of a diversity of stakeholders (notably landowners and land users). It also encompasses a new way of governance: the management of floods, therefore, needs to shift from a one-sided compounding technocratic and predominantly hierarchic top-down perspective on floods towards a more inclusive, horizontal, bottom-up, interactive, spatial perspective that takes multiple stakeholders and multiple issues into account (Edelenbos et al., 2013). The departing point and extent of this shift differ in various countries. In the Netherlands, for example, locally rooted governance is more established than in some other countries (e.g. Eastern Germany) (Eerd et al., 2014).

Not all measures of resilient flood risk management can be expected to be achieved without conflict. Moreover, such measures of resilient flood risk management contradict, at their core, the values and expectations shaping the relationship between citizens and public administration; citizens – not only in the Netherlands – expect public administration to prevent disasters (Hartmann and Albrecht, 2014; Reinhard, 2008). Flood protection of cities is usually considered to be a governmental task (Barraqué, 2014). Such tensions ask for a strong legitimacy of interventions for (resilient) flood risk management. Moreover, when considering policy-and decision-making a more collaborative and discursive process-new forms for obtaining legitimacy are necessary.

This contribution discusses the tensions of legitimacy in flood risk management resulting from the claim for more flood resilience. To understand these tensions, the concept of legitimacy itself is discussed beforehand (Section one). In the next part, the concept of legitimacy is introduced to the resistance-orientated flood protection approach (Section two). In this section, the theoretical framework is explained using an elaborated literature review. Further on, the erosion of legitimacy components in the resistance approach are discussed (Section three). Reference is made to empirical research conducted in the Netherlands in 2014. Eight water management experts of the water boards, Deltares and municipalities have been interviewed about issues of flood risk management and its legitimacy. Findings have been validated in reference to their professional experience with projects with issues of legitimacy.

The interviews were thereby used to link theory and practice. In the final part, the claim for an extra form of legitimacy is proposed to extend the legitimacy of flood risk management (Section four).

The concept of legitimacy

The concept of legitimacy is a political-philosophical discussion. Legitimacy is linked to the idea of democracy, and a rather straightforward definition of democracy is provided by Held (2006, p. 1): 'democracy is a form of government where the people rule'. But what is meant by 'the people' and 'the government'? Just to put it into context, there are generally two perspectives on democracy, the *substantive* perspective where democracy is a construct based on certain values. It is a society of mutual relationships between people on different levels, which together form a part of the democracy. Differences between democracies are the result of a variety in value judgements concerning the essence of democracy (MacPherson, 1977). An *instrumental* perspective is based on the vision that democracy is an instrument to choose and authorize governments, legislation and political decision-making. In this sense, the form of democracy needs to be practicable for the possibilities and needs of the people. Importantly, democracy requires general conformity and support to function (MacPherson, 1977). Thus, at the core, the concept of democracy is about a rightful authority, where political equality, moral self-development, and the general interest are preconceived. Decisions are therefore binding, whereas all interests are included, so that social relevance, satisfying of wishes and efficiency of decisions are offered to all (Held, 2006).

According to Luhmann (1975, p. 25) legitimacy is about a 'generalised willingness to accept decisions, whereof the content is unknown, with a certain margin.' Benhabib (1996, p. 68) defines legitimacy as a 'result of free and unlimited deliberation'. Schmitter (2001) defines legitimacy as a certain shared expectation between actors within a collaborative asymmetric power relation. In this sense, actions of the government are accepted by the governed. In other words, they are convinced that those actions are in line with predefined norms. Suchman (1995, p. 574) defines legitimacy as 'a generalized perception or assumption of desired actions, meaningful and right actions of one entity within a socially constructed system of norms, value, beliefs and definitions.' Thus, we can conclude that legitimacy converts power into authority and thereby leads to an obligation of obedience and the right to govern.

In practice, legitimacy is obtained when decision-making is based on adequate information gained through research and consultation with stakeholders. Based thereon, an honest, just and balanced consideration between the public interest and the private stakeholders' interests is made (van Buuren et al., 2013). In fact, this means informing citizens about decision-making and offering them an opportunity to give their opinion and formally express their interests. Thus, considering democratic legitimacy, there are three sources: Accountability, voice and deliberation (van Buuren et al., 2012). *Accountability* means that government representatives must answer to citizens for their decisions and decision-making processes. Citizens can hold representatives responsible; in this sense, it gives them a sense of protection. *Voice* is a legitimacy source when citizens make themselves heard in the decision-making process and make use of opportunities to influence decision-making (van Buuren et al., 2012). People tend to feel treated fairly when they have the opportunity to hand in suggestions for solving conflicts or problems (Tyler, 2000). *Deliberation* is related to the organisation of a process. The procedures or 'the rules of the game' outline how many opportunities for involvement are offered. However, this is rather complex since rules and procedures are both written and unwritten and can change or emerge during the process (Edelenbos, 2005).

Contemporary policy-making is taking place in a network of private and public interest (Mees et al., 2014). This governance network is a multi-layered system and functions as an extension of the democracy (Sørensen, 2002). A governance network view implies a redefinition of the democratic legitimacy sources. *Accountability* is more diffuse and shared between different stakeholders within informal network relations (van Buuren et al., 2012). *Voice* is more complex because of the multitude of stakeholders and the absence of legislation. On the other hand, more opportunities exist for formal and informal contribution of voice in networks when compared to the (formal) democracy. *Deliberation* follows from voice. The lack of a procedural structure is the consequence of an institutional void. The interaction between stakeholders takes places in ad hoc meetings (van Buuren et al., 2012). Thus, the establishment of legitimacy in a network is different from the routine of democratic legitimacy. In a governance legitimacy network, multiple democratic thoughts combined do not necessarily lead to one unified democratic thought (Esmark, 2007, as cited by van Buuren et al., 2013). Indeed, networks exist of multiple government institutions, and, more importantly, they also include other stakeholders and/or interest groups. Furthermore, a governance network also holds other forms of legitimacy when compared to those of the democracy. Therefore, acquiring legitimacy in a governance network is realized through a three-step procedure: input, throughput and output (Mees et al., 2014; van Buuren et al., 2013). 'Step' suggests that they are sequential, but in different policy fields there can be different emphasises on those three types of legitimacy (as shall be discussed below).

Input legitimacy is a model of classic democracy linked to the social contract which is, for instance, described by Thomas Hobbes' Leviathan where members of society giver their power to decide to an institution (Davy, 1997; Scharpf, 1997; van Buuren et al., 2012). Input legitimacy justifies policies when governmental action is enacted by representative, authorized and accountable institutions. These institutions are embedded in the democratic system and receive their legitimacy through the respective political system.

Transparency in the design of the process enables input legitimacy. Furthermore, input legitimacy increases when more stakeholders are included in policy construction and the political debate.

Throughput legitimacy considers the quality of rules and procedures for decision-making and justice and fairness of the process as a whole (Bekkers and Edwards, 2007; Mees et al., 2014). Actions of government are legitimized through active participation of stakeholders and citizens in a process characterized by transparency, accountability and inclusiveness (Schmidt, 2013). Thus, throughput legitimacy is orientated on the interactive process of involving all stakeholders and citizens in decisions and the decision-making (Coenen et al., 2001).

Output legitimacy is warranted when the outcomes of the process reflect the input of stakeholders in the previous stages (Scharpf, 1997). In other words, the result of governmental actions justifies the measures (Schmidt, 2013). Output legitimacy concerns the perception of effectivity of achieving the policy goal; it does not have to mean an actual solution to issues (Biermann and Gupta, 2011; van Tatenhove, 2011). There is consensual agreement of goals and values are within the public interest.

Briefly summarized, *input legitimacy* is assessed based on criteria such as authorization, representation, and accountability; *output legitimacy* judges the policy results for citizens or stakeholders; and *throughput legitimacy* is about the inclusiveness and openness to consulting with citizens (or stakeholders) (Schmidt, 2013).

Legitimacy of resistance-oriented flood protection in the Netherlands

Historically, in the Netherlands, strong water management authorities were required in order to maintain 'dry feet' (Hartmann and Spit, 2016).

Moreover, the economic purpose of water engineering was predominant: flood protection for enabling agriculturally fertile floodplains, regulating discharge, shipping and increasing the value of riparian land (Nisipeanu, 2008). Without these resistance-based flood protection measures, approximately two-thirds of the most densely populated part of the Netherlands would flood every day (van Stokkom et al., 2005). This has created very strong and well-established water engineering institutions in the Netherlands (Hartmann and Driessen, 2013). Until today, resistance-based flood protection measures are the dominant approach to dealing with floods (Offermans et al., 2011). Derived from the traditional thought that water should be kept out, for decades, investments were made in the improvement of water embankments and dykes (van Buuren et al., 2012). So, Dutch resistance-based flood protection rests on strong institutions and on their promise to defend citizens and their land from floods. Dutch water managers derived a prominent position from the responsibility to provide flood protection through water engineering (Reinhard, 2008). The importance of this task exemplifies the empowerment of these institutions with a clear aim by the political system (Hartmann and Spit, 2016). An example of such an institution is 'Rijkswaterstaat' or the Dutch Directorate-General, a strong central institution for water-related issues. It governs and initiates water-related issues with a 'hegemony of state' (Wiering and Crabbé, 2006, p. 99); also in other countries, water institutions traditionally rest on relatively strong institutions (Hartmann and Driessen, 2013; Moss, 2004; Nisipeanu, 2008). At the local level the oldest democratically elected bodies in the Netherlands – the water boards, are responsible for water control, water quantity and water quality issues (Heer et al., 2004). The water boards were first established in the thirteenth-century and are characterized by their bottom-up approach to water management (van Steen and Pellenbarg, 2004). These are local authorities that have evolved from bottom-up initiatives.

Water engineering provides sharp boundaries, separating areas that will be protected from areas that are subject to flooding (floodplains). The sharply drawn inundation zones in flood risk maps are publically interpreted as lines where the risk of flooding seems to end, and for many local decision-makers, such lines mean that the areas beyond the lines are 'flood risk free' (Loucks et al., 2008). The promise to keep the water out rests on strong technical flood defence systems. Also in many other countries, this is clearly the predominant approach to floods (Moss and Monstadt, 2008; Saurí-Pujol et al., 2001), but in the Netherlands, because of the exposure to flood risk and the vulnerability, this approach is brought to its extreme (Warner et al., 2012). Precise calculations, hydraulic models, and empirical data are the basis for the size and shape of technical flood defence constructions – particularly for dykes (Patt and Jüpner, 2013). In water engineering, decisions are justified via measurable data and scientific proof count (Hartmann and Driessen, 2013).

The dominance of technical expertise in engineering is deeply rooted, not only in cultural beliefs and in the practices of water authorities (Wesselink, 2007), but also in Dutch water laws (Gilissen et al., 2009). Such traditional views of risk management stress the primacy of scientific knowledge (Brown and Damery, 2002), neglecting the social and political dimension of risk awareness and acceptance (Hartmann and Driessen, 2013): 'A decision is legitimate when it is based on the best possible scientific assessment' (Larsson, 2014, p. 35); the key actor is thus the (water) expert. In conclusion, traditional flood protection is legitimized by the output it produces: dry feet.

This has led to a very strong and long-lasting tradition of a resistance-based approach of water engineering in the Netherlands (Hartmann and Driessen, 2013). Responsibility for national flood protection (along the large rivers and on the coast) in the Netherlands lies with government institutions. The provision of flood protection has always been the responsibility of the state (Reinhardt, 2008). It is the task of the government to make and keep the land inhabitable and to protect and to improve the environment through spatial intervention. The Water Act (2009), the Water Board Act (1991), the Spatial Planning Act (2008), Spatial Planning Resolution (2008), the Delta Act (2011) exemplify government water policy. Other relevant water-related policies in the Netherlands include the flood protection program (*Hoogwaterbeschermingsprogramma [HWBP] 1) and 2*) and the Management Agreement Water *(Bestuursakkoord Water)* to further delineate responsibilities for executing flood protection measures to the involved government institutions.

The legitimacy of interventions by those strong water institutions in the Netherlands rests on a historically grown input legitimacy. This input legitimacy provides the basis for the implementation of policy goals via rules and regulations (Hartmann and Albrecht, 2014). Finally, traditional resistance-oriented flood protection in the Netherlands is sustained by a combination of input-legitimacy and output-legitimacy.

Changing legitimacy in flood risk management

Until today, dykes in the Netherlands are continuously heightened and strengthened. Wiering and Immink (2006) state that there is a 'control paradox' when considering the improvement of water embankments, which Hartmann described as a lock-in situation in the social construction of the floodplains (Hartmann, 2011). This is also called the dyke dilemma (Hartmann and Spit, 2016). The improvement of water embankments (e.g. dykes) leads to a perception of increased safety. As a result, the land use behind the dyke intensifies (Hartmann, 2011). This relationship of land use and flood protection is part of a robust social construction in floodplains (Hartmann, 2011; Figure 6.1) that finally contributes to increasing flood risks (Tempels and Hartmann, 2014).

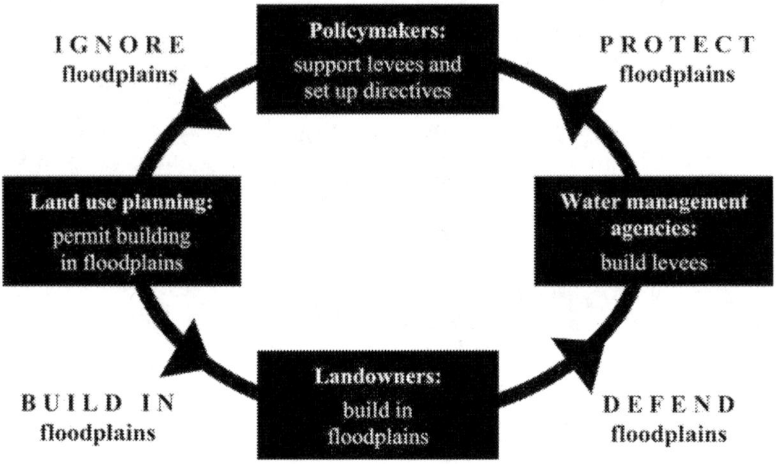

Figure 6.1 The social construction in the floodplains.
Source: Hartmann, (2011).

In other words, dyke improvement is sufficient for a certain amount of time and certain norms on flooding and high water levels. Thus, these kinds of flood prevention measures inherently imply future dyke improvement.

Dirven et al. (2002) states that the water system as a whole has become a kind of 'wicked problem' (Rittel and Webber, 1973). This means that modern flood risk management can be described as significantly complex in terms of interrelated actions and measures, structural uncertainty with respect to forecasting and modelling, and due to the diversity of interests and stakeholders, it is inherently normative. Accordingly, the mode of governance needs to respond to these characterizations (van der Brugge et al., 2005).

The above dyke dilemma and social construction of the floodplains shows that water management and land-use planning are dependent on each other. On the one hand, land-use planning is part of the problem in flood risk management, because planners allocate vulnerable land uses to flood-prone areas (Hartmann, 2011); on the other hand, land-use planning is essential for the implementation of resilient flood risk management, because the measures need to be implemented in the area, not only on small strips along the river. This is denoted as the spatial turn in flood risk management (Hartmann and Spit, 2016).

How input legitimacy is challenged

This ambivalent role of land-use planning makes the collaboration between water engineers and land-use planners difficult. On top of that, both institutions pursue fundamentally different modes of governance (Hartmann and Driessen, 2013; Moss, 2004, 2009). The different modes of governance between water management and land use planning can best be understood with the analytical distinction in sectoral and facet planning (Spit and Zoete, 2006). Sectoral planning concerns a part of a government institution that focuses on the most effective and efficient way of programming, for instance, water management (Hartmann, 2011). Alternatively, facet planning involves the integration of all government tasks from a certain kind of policy, for example, land use planning of the environment. Resilient flood risk management requires reconciliation and coordination between the different sector and facet policies (Spit and Zoete, 2006). This undermines the input legitimacy of water authorities described earlier.

However, the integrative turn in water management is not simple. Kuijpers and Glasbergen (1990) stated that there has been synchronization in policy and control tasks between different layers of the government in the Netherlands. The term integral water management appeared for the first time in the 'Third Note on Water Management' *(Derde Nota Waterhuishouding)* (Kienhuis et al., 1993). Whether there is really synchronization between land use planning and water management has been discussed frequently in academic literature in the past decades (Kienhuis et al., 1993; Wiering and Immink, 2006; Wolsink, 2006; Woltjer and Al, 2007). Hindering factors for such synchronization are the hiatus between strategic policy visions and the implementation in practice: "Integrative is also fashion-term" one manager at the regional water board Hollandse Delta explained. Government institutions are increasingly looking outwards to other institutions and stakeholders. But the governance structure of the water management arena does not seem suitable for more collaboration with and participation of stakeholders (Wolsink, 2006).

How output legitimacy is challenged

Also, the output legitimacy for resistance-oriented flood protection has diminished: agreement in the scholarly debate and practice on that dykes cannot be heightened and strengthened infinitely has increased (Wiering and Driessen, 2001). Besides this technical argument, the growing awareness of the values of the landscape, nature and culture also plays a role: "From our water board perspective, we often focus too much on the most optimal engineering instead of taking also other issues into account" (manager at the regional water board Rivierenland).Especially relatively recent flood disasters (i.e. 1993, 1995, 1998, 2003) have changed the way the Dutch think of water management (Hidding and van der Vlist, 2003; Neuvel and van der Knaap, 2010; van Stokkom et al., 2005; Warner et al., 2012). These disasters put forward the notion that drainage basins are not bound to stringent structures imposed by human intervention (Warner et al., 2012). An example of this alternation of thinking of water management in the

Netherlands is the policy change with the 'Room for the River' programme from 2001 as an ad-hoc response to the events of 1993 and 1995 (Rijke et al., 2012; van der Brugge et al., 2005). These events have led to an increased public, political and professional awareness of the limited possibilities to control nature and water using only technical measures (Rijke et al., 2012). In the past, the focus was on challenging flooding and high water levels as solely water issues without compromise in a more interest- and representation-based democracy. Today's water management is perceived as a public and political discussion about certain spatial issues, wherein water is one of the components. This also implies a shift in the perception of flood risk – whereas traditional flood protection was oriented on the probability of events (i.e. flood recurrence intervals), current flood risk management emphasizes the consequences of floods (i.e. focus on resilience and vulnerabilities). In this way, the borders between land use functions and water functions are fusing (Wiering and Immink, 2006). Also the type of measures and therefore the output of flood risk management is changing.

Alongside governmental and/or political obstacles in water management, there is also a fundamental change in the realisation of the water policy due to societal changes. The process of policy development, implementation and decision-making have also changed. Traditionally, keeping the water at a distance, prevention, has been a dominant rational engineering approach or 'command and control' approach (Wolsink, 2006). Since the paradigm shift with the 'Room for the River' *(Ruimte voor de Rivier)* programme, interactive policy making and implementation have become tools to satisfy the urgency for actions and to hasten the throughput time of legal procedures (Wiering and Driessen, 2001). Stakeholders demand to be involved in informal ways, as a project leader at a regional water board affirmed: "the context works completely different than ten-years ago. What we can observe is that it is changing towards more demanding citizens and easier access to information. We have to deal with this context" (project leader at Waterschap Vallei en Veluwe). These developments lead to new questions within the water management arena. An important issue is the role of legitimacy in this new kind of water management. Water managers try to identify their new role in this new way of thinking – "We need to get rid of the fear that people intervene in our plans", confirmed an interviewee at the regional water board Rivierenland. Since a paradigm shift in water management inevitably influences the source for acquiring democratic legitimacy.

Conclusion: the emergence of throughput legitimacy

Our interviews with stakeholders all over the Netherlands confirmed a change in the way water management and the management of floods, in particular, has been gradually changing over the past decades: there is a shift from a predominantly interest-and representation-based perspective on legitimation towards a more inclusive, horizontal, bottom-up, interactive perspective that takes multiple stakeholders and multiple issues into account (i.e. a new perspective of governance regarding the management of floods). In other words, an evolvement from resistance-based flood protection to a more resilient flood risk management paradigm, which challenges the common way of legitimization. Input and output legitimacy are complemented by an extra component of throughput-legitimacy. In contrast to the democratic legitimacy of input (equal rights of influence) and output (effective policy goal achievement), throughput complements the justice and fairness component of the process in flood risk management. In other words, throughput legitimacy focuses on the quality of a deliberative process through reviewing the cooperation between actors in terms of problem analysis, the development of possible solutions and final policy decisions (Berry et al., 1993; Dryzek, 2000).

To what extent throughput legitimacy can become a substitute for the other forms of legitimacy, or rather complementary to them, needs to be further monitored. However, it is unlikely that the other forms of legitimacy diminish completely because traditional forms of flood protection will most likely not be abolished. Resilient flood risk management still needs dykes and expertise from traditional water management institutions. And interventions cannot always be justified and conflicts prevented or resolved by process-oriented throughput legitimacy alone. But the above discussion reveals that the need and trend towards resilience add new aspects of legitimacy: input and output legitimacy can barely provide sufficient support for measures of resilient flood risk management. Therefore, throughput legitimacy is necessary to obviate the shortcomings of input and input legitimacy with resilient flood risk management approach.

To determine the consequences for legitimacy of both resistant and resilient approaches in flood risk management, future research needs to make use of the evaluation of instruments and methods where legitimacy issues are concerned. This implies, for instance, reviewing participation processes, governance schemes, or the consequences of the new legislation for flood risk management.

References

Barraqué, B. (2014). The common property issue in flood control through land use in France. *Journal of Flood Risk Management*. doi:10.1111/jfr3.12092.

Begum, S., Stive, M. J. F., and Hall, J. W. (Eds.). (2007). *Flood risk management in Europe: Innovation in policy and practice*. Dordrecht: Springer.

Bekkers, V. J. J. M., & Edwards, A. (2007). Legitimacy and democracy: A conceptual framework for assessing governance practices. In V. J. J. M. Bekkers (Ed.), *Governance and the democratic deficit: Assessing the democratic legitimacy of governance practices* (pp. 35–60). Burlington, VT: Ashgate.

Benhabib, S. (Ed.). (1996). Democracy and difference: Contesting the boundaries of the political, 31. Princeton, NJ: Princeton University Press.

Berke, P. R., & Campanella, T. J. (2006). Planning for postdisaster resiliency. *The ANNALS of the American Academy of Political and Social Science*, *604*(1), 192–207. doi:10.1177/0002716205285533.

Berry, J. M., Portney, K. E., & Thomson, K. (1993). *The rebirth of Urban democracy*. Washington, DC: Brookings Institution.

Biermann, F., & Gupta, A. (2011). Accountability and legitimacy in earth system governance: A research framework. *Ecological Economics*, *70*(11), 1856–1864. doi:10.1016/j.ecolecon.2011.04.008.

Brown, J. D., & Damery, S. L. (2002). Managing flood risk in the UK: Towards an integration of social and technical perspectives. *Transactions of the Institute of British Geographers*, *27*(4), 412–426. doi:10.1111/1475-5661.00063.

Coenen, F., Peppel, R., & Woltjer, J. (2001). De evolutie van inspraak in de Nederlandse planning. *Beleidswetenschap*, *15*(4), 313–332.

Davy, B. (1997). *Essential injustice: When legal institutions cannot resolve environmental and land use disputes*. New York: Springer.

De Bruijn, K. M. (2005). *Resilience and flood risk management: A systems approach applied to lowland rivers*. Delft: Delft University Press.

Dirven, J., Rotmans, J., Verkaik, A. P. (2002). *Samenleving in transitie: een vernieuwend gezichtpunt*. Retrieved from www.innovatienetwerk.org.

Dryzek, J. S. (2000). *Deliberate democracy and beyond: Liberals, critics, contestations*. Oxford: Oxford University Press.

Edelenbos, J. (2005). Institutional implications of interactive governance: Insights from Dutch practice. *Governance*, *18*(1), 111–134.

Edelenbos, J., Bressers, N., & Scholten, P. (Eds.). (2013). *Water governance as connective capacity*. Burlington, VT: Ashgate.

Eerd, M. C., Wiering, M., & Dieperink, C. (2014). Exploring the prospects for cross-border climate change adaptation between North Rhine-Westphalia and the Netherlands. *Utrecht Law Review*, *10*(2), 91–104.

Esmark, A. 2007. Democratic accountability and network governance - Problems and potentials. In E. Sørensen & J. Torfing (Eds.), *Theories of democratic network governance* (pp. 274–297). Basingstoke: Palgrave.

Gilissen, H., van Rijswick, M., & van Schoot, T. d. (2009). *Water en ruimte: De bescherming van watersysteembelangen in het ruimtelijk spoor*. Amsterdam: Berghauser Pont Publishing.

Grünewald, U. (2005). Vom Hochwasser-'Schutzversprechen' zum 'Hochwasser-Risikomanagement'. In R. Jüpner (Ed.), *Hochwassermanagement* (pp. 5–22). Aachen: Shaker.

Hartmann, T. (2011). *Clumsy floodplains: Responsive land policy for extreme floods*. Farnham: Ashgate.

Hartmann, T., & Albrecht, J. 2014. From flood protection to flood risk management: Condition-based and performance-based regulations in German water law. *Journal of Environmental Law*, *26*(2), 243–268. doi:10.1093/jel/equ015

Hartmann, T., & Driessen, P. (2013). The flood risk management plan: Towards spatial water governance. *Journal of Flood Risk Management*. doi:10.1111/jfr3.12077.

Hartmann, T., & Spit, T. (2016). Legitimizing differentiated flood protection levels–Consequences of the European flood risk management plan. *Environmental Science & Policy*, *55*, 361–367. doi:10.1016/j.envsci.2015.08.013.

Heer, J. d., Nijwening, S., Vuyst, S. de, van Rijswick, M., Smit, T., & Groenendijk, J. (2004). *Towards integrated water legislation in The Netherlands: Lessons from other countries*. Retrieved from www.uu.nl/.

Held, D. (2006). *Models of democracy*. Stanford, CA: Stanford University Press.

Hidding, M., & van der Vlist, M. (2003). *Ruimte en water, Planningsopgaven voor een rode delta*. Den Haag: Sdu uitgevers.

Holling, C. S. (1973). Resilience and stability of ecological systems. *Annual Review of Ecology and Systematics*, *4*(1), 1–23. doi:10.1146/annurev.es.04.110173.000245.

IKSR. (2002). *Hochwasservorsorge Maßnahmen und ihre Wirksamkeit*. Retrieved from www.iksr.org/.

IPCC. (2014). Climate Change 2014: Impacts, Adaptation, and Vulnerability: IPCC WGII AR5 Chapter 23. Retrieved from www.ipcc.ch/report/ar5/wg2/.

Kienhuis, J. H. M., Westerwoudt, T. W., van der Wal, J. T., & Berge, A. P. (1993). *Het waterschap van oud naar nieuw [The water authority from old to new]*. Delft, the Netherlands: Hoogheemraadschap van Delfland. Leiden: Drukkerij Groen bv.

Kuijpers, C. B. F., & Glasbergen, P. (1990). Perspectieven voor integraal waterbeheer: een bestuurskundige analyse ten behoeve van de uitwerking van integraal waterbeheer. 'S Gravenhage: SDU uitgeverij.

Larsson, S. (2014). *Law and spatial planning: Socio-legal perspectives on the development of wind power and 3G mobile infrastructures in Sweden*. Karlskrona: Blekinge Institute of Technology.

Loucks, D. P., Stedinger, J. R., Davis, D. W., & Stakhiv, E. Z. (2008). Private and public responses to flood risks. *International Journal of Water Resources Development*, *24*(4), 541–553. doi:10.1080/07900620801923286.

Luhmann, N. (1975). *Legitimation durch Verfahren*. Luchterhand: Neuwied-Berlin.

MacPherson, C. B. (1977). *The life and times of liberal democracy*. Oxford: Oxford University Press.

Mees, H. L., Driessen, P. P., & Runhaar, H. A. (2014). Legitimate adaptive flood risk governance beyond the dykes: The cases of Hamburg, Helsinki and Rotterdam. *Regional Environmental Change*, *14*(2), 671–682. doi:10.1007/s10113-013-0527-2.

Moss, T. (2004). The governance of land use river basins: Prospects for overcoming problems of institutional interplay with the EU Water Framework Directive. *Land Use Policy*, *21*(1), 85–94. doi:10.1016/j.landusepol.2003.10.001.

Moss, T. (2009). Zwischen Ökologisierung Gewässerschutz und Kommerzialisierung der Wasserwirtschaft: Neue Handlungsanforderungen an Raumplanung und Regionalpolitik. *Raumforschung und Raumordnung*, *67*(1), 54–68.

Moss, T., & Monstadt, J. (2008). *Restoring floodplains in Europe: Policy contexts and project experiences*. London: IWA Publishing.

Neuvel, J. M. M., & van der Knaap, W. (2010). A spatial planning perspective for measures concerning flood risk management. *Water Resources Development*, *26*(2), 283–296. doi:10.1080/07900621003655668.

Nisipeanu, P. (2008). Tradition oder Fortentwicklung? Wasserrecht im UGB. *Natur und Recht*, *30*(2), 87–97.

Offermans, A., Haasnoot, M., & Valkering, P. (2011). A method to explore social response for sustainable water management strategies under changing conditions. *Sustainable Development*, *19*(5), 312–324. doi:10.1002/sd.439.

Patt, H., & Jüpner, R. (Eds.). (2013). *Hochwasser Handbuch: Auswirkungen und Schutz*. Heidelberg: Springer.

Petrow, T., Thieken, A. H., Kreibich, H., Merz, B., & Bahlburg, C. H. (2006). Improvements on flood alleviation in Germany: Lessons learned from the Elbe flood in August 2002. *Environmental Management*, *38*(5), 717–732. doi:10.1007/s00267-005-6291-4.

Plate, E. J. (Ed.). (2001). *Naturkatastrophen: Ursachen, Auswirkungen, Vorsorge; mit 31 Tabellen*. Stuttgart: Schweizerbart.

Reinhardt, M. (2008). Identität und Zukunft des Wasserrechts als Bestandteil eines Umweltgesetzbuchs. *Zeitschrift für Umweltrecht*, *7–8*, 352–357.

Rijke, J., van Herk, S., Zevenbergen, C., & Ashley, R. (2012). Room for the river: Delivering integrated river basin management in the Netherlands. *International Journal of River Basin Management*, *10*(4), 369–382. doi:10.1080/15715124.2012.739173.

Rittel, H. W., & Webber, M. M. (1973). Dilemmas in a general theory of planning. *Policy Sciences*, *4*(2), 155–169.

Saurí-Pujol, D., Roset-Pagès, D., Ribas-Palom, A., & Pujol-Caussa, P. (2001). The 'escalator effect' in flood policy: The case of the Costa Brava, Catalonia, Spain. *Applied Geography*, *21*(2), 127–143. doi:10.1016/S0143-6228(01)00003-0.

Schanze, J. (2006). Flood risk management-a basic framework. In J. Schanze, E. Zeman, & J. Marsalek (Eds.), *Flood risk management. Hazards, vulnerability and mitigation measures* (pp. 149–167). Dordrecht: Springer.

Scharpf, F. W. (1997). *Games real actors play: Actor-centered institutionalism in policy research. Theoretical lenses on public policy*. Boulder, CO: Westview Press.

Schmidt, V. A. (2013). Democracy and legitimacy in the European Union revisited: Input, output and 'throughput'. *Political Studies*, *61*(1), 2–22. doi:10.1111/j.1467-9248.2012.00962.x.

Schmitter, P. C. (2001). *What is there to legitimize in the European Union... and how might this be accomplished?* Vienna: Institute for Advanced Studies.

Sørensen, E. (2002). Democratic theory and network governance. *Administrative Theory & Praxis*, *24*(4), 693–720.

Spit, T. & Zoete, P. (2006). *Ruimtelijke ordening in Nederland, een wetenschappelijke introductie in het vakgebied*. Den Haag: Sdu Uitgevers.

Stead, D. (2014). Urban planning, water management and climate change strategies: Adaptation, mitigation and resilience narratives in the Netherlands. *International Journal of Sustainable Development & World Ecology*, *21*(1), 15–27. doi:10.1080/13504509.2013.824928.

Suchman, M. C. (1995). Managing legitimacy: Strategic and institutional approaches. *Academy of Management Review*, *20*(3), 571–610.

Tempels, B., & Hartmann, T. (2014). A co-evolving frontier between land and water: Dilemmas of flexibility versus robustness in flood risk management. *Water International*, *39*(6), 872–883. doi:10.1080/02508060.2014.958797.

Tyler, T. R. (2000). Social justice: Outcome and procedure. *International Journal of Psychology*, *35*(2), 117–125.

van Buuren, A., Klijn, E. H., & Edelenbos, J. (2012). Democratic legitimacy of new forms of water management in the Netherlands. *International Journal of Water Resources Development*, *28*(4), 629–645.

van Buuren, A., Driessen, P., Teisman, G., & van Rijswick, M. (2013). Toward legitimate governance strategies for climate adaptation in the Netherlands: Combining insights from a legal, planning, and network perspective. *Regional Environmental Change*. doi:10.1007/s10113-013-0448-0.

van der Brugge, R., Rotmans, J., & Loorbach, D. (2005). The transition in Dutch water management. *Regional Environmental Change*, *5*(4), 164–176.

van Steen, P.J.M. & Pellenbarg, P.H. 2004. Water management challenges in the Netherlands. *Tijdschrift voor Economische en Sociale Geografie*, *95*(5), 590–599.

van Stokkom, H. T., Smits, A. J., & Leuven, R. S. (2005). Flood defense in The Netherlands. A new era, a new approach. *Water International*, *30*(1), 76–87. doi:10.1080/02508060508691839.

van Tatenhove, J. (2011). Integrated marine governance: Questions of legitimacy. *Maritime Studies*, *10*(1), 87–113.

Vogt, M. (2005). Hochwassermanagement und räumliche Planung. In R. Jüpner (Ed.), *Hochwassermanagement* (pp. 97–118). Aachen: Shaker.

Warner, J. F., van Buuren, A., & Edelenbos, J. (2012). *Making space for the river, governance experiences with multifunctional river flood management in the US and Europe*. London and New York: IWA Publishing.

Wesselink, A. (2007). Flood safety in the Netherlands: The Dutch response to hurricane Katrina. *Technology in Society*, *29*(2), 239–247. doi:10.1016/j.techsoc.2007.01.010.

Wiering, M. A., & Crabbé, A. (2006). The institutional dynamics of water management in the low countries. In B. Arts & P. Leroy (Eds.), *Institutional dynamics in environmental governance* (pp. 93–114). Dordrecht: Springer.

Wiering, M. A., & Driessen, P. P. (2001). Beyond the art of diking: Interactive policy on river management in The Netherlands. *Water Policy*, *3*(4), 283–296. doi:10.1016/S1366-7017(01)00075-7.

Wiering, M. A., & Immink, I. (2006). When water management meets spatial planning: A policy-arrangements perspective. *Environment and Planning C*, *24*(3), 423.

Wolsink, M. A. (2006). River basin approach and integrated water management: Governance pitfalls for the Dutch Space-Water-Adjustment Management Principle. *Geoforum*, *37*(4), 473–487. doi:10.1016/j.geoforum.2005.07.001.

Woltjer, J., & Al, N. (2007). Integrating water management and spatial planning: Strategies based on the Dutch experience. *Journal of the American Planning Association*, *73*(2), 211–222. doi:10.1080/01944360708976154.

7 Flood groups in England

Governance arrangements and contribution to flood resilience

Steven Forrest, Elen-Maarja Trell and Johan Woltjer

Introduction

Flooding is a very real and present threat in European countries, which experienced 215 coastal, river and flash flood events from 2004 to 2014 causing 1,021 deaths (Guha-Sapir et al., 2015). This has affected over 5.8 million people and resulted in over €45 -billion in damages (Guha-Sapir et al., 2015). Climate change is also expected to lead to an increase in the frequency and intensity of future flooding and flood-related damage in Europe (Alfieri et al., 2015; EEA, 2012).

In light of the above, it is clear that flooding is an issue that requires immediate attention, especially in countries that have recently suffered severe flooding and are expected to face worse floods in the future, such as England (EA, 2009). Flooding has become a more prominent issue in England since severe floods in Boscastle (2004), Carlisle (2005), Hull (2007), Cumbria (2009) and the more recent 'Winter floods' (2013/2014 and 2015). The impact of these recent flood events has raised the profile of flooding and led to a greater scrutiny of the work of flood authorities and the funding allocated to flood risk management by the government (Priestley and Allen, 2016; Thorne, 2014). Research into these recent flood events has challenged existing beliefs about flood risk management in England, including the current national governance systems for floods and the use of "large-scale flood defences as the most effective intervention approach" (White, 2013:107).

At the same time, there has been an ongoing paradigm shift in flood risk management from *resistance* and 'keeping water out' towards 'living with water' and the idea of increasing flood *resilience* through "more strategic, holistic and long-term" approaches (Scott, 2013:103). This shift towards flood resilience is evident in England through the *Making Space for Water* strategy (Defra, 2005), which emphasises an attempt to live with water (Johnson and Priest, 2008; Meijerink and Dicke, 2008). In disaster management literature, resilience is traditionally understood as the ability of social systems to absorb/resist shocks without losing their ability to function and then to recover and 'bounce-back', although more recent interpretations are increasingly including the ability of social systems to adapt and transform (i.e. 'bounce-forward') (Davoudi, 2012; Masterson et al., 2014; Restemeyer et al., 2015; Tierney, 2014). Thus, while the *resistance* approach focuses on flood hazard control measures, the *resilience* approach also acknowledges the possibility of a flood to occur and the need to address that possibility through policy measures throughout different levels of government.

Alongside the transition in flood risk management from resistance to resilience is a change in the roles and responsibilities between the state, market and civil society. There is a greater emphasis on increasing public participation and local input in flood risk management to transform members of the public into "active risk managers" who take a greater role in solving flooding issues and contributing to flood resilience (Johnson and Priest, 2008; Kuhlicke and Steinführer, 2013:115). In England, this emphasis is highlighted in documents such as the *Making Space for Water* strategy (Defra, 2005), the *Pitt Review* (Pitt, 2008), and the *Flood and Water Management Act* (UK Government, 2010). Importantly, recent national efforts to increase community-level resilience to flooding in England include the *Flood Resilience Community Pathfinder Scheme 2013–2015* by the UK Department for Environment, Food and Rural Affairs (Defra) (Twigger-Ross et al., 2014). This scheme emphasized civil society's role in flood resilience and specifically supported interventions to increase community resilience to flooding (ibid). It also functioned as a driver for the creation of flood groups (ibid). The evidence suggests that due to climate change the communities will indeed need to "become better prepared and more resilient to flood events" in the future (O'Brien et al., 2014:8). This is seen in 'resilience-building' grey literature in the UK, which repeatedly advocates increasing levels of self-reliance in communities (Davoudi, 2012). These increases in self-reliance can be perceived as constructive as officials are supporting "stewardship of lay people" (Schelfaut et al., 2011:831) and this could enable communities to become better prepared and more flood resilient. However, the focus on self-reliance can be accompanied by a corresponding decline in the role of the government (Davoudi, 2012) with responsibilities passed on to community and voluntary (flood) groups. Therefore, the increasing focus on *resilience* within flood risk management practice/policy-making necessitates a better understanding of the capacities of communities on a local level.

As illustrated above, some attention has been given to involving the community in flood risk management. However, the role that civil society can play within flood resilience and the actual capacities of a community to take on such a role are not well documented (Van der Vaart et al., 2015). To contribute to the understanding of the role of civil society in flood risk management and in community resilience to flooding, this chapter focuses on exploring flood groups. These are becoming more common and established in England: in the past decade, the number of flood groups has increased from "more than fifty" (Defra, 2004:99) to over 221 in England (NFF internal database, 2015). This rise in prominence indicates a shift in the flood risk management landscape. Despite this, there is no concrete definition of what constitutes a 'flood group'. Existing academic literature and government documentation consider all forms of community groups working on flood issues as 'flood groups', which makes comparisons, generalisations and pinpointing the potential role of flood groups a challenge. In addition, the mere existence of flood groups may not by definition mean that they have an impact on flood resilience, although previous research suggests that they contribute towards it (see Geaves and Penning-Rowsell, 2015). This chapter argues that to make valid statements regarding the potential role of flood groups in community flood resilience, more needs to be known about their formation, membership, position in the local flood risk management landscape and activities.

By focusing on developing a working definition of flood groups in England, and by analysing their governance arrangements, this research aims to shed light on their potential influence on community resilience to flooding. The chapter first discusses resilience in relation to flooding at a local level and develops a framework to analyse the influence of flood groups on community resilience to flooding. Second, it provides information on England's current flood risk management landscape. Third, the research methodology is introduced. Fourth, the chapter presents and discusses the findings whilst reflecting on the influences of flood groups and offering insights into the wider implications of this research.

Flood resilience

Over the last few decades, the policy discourse on flood risk management in many countries has been moving from a focus on large-scale engineering-based systems towards a more holistic *flood resilience* approach (Schelfaut et al., 2011; Scott, 2013). This latter approach acknowledges that floods cannot always be prevented, but their impacts can be reduced. It also understands and accepts that uncertainty is present in any flood risk management endeavour and acts on a "more integrated and precautionary basis" (White, 2013:110). Furthermore, in disaster studies, the analysis of resilience has seen the level of the local community as "an appropriate level at which to take action" (Coates, 2015:2). This focus on the community level and community resilience has also been evident at the global level (e.g. the 2009 Global Platform for Disaster Risk Reduction) and in resilience definitions by the United Nations International Strategy for Disaster Risk Reduction (Schelfaut et al., 2011).

Community resilience to flooding

'Community resilience to flooding' examines flood resilience at the local level and places the community and its resilience to flooding at the heart of the analysis. When placing community at the centre of the analysis, one unavoidably must pay attention to (often romanticised) assumptions connected to the notion of 'community'. These include the power relations present on the local level as well as the connected issues of "justice and fairness", both of which may influence resilience (Coates, 2015; Davoudi, 2012:306; Fainstein, 2015). Variations in the distribution of capacities over community members are inherent to resilience-thinking. Increasing 'community' resilience may not necessarily benefit all community groups equally (Fainstein, 2015; Wilson, 2012) with certain groups potentially being excluded or affected unevenly (Davoudi, 2012). This exclusion may exist before any activities to enhance resilience are undertaken when decision-makers define the 'community' (Porter and Davoudi, 2012). Ideally, the term 'community' would include and represent all social groups affected by flooding. However, in practice, the representativeness of flood groups is likely to selectively influence whether the flood groups are improving community resilience for everybody or only for those included in the flood group and its decision-making processes. Therefore, this research incorporated issues of representativeness and inclusion into the analysis of the flood groups.

In the disaster-related literature, community resilience is often conceptualised as a network of different capacities that can be accessed and harnessed by communities (e.g. Cutter et al., 2008, 2010; Forrest et al., 2014; Masterson et al., 2014; Norris et al., 2008). Such conceptualisations suggest that communities can become more resilient by developing and increasing these capacities. Norris et al. (2008) proposed four central capacities for community resilience to disasters in general: community competence, social capital, information and communication, and economic development. Cutter et al. (2008) developed a place-based model for resilience to 'natural' disasters and propose six indicator categories of community resilience: social, institutional, community competence, ecological, infrastructure, and economic. The framework by Cutter et al. (2008) has recently been used to measure community resilience to flooding in England as part of Defra's *Flood Resilience Community Pathfinder Scheme 2013–2015* (Forrest et al., 2014). Masterson et al. (2014) used four capitals (social, physical, human and economic) that together describe what they term 'community capacity' to deal with disasters.

There are common elements within the above frameworks, such as the community's internal social capital and external social connectedness and capabilities, the condition of the natural/built environment (i.e. ecological capital, infrastructure capital and physical capital), the characteristics of individuals in the communities (i.e. human capital and community competence), and the economic resources accessible to the community (i.e. economic development and economic capital). This chapter adapts and builds upon these common elements to analyse how flood groups in England have influenced community resilience to flooding in terms of 'community capacity' as defined by four capitals: social, natural/built environment, human, and economic. These capitals relate to the ways that the community is resilient to (i.e. prepares for, withstands, responds to, recovers from, adapts to, and transforms in response to) flooding.

Understanding community capacity

Community capacity is understood in this chapter as the "sum of the individual and organisational capacities within a community" and their collective ability to achieve "community goals" (Masterson et al., 2014:36). In this context, the focus is on how the flood groups affect these capacities, within the four capitals, to influence community resilience to flooding. Therefore, to understand community capacity it is relevant to explore the four constituent capitals and the ways these capitals are operationalised for this chapter in more detail (see Table 7.1).

Social capital expresses the extent to which individuals interact with one another within a community and how the community's internal social networks and structures, as well as external formal/informal institutional structures and support, influence how individuals engage with flooding (Cutter et al., 2008; Masterson et al., 2014). The relationships between the community and local flood authorities, such as "emergency planners, voluntary sector and local responders" (Twigger-Ross et al., 2014:11), and the institutional structures that exist in the community are important for flood resilience. Individuals and communities with highly developed social networks and institutional structures may have greater access to support and resources to increase flood resilience. The information and communication capacity of a community is important in the case of emergencies (Norris et al., 2008) and informal social networks can act in collaboration with official flood warning systems (Parker and Handmer, 1998). The ability of a community to organise itself, access information and work together (i.e. their community competence) is also important to consider as it will affect their ability to engage with flood issues (Norris et al., 2008).

Table 7.1 Understanding and specifying community capacity in terms of the four capitals

Capital	*In this chapter*
Social	Focuses on how individuals within a community interact with one another and how the community interacts with local flood actors in relation to flood issues
Natural/built environment	Focuses on temporary and permanent changes to the local physical landscape and on rules imposed on changing the landscape (spatial planning) in relation to flood issues
Human	Focuses on the individual's ability to engage with flood issues
Economic	Focuses on the economic resources available for individuals and the community to better engage with flood issues

Source: Authors.

Natural and built environment capital describes the level to which the spatial planning policies and physical characteristics of the local context support the community's resilience to flooding. Natural environment measures already taken at the catchment level can include upstream land management that supports flood risk mitigation, such as the use of wetlands as a natural flood buffer and woodland for flood attenuation (UK NEA, 2014). The built environment 'indicator' includes the amount of pervious structures within a community, land zoning policies for flood risk, and the resilience of critical facilities (Cutter et al., 2008; Masterson et al., 2014). The built environment also describes permanent and temporary physical flood measures that reduce and manage flood risk such as embankments, river widening and dredging, and temporary barriers.

The key difference between human and social capital as operationalised in this chapter is the explicit focus of human capital on the *individuals* and their current and potential capability to individually engage with flooding. When evaluating community resilience to flooding it is relevant to pay attention to the general health and well-being on the individual level (Masterson et al., 2014) as individuals with ill-health or disabilities may be less resilient to flooding than the overall community. The level of education, knowledge and skills of the individuals within a community are further characteristics differentiating the flood resilience of individuals within a community and should be considered, especially when aiming to understand vulnerabilities within a community (Cutter et al., 2008; Masterson et al., 2014).

Economic capital refers to economic resources (Masterson et al., 2014) of both the individual and community, such as homeownership, employment rate (Cutter et al., 2014) and community funds. Additional influential economic indicators include the equitable distribution of wealth (Cutter et al., 2008; Norris et al, 2008) and the uptake of flood insurance as a means of spreading the risk (Botzen and van den Bergh, 2008). These resources can influence the extent to which they are able to be resilient to flooding, especially in terms of preparing for floods and for post-flood recovery.

England's flood risk management landscape

According to the House of Commons (2015), approximately 2.4-million properties in England are at risk from fluvial flooding, 3-million from pluvial flooding and 600,000 are at risk from both. In order to deal with the risks, several actors, sectors and policy documents interact and intersect with each other in what this chapter terms the '*flood risk management landscape*'. In the context of England, Defra is responsible for national and strategic emergency planning for flooding, whilst the Environment Agency (EA) is responsible for implementing flood risk management works and issuing flood warnings (i.e. the 'boots on the ground'). Additional primary flood actors in England include water and sewerage companies, highway authorities, the Met Office, the Flood Forecasting Centre, the National

Flood Forum (NFF), Public Health England, Regional Flood and Coastal Committees, Internal Drainage Boards, coastal erosion risk management authorities, Lead Local Flood Authorities (LLFAs), local resilience forums and local councils.

Meijerink and Dicke (2008) found a general shift towards decentralisation in flood risk management in many countries with governments seeking to share flood risks with other actors. It is particularly true in England's flood risk management landscape where an ongoing trend towards local level involvement/action and the sharing of flood risk between multiple non-state actors, such as the local communities, can be detected. England's *Making Space for Water* strategy (Defra, 2004) highlights the importance of people at risk of flooding being involved in flood issues in their area through 'flood action groups'. The strategy also places greater responsibility on the public to "manage their own flood risk" (Johnson and Priest, 2008:520) and envisions them being more aware of flood risks and "empowered to take suitable actions themselves where appropriate" (Defra, 2004; Defra, 2005:14).

The *Pitt Review* (Pitt, 2008), an independent review into the management of the 2007 floods in England, also encourages connecting local groups with local organisations. The review included input from several flood groups, which shows that flood groups were consulted and contributed to this influential document. The *Flood and Water Management Act* (UK Government, 2010) named LLFAs as responsible for local flood risk management. These LLFAs are encouraged to involve and consult the local community on local flood risk management issues (Local Government Association, 2012). The *National Flood and Coastal Erosion Risk Management Strategy for England* (EA and Defra, 2011), created as a requirement of the *Flood and Water Management Act*, also focuses on increasing the involvement of the community in flood risk management. Overall, the shift towards flood resilience in England seems to have been accompanied by a decentralisation in flood risk management and an increased focus on the local level, especially on citizen involvement and responsibility.

Methodology

To understand the governance arrangements and potential influence of flood groups on the four capitals presented in Table 7.1, data were collected from national actors working with local flood groups and associated local actors. Semi-structured interviews were held with national actors in Defra (2 interviewees), the EA (1), the NFF (1) and the Association of Drainage Authorities (1) to gain their perspectives on local flood groups.

An online survey provided data on the governance arrangements of flood groups and their influence on community resilience to flooding. It was distributed to 221 flood groups across England and completed by forty groups; a further inspection of the low response rate found that the flood groups were being inundated by data requests from academics (and other bodies) and had to prioritise which ones to respond to. The NFF provided additional legitimacy to the research and functioned as a 'gatekeeper' to access and distribute the surveys to the flood groups. However, it meant that the survey missed flood groups with no links to the NFF.

The survey data and recommendations by national level interviewees were used to identify six flood groups for further research. These groups were selected based on following considerations: It was important that the selected flood groups had existed over a sufficient period (>1 year) for governance arrangements to have developed and for activities to have been undertaken. Since the research focused on public involvement it was also important to select flood groups that consisted primarily of members of the public with an interest in flooding but without a paid position with a formal flood actor. The position of these flood groups in the local flood risk management landscape was important to understand in order to identify where they were influencing community resilience to flooding and how they were affecting existing local flood actors, especially local flood authorities. Therefore, the flood groups needed to have links with local flood authorities (i.e. local government) and other local actors. These considerations resulted in the following criteria being applied to the survey data to identify appropriate flood groups that: (i) were established over 1-year ago, (ii) had a membership consisting of more than 75% members of the public, (iii) worked with other local actors and (iv) worked with the local council. The six groups selected are represented in Table 7.2.

Table 7.2 Details of the selected flood groups. *The Todmorden group operated from 2000–2003 before reconvening in 2012

Flood group	*i) Date established*	*ii) Public membership*	*iv) Local actors that they work with*
Hebden Bridge Flood Action Group	2012	100%	Local council; EA; Other flood groups
Mytholmroyd Flood Group	2014	100%	Local council; EA; Other flood groups
Garforth Flood Support Group	2013	94%	Local council; EA; Other flood groups; Water company
Bodenham Flood Protection Group	2008	100%	Local council; EA; Other flood groups
Todmorden Flood Group	2000–2003; 2012*	80%	Local council; EA; Other flood groups; Local community groups
Much Wenlock Flood Action Group	2007/2008	100%	Local council; EA; Other flood groups; NFF; Water company; Emergency services

Source: Authors.

A number of semi-structured interviews were undertaken with representatives of these six flood groups and, in the latter two cases, with the local council and the EA representatives that worked with the flood groups. The national interviewee for the EA also represented the Cornwall Community Flood Forum (CCFF) and was also interviewed about this non-NFF flood group. These interviewees were also asked to map the stakeholders that they worked with and to describe their relationships with them. Several also provided additional documentation (e.g. community flood plans) from their flood groups. All interviews were transcribed and coded thematically. The interview data were supplemented by an analysis of the flood groups' documentation provided by interviewees and from desk-based research.

Findings and discussion

Flood groups: a working definition

This research identified 221 flood groups currently active in England. These groups ranged from community flood 'forums', 'committees' and 'action groups' that exclusively focus on flooding to groups that focus on flooding in addition to wider community issues, such as parish councils and residents' associations.

All of the flood groups interviewed aimed to build flood-related community capacity, with the majority also aiming for self-sufficiency (similar to findings by Harries, 2009; Waylen et al., 2011). The flood groups also aimed to increase local flood risk communication, which has been previously identified in such groups across the UK (by McCarthy and Tunstall, 2008; Scott Wilson Kirkpatrick and Co Ltd et al., 2003).

The flood groups interviewed in this research made varying contributions to flood risk management and resilience. The survey and interview data showed that several flood groups were action-orientated and focused on measures to reduce flood risk (e.g. clearing out ditches in Bodenham and creating temporary water storage areas in Garforth). Some of these flood groups also focused on actions to reduce the consequences of flooding (e.g. flood stores in Todmorden to Hebden Bridge) and to support flood recovery (as similarly found by Andrew, 2012; Twigger-Ross et al., 2011). Flood groups were also found to be involved with advocacy activities that ranged from discussing local flood issues (e.g. Bodenham, Todmorden, Hebden Bridge and Mytholmroyd) to actively pressuring and seeking to influence (i.e. lobby) authorities on local flood issues (e.g. the development of flood attenuation ponds in Much Wenlock and planning application objections in most interviewed flood groups). This supports previous research that identified flood groups lobbying for local flood defence schemes (Thaler and Priest, 2014) and campaigning for local flood issues (Geaves and Penning-Rowsell, 2015; Neill and Neill, 2012; Thaler and Priest, 2014; Twigger-Ross et al., 2011). Despite previous research indicating their contribution towards the independent scrutiny of previous local flood events (McCarthy and Tunstall, 2008), this was not identified in this research.

It is important to note that the activities of flood groups are flexible and groups may change over time (interview EA, 2015). These changes may be expressed in the activities conducted, with flood groups moving from action to advocacy or vice-versa, and in the types of local flood actors that they work with.

Interview data with some input from literature was used to create a working definition of a 'flood group' that forms a starting point for data analysis in this chapter:

> A flood group is primarily made up of a group of individuals with a personal interest in local flood issues who frequently meet with one another in specific flood group meetings to discuss flood-related issues in a specific geographical area. In addition to meeting, a flood group is often involved in action and/or advocacy on flood-related issues in their local area. Importantly, the individuals comprising a flood group form a shared identity that arises from having been affected by a shared flood event, by having a shared local flood source and/or a shared local geographical area at risk of flooding.

Formation and membership

All the flood groups interviewed were formed after flood events, which is a common narrative in England (O'Brien et al., 2014). The scale of flood disturbance also influenced whether a flood group was formed or not (Geaves and Penning-Rowsell, 2015). In addition to recent flood experiences, interviews reported a variety of drivers that supported the formation of the interviewed flood groups, such as support from the local parish council (e.g. Bodenham), local referendums and from local politicians (e.g. Much Wenlock). Interviews with flood groups and local flood authorities indicated that it was necessary to have a community demand and interest in having a flood group. Thus, flood group formation was typically a bottom-up process which cannot be forced onto communities in a solely top-down manner. However, the findings indicate that flood authorities could encourage the formation of flood groups by providing stimuli such as financial support (e.g. The Defra *Flood Resilience Community Pathfinder Scheme* in Todmorden, Hebden Bridge, Mytholmroyd and CCFF).

All the flood groups interviewed were comprised of volunteers who could be classified into permanent or convergent volunteers based on the frequency of their volunteering. Permanent volunteers were part of the flood group throughout the year and involved themselves in the ongoing organisation and activities of the group. Conversely, convergent volunteers may have had no previous links to local flood risk management, but volunteered during flood emergencies (interview EA, 2015). Some flood groups had access to large numbers of convergent volunteers that signed up to the flood group or to other community groups (e.g. the Todmorden group had access to approximately 200 convergent volunteers).

The role and emergence of so-called 'local leaders' and other influential individuals have been found to be important in the formation and activities of civil society groups in a range of settings (Salemink and Strijker, 2015; Terluin, 2003; Twigger-Ross et al., 2011). The flood groups were also found to have such 'key members': influential residents, who were prepared or able to put time and effort into organising the flood group. Similarly, to the interviewee quoted below, all the interviewed flood groups acknowledged that without their key members they would have been unlikely to have formed and developed to their current levels (cf. O'Brien et al., 2014; Salemink and Strijker, 2015):

> Flood groups that are successful, there's usually a nucleus, someone who really cares and has respect in that community, and I think that you get luck [in] finding that person and you can't appoint someone to this position...as authorities we can't find these people, but if you provide the right stimulus then you'll have these people appear.
>
> Defra interviewee, 2015

However, key members could also have a negative impact upon flood groups. In one flood group, personal disputes between key members and partner organisations dictated the relationship between the whole flood group and the 'external' organisation. In another flood group, such disputes resulted in the deliberate exclusion of individuals from the group. Findings by Coates (2015) provide a similar warning that flood groups centred on key members may deter other individuals in the wider community from joining and not be representative of the wider community.

Representation, exclusion and potential marginalisation

Power relations need to be examined when researching into resilience (Davoudi, 2012), especially community resilience, and the associated issues of "resilience from what, to what, and *who gets to decide*" (Porter and Davoudi, 2012:331, emphasis added). The last part of 'who gets to decide' is important as those involved in the decision-making can define the boundaries of their 'resilience work' and outline the priorities, which may lead to the exclusion of other perspectives (Davoudi, 2012). In the flood groups interviewed, the permanent members decided on the activities to be undertaken and defined the desired outcomes. Therefore, the representativeness of the permanent members is important to ensure decisions accurately reflected the community.

Several national interviewees suggested that the flood groups were *always* 'representative' of the community as those who want to join can. However, this representativeness should not be taken for granted as there may be individuals that are excluded (Davoudi, 2012), if not purposefully then perhaps inadvertently. Some flood groups interviewed attempted to be representative of the community by creating elected area representatives (e.g. Bodenham) and street wardens (e.g. Todmorden).

At the same time, members of the community were excluded by some of the flood groups interviewed. Interviewees argued that some individuals became excluded because of differences of opinion during meetings with flood groups and local flood authorities. These differences were in how permanent flood group members interacted with local flood officials. For example, in the aftermath of the 2013/14 UK floods, public criticism was directed towards the government and EA for a lack of river maintenance and farmers for inappropriate land management techniques (Thorne, 2014). It was evident from the interviews that, in a similar vein, some individuals in the flood groups blamed the government and local flood officials for failures in dealing with past flood events whilst others did not. These differences led to tensions within the flood groups and made consensus-building difficult. The sharp criticism from these individuals at flood group meetings was also perceived as straining the relations with local flood officials. Furthermore, in two flood groups interviewed, the individuals were excluded by personal decisions to leave the flood group, and no longer attend flood group meetings, as they did not agree with the direction that the flood group was taking in working with their local flood officials. Although this exclusion was beneficial for consensus-building within the flood group and collaboration efforts with local flood officials, it did marginalise certain individuals at risk from flooding.

Inadvertent exclusion may also occur due to the voluntary nature of flood groups. They are formed of volunteers and this introduces a selective aspect to their membership, which has implications for their representativeness. Recent research found that flood and coastal risk management volunteers in England tended to be older (i.e. above 50-years-old) individuals, with few volunteers from poorer backgrounds and with little ethnic diversity (Edwards et al., 2015). Whilst this research did not explore individual background and ethnic diversity, it did support findings about volunteer age. For example, certain flood groups (e.g. Bodenham and Garforth) were predominantly formed of older people and retirees with younger residents being too busy with their families or too tired to attend meetings after work (interview Bodenham, 2015). There was recognition of the need for younger residents to be involved in these groups to sustain them. However, this type of inadvertent exclusion and potential marginalisation was outside the control of flood groups. Several reported experiencing difficulties in recruiting new members and keeping them engaged due to widespread public apathy towards flooding, residents purposely avoiding dealing with flood risk or not wanting to admit having been flooded due to fears about the negative impacts on property prices and flood insurance policies. Such factors could be barriers to community-led schemes in achieving community resilience to flooding.

Flood groups in the local flood risk management landscape

The emergence of flood groups adds a "new element" to the existing governance arrangements for flood risk management at the local level (Geaves and Penning-Rowsell, 2015:1). The flood groups interviewed worked with a range of actors in the local flood risk management landscape (see Figure 7.1). These actors shared resources with the flood groups: physical resources (e.g. meeting rooms, staff members), financial resources, and knowledge and ideas. Knowledge and ideas were the most common resource shared, especially by the County Council, Local/Parish Council and the EA, whilst financial resources were rarely shared. However, financial support was given in the form of small loans (e.g. Bodenham) and through local community funds (e.g. Garforth). The ability of flood groups to access community funds that were not available to local flood authorities is an example of how they add value to the local flood risk management landscape.

The flood groups were also found to have opportunities to influence other actors in the local flood risk management landscape: they were often asked to consult on the plans/documents of the County Council (13 groups), Local/Parish Council (15) and the EA (15), and to support the designing and drafting of their documents (see Figure 7.1). The fact that these important actors interacted with the flood groups in these ways suggests that the groups were established and visible enough in the local context to contribute on flood-related issues. The flood groups also worked with the Emergency Services (police, fire and ambulance service), flood consultants, landowners, village magazines, internal drainage boards, other community groups, universities, Network Rail and Defra ('Others' category). This shows that the flood groups interacted with a broad range of actors and included other specific local organisations, but that these interactions varied considerably across the flood groups.

The roles and responsibilities of the state/local flood authorities and civil society/the flood groups were important to understand further especially considering research suggesting that civil society involvement could lead to a decline in state support (Davoudi, 2012). Many of the flood groups saw themselves as intermediaries between the community and the local flood authorities. National interviewees also viewed the flood groups in this way and as a conveyer of local knowledge. The flood groups did not see themselves as replacing or taking responsibilities from existing actors. There was evidence of local flood officials, from the EA and LLFAs, going beyond their assigned duties by attending extra meetings and providing expertise to support the flood groups interviewed.

Interviews found that flood groups offered added value within the local 'flood risk management landscape' in the form of information resources embedded in local knowledge, experiences and engagement. They contributed by sharing local knowledge on their local area and, for example, its

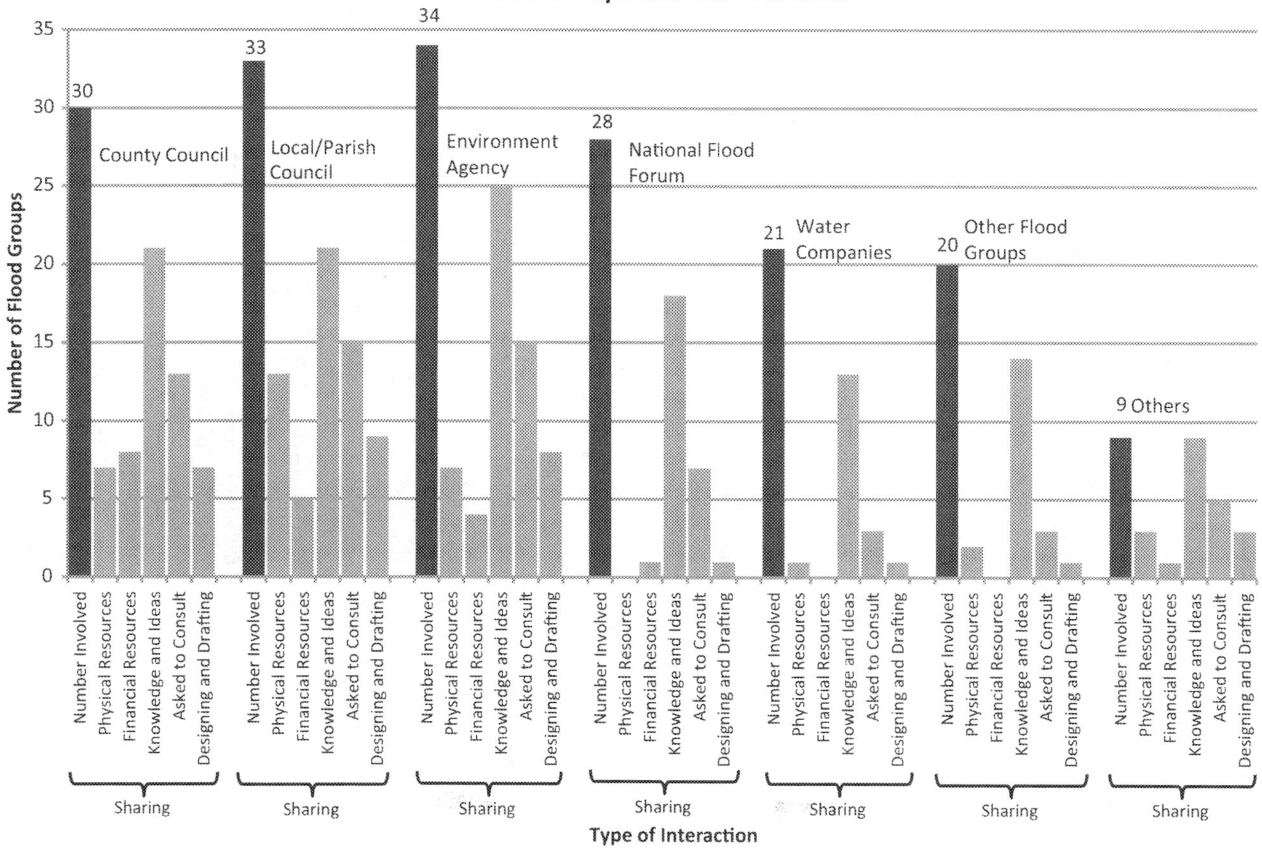

Figure 7.1 Flood groups and their relationships with other local actors (first column represents the number of flood groups working with the named local actor; some groups had several types of interaction with each local actor; n=36).

Source: Authors.

drainage system (interview Much Wenlock, 2015), past flood and rainfall data, and river and road ownership (interview Todmorden, 2015). Their input was able to correct EA data on previous flooding and help fill existing knowledge gaps. It was also reported by flood group members and national interviewees that residents were more willing to talk to, and respect, key members in local flood groups than local officials:

> People will talk to us because they know us, they recognise our faces, we've been to school with them – people come to talk to us because we're not the council, we're not the EA and that's how we find out more things.
>
> Todmorden flood group interviewee, 2015

However, in some cases, actors also withheld from interacting with flood groups, despite appeals by the flood groups themselves (e.g. Yorkshire Water in Todmorden). Reasons for not interacting with the flood groups included the perception that there were better avenues for engaging with local flood risk management.

Influence of flood groups on community resilience to flooding

Based on findings from empirical data, Table 7.3 presents an overview of activities through which the flood groups influenced community capacity and resilience to flooding. Not all the activities can be solely classified under one category and there are also hybrid links between some categories.

Social capital

The findings indicate that flood groups influenced the social capital of these communities in terms of their internal social networks and structures, community competence, information and communication, and external institutional structures and support.

Interviews suggested that flood groups maintained and created new social connections by organising social events in the community (interview Bodenham, 2015; interview Garforth, 2015). Internal communication structures were created to support the dissemination of flood warnings (e.g. telephone trees in Much Wenlock and Hebden Bridge) and new governance structures to connect residents and flood groups (e.g. the area representative system in Bodenham). These were examples of community competence (Norris et al., 2008). Interviews suggested that flood groups created and developed links between the community and external institutions such as the EA.

Table 7.3 Flood group activities, based on interview and survey data

Community capacity	*Activity*
Social capital	Shared knowledge with neighbouring communities Supplied data for local council flood models Provided knowledge on which drains and 'pinch points' to watch during heavy rainfall Created community flood plans Created and supported flood warning systems Reported river blockages Conducted village sewer surveys Installed and tested flood sirens with flood authorities Developed more coordinated approaches and partnership plans across different flood actors Conducted joint flood exercises with local councils and the EA Provided flood recovery support to neighbours
Natural/built environment capital	Objected (and forced changes) to new building developments that would increase flood risk Integrated flood risk management and spatial planning Encouraged flood risk management to appear in land use plans Cleared and maintained ditches and watercourses Erected flood walls and barriers (property-level protection) Operated flood pumps Developed temporary water storage areas Created community flood stores with post-flood equipment Led catchment based approaches
Human capital	Aimed to increase flood knowledge and risk awareness in general Started education initiatives on current and future flood risk for citizens and schools Formed community support networks to help vulnerable people during and after flooding Aimed to reduce deprivation and increase health and well-being in communities
Economic capital	Provided flood insurance help and advice Undertook community fundraising for flood mitigation and recovery measures Attracted funding for property level protection measures and early warning systems Accessed local community funds

Source: Authors.

Natural/built environment capital

According to our survey, flood groups were found to influence natural and built environment capital through maintenance measures, temporary physical measures and through spatial planning. For example, the Bodenham flood group maintained and improved the efficiency of water infrastructure by cleaning out watercourses and blocked culverts, in effect replicating the tasks of authorities. While this example shows flood groups taking action to solve flood risk problems themselves, it also raises wider questions about flood risk management responsibilities. The flood group, in carrying out this maintenance, showed signs of an expanding civil society and community involvement in owning their flood risk. However, it could also be an indication of local government/authorities 'reallocating' their duties to maintain watercourses to unpaid members of the public (see also Geaves and Penning-Rowsell, 2015).

Temporary physical measures such as demountable barriers, flood stores containing post-flood recovery equipment (e.g. Garforth, Hebden Bridge, Mytholmroyd and Todmorden) and water-sacks are examples of flood group actions taken to increase both local flood resistance and resilience. These demountable barriers and water-sacks focus on withstanding and resisting flooding and occur at the neighbourhood and individual property level respectively. However, the creation of flood stores represents an acknowledgement that some flooding is inevitable and illustrates a focus on reducing the consequences of flooding.

Flood groups also influenced spatial planning in their communities from both a physical and policy-making level. For instance, at the physical level, the Garforth flood group raised a bund around a playing field and secured agreement for its use as a temporary water storage area when flooding was predicted. In terms of policy-making, flood groups (e.g. Much Wenlock) could influence the content of their local 'neighbourhood plan', a statutory document that strongly influences local planning, to include certain local flood issues in future developments. This influence may alter the perception that future policy-makers have of local flood issues and affects the type of developments that can be undertaken in the future. The flood groups also maintained a critical eye on local planning applications for new developments and raised flood-related concerns with local councils and the EA (e.g. Much Wenlock, Garforth, Bodenham and Todmorden). In some cases, they have managed to force changes to new developments, but in others, their views have been considered but outweighed by other concerns.

Human capital

Flood groups influenced human capital through their impacts on individual flood awareness and in supporting those deemed more vulnerable to flooding. They also provided emotional support to flood victims and acted *"as a shoulder to cry on*" (interview Bodenham, 2015), which is important as flood events can have a significant impact on the mental health and wellbeing of those affected (Tapsell and Tunstall, 2008).

It is difficult to specifically estimate the extent to which flood awareness and knowledge increased as a direct result of the flood groups' activities. However, it is possible to state that flood groups maintained awareness of local flood issues by handing out leaflets, publishing in newspapers, producing YouTube videos, and providing personalised flood plans with contact information. Further efforts to increase local flood knowledge were made using flood group websites, an online training module and by working in schools (e.g. CCFF). Such efforts can also be argued to influence the community and to increase social capital. The existence of the flood groups also served as a reminder to local people of past flooding and of the current flood risk.

Flood groups also supported the more vulnerable, described by the groups interviewed as the elderly, infirm, those with young children, new residents to the area, and residents that are away during a flood and cannot protect their homes. The flood groups organised equipment and helped erect property-level protection measures for these groups of people, with Bodenham having a 'buddy system' that paired residents together so that they can support one another during flood events (related to internal social networks and structures as part of social capital).

Economic capital

The flood groups interviewed attempted to influence economic capital by lobbying decision-makers and organisations to invest money into their communities to protect them against flooding (interview EA, 2015). Interviewees reported that fundraising (by member subscriptions or from accessing community grants) by flood groups also increased the economic capital available for local flood risk management activities (i.e. community funds). Flood group members without fundraising skills could potentially become marginalised (Geaves and Penning-Rowsell, 2015), although at least one flood group interviewed was aware of this and included individually-tailored tasks to avoid this form of exclusion.

Flood groups were found to both positively and negative influence availability and cost of flood insurance in the community. On the positive side, flood groups could act as an official voice and talk directly to insurance companies when residents had been refused flood insurance cover, which was successful in several cases. Key members were also able to use their strong personal relationships with influential individuals to gain access to heads of insurance companies and insurance brokers, and lists of potential flood insurers to distribute to their residents.

Homeowners can have difficulty in obtaining flood risk insurance or face increases in the premiums associated with such policies if they are perceived to be at flood risk (Lamond et al., 2009). Flood insurance premiums are determined by flood risk maps, but these maps are not always reliable in areas where data on previous flooding is incomplete. On the negative side, in one flood group (name withheld), it was reported that several insurance agencies noticed that some properties were at risk of flooding based on the flood group's work and this led to an increase in insurance policy prices. Such outcome represents a common fear of residents, affecting their willingness to acknowledge their own flood risk and in some cases discouraging them from installing visible property-level protection measures.

Community capacity and flood groups

The influence of the flood groups interviewed is typically based on the expansion of existing social capital, following flooding events, through networks of volunteers and facilitated by institutional support. Interventions are focused to a large extent on knowledge exchange, on the local area or on gaining financial support, and interactions around small-scale maintenance-oriented activities.

The influence of flood groups on natural/built environment capital was primarily restricted to smaller, less resource-intensive maintenance and local building protection activities as opposed to larger-scale, more resource-intensive activities such as greening of the landscape and the implementation of water-sensitive urban design. The focus on smaller activities is due, in part, to the fact that they are comprised of volunteers and run as voluntary groups with limited resources. However, a few groups interviewed also carried out more extensive activities such as an attempt to change the local landscape by developing temporary water storage areas and another to influence future urban planning by contributing to long-term strategic development plans.

Human capital influences were typically focused on increasing public flood risk awareness and supporting those that are identified as vulnerable by the flood group. The perceptions of 'who is vulnerable and why' are influenced by local flood authorities and the flood group membership, which increases the importance attached to issues of representativeness and inclusion within the flood groups themselves. The flood groups are also influencing economic capital, albeit to a lesser extent, by increasing levels of social protection through fundraising and from working to ensure insurance coverage. However, the influence of flood group activities on reducing flood insurance premiums is still low due to doubts from insurers over flood group effectiveness in increasing flood resilience and reducing potential flood losses.

Conclusions

This chapter focused on the influence and potential role of civil society, through flood groups, on community resilience to flooding in England. While flood groups in England are increasing in number and carrying out a diverse range of activities, there is limited research available on the nature of such flood groups and their potential influence on community resilience to flooding. The goal of this research was to provide a working definition for flood groups, introduce their governance arrangements and explore the ways the groups might influence community resilience to flooding. A survey with 40 flood groups and semi-structured interviews with national actors and six selected flood groups provided a basis for reaching these goals.

The flood groups interviewed were all formed in response to a flood event and were predominantly made up of members of the public living in the affected areas with an interest in flooding but without a paid position with a formal flood actor. The flood groups were found to actively interact with other formal flood risk management actors. This chapter discussed the role of these flood groups on community resilience to flooding via their influence on: the community's social connectedness (social capital), the spatial planning and physical characteristics in the community (natural/built environment capital), the capabilities of individuals (human capital), the economic resources available in communities (economic capital).

The flood groups interviewed were predominantly contributing to expanding community's social capital and connections with institutions as well as supporting vulnerable individuals and raising flood risk awareness (human capital). The research suggests a focus on knowledge exchange by the flood groups interviewed. Their influence on natural/built environment capitals was restricted to smaller, less resource-intensive activities, which were strongly dependent on the local context and limited by resource availability. More extensive flood resilience activities such as greening of urban areas or advancing water-sensitive urban design were relatively ignored by the flood groups interviewed and surveyed. However, some more strategic activities such as the development of temporary water storage areas and contributing to long-term strategic plans were undertaken by some flood groups. The influence of the flood groups on economic resilience was limited to fundraising and supporting citizens in gaining flood insurance.

When discussing the contribution of flood groups to community resilience to flooding, the findings of this research highlight that it is important to be critical towards the extent to which a community can be fully represented by community groups (Coates, 2015; Wilson 2012). Flood groups were indeed found to not always represent the full community they intended to represent. Some of the flood groups interviewed included mainly older individuals and retirees, partly due to the voluntary nature of the groups. Community members without the time to volunteer or individuals with different perspectives were excluded. However, some flood groups seemed to be aware of these issues and some were attempting to ensure broader representation and maximising representativeness.

The increasing importance of the concept of resilience in flood risk management alongside the increasing emphasis on self-reliance of communities, via flood groups among other things, in government policies raises questions about whether the state is retreating from its existing responsibilities and reallocating accountability (Davoudi, 2012; Geaves and Penning-Rowsell, 2015). This research found indications of local government retreating (e.g. in relying on voluntary flood groups to maintain local watercourses), but also of the local state going beyond their assigned duties (e.g. by providing additional time and expertise to support the flood groups).

To conclude, this chapter has found that there is value in being receptive to flood groups within the local flood risk management landscape. The following summarises the ways that flood groups were successful in adding value to the local flood actors, the community itself and the individuals within the community: Firstly, they acted as an important local knowledge resource and provided information that local flood actors would not have otherwise been able to access. Secondly, they allowed the community to have a role in the prioritisation and decision-making processes relating to local flood risk management activities. Thirdly, the flood groups played an important role in activating local individuals and creating active flood risk managers, either by being members of or interacting with the flood groups. Fourthly, their existence also acts as an informal reminder of current local flood risk. This influence on flood risk awareness could be especially useful for countries with high flood risk but relatively low public flood risk awareness, such as in the Netherlands. These four ways in which the flood groups added value can also be useful to other countries that are exploring approaches to increase citizen involvement in local flood risk management to support the transition from technocratic, top-down governance approaches to more bottom-up, citizen supported approaches to flood resilience.

Acknowledgements

We would like to thank the members of Hebden Bridge Flood Action Group, Mytholmroyd Flood Group, Garforth Flood Support Group, Bodenham Flood Protection Group, Todmorden Flood Group, and Much Wenlock Flood Action Group for sharing their experiences with us. We would also like to thank interviewees from Defra, the Environment Agency, the Association of Drainage Authorities, and the National Flood Forum for allowing us to interview them. Additional thanks go to the NFF for allowing us access to their data on flood groups and for distributing our online survey through their networks. We would also like to thank Hannah Tankard, Tarandeep Jagdev, dr. Katya Brooks and the two anonymous reviewers for their feedback on earlier versions.

References

Alfieri, L., Burek, P., Feyen, L. & Forzieri, G. (2015) Global warming increases the frequencies of river floods in Europe. *Hydrology and Earth System Sciences Discussions*, 12, 1119–1152.

Andrew, R. (2012) Building community resilience. *Proceedings of the Institution of Civil Engineers*, 165(6), 59–64.

Botzen, W.J.W. & van den Bergh, J.C.J.M. (2008) Insurance against climate change and flooding in the Netherlands: Present, future, and comparison with other countries. *Risk Analysis*, 28(2), 413–426.

Coates, T. (2015) Understanding local community construction through flooding: The conscious community' and the possibilities for locally based communal action. *Geography and Environment*, 2(1), 55–68.

Cutter, S.L., Barnes, L., Berry, M., Burton, C., Evans, E., Tate, E. & Webb, J., (2008) A place-based model for understanding community resilience to natural disasters. *Global Environmental Change*, 18, 598–606.

Cutter, S., Burton, C.G. & Emrich, C.T. (2010) Disaster resilience indicators for benchmarking baseline conditions. *Journal of Homeland Security and Emergency Management*, 7(1), 1–15.

Davoudi, S. (2012) Resilience: A bridging concept or a dead end? *Planning Theory & Practice*, 13(2), 299–307.

DEFRA (2004) *Making space for water-developing a new government strategy for flood and coastal erosion risk management in England (Consultation Document)*. London: UK Department for Environment, Food and Rural Affairs.

DEFRA (2005) *Making space for water-taking forward a new government strategy for flood and coastal erosion risk management in England (Government response March 2005)*. London: UK Department for Environment, Food and Rural Affairs.

EA (2009) *Flooding in England: A National Assessment of Flood Risk*. Bristol: Environment Agency.

EA and Defra (2011) The national flood and coastal erosion risk management strategy for England www.gov.uk/government/uploads/system/uploads/attachment_data/file/228898/9780108510366.pdf (Date Accessed: 1st November 2015).

Edwards, D., O'Brien, L., Ambrose-Oji, B. & Morris, J. (2015) *Issues and options concerning FCRM volunteering (Report – SC120013/R4)*. Bristol: Environment Agency.

EEA (2012) *Climate change, impacts and vulnerability in Europe 2012 (EEA Report No 12/2012)*. Copenhagen: European Environment Agency.

Fainstein, S. (2015) Resilience and justice. *International Journal of Urban and Regional Research*, 39, 157–167.

Forrest, S., Orr, P., Twigger-Ross, C. & Brooks, K. (2014). Translating Resilience from Theory to Practice. *Paper presented at 2nd International Conference on Urban Sustainability and Resilience*, London. November 2014.

Geaves, L.H. & Penning-Rowsell, E.C. (2015) 'Contractual' and 'cooperative' civic engagement: The emergence and roles of 'flood action groups' in England and Wales. *AMBIO 2015*, 44, 440–451.

Guha-Sapir, D., Below, R. & Hoyois, Ph. (2015) EM-DAT: International Disaster Database – www.emdat.be – Université Catholique de Louvain – Brussels – Belgium. Search Terms: "Continent-Europe"; Year – "from 2000 until 2014"; Disaster classification – "Natural" > "Hydrological" > "Coastal Flood", "Flash Flood", "Riverine Flood". Search conducted on 16 February 15.

Harries, T. (2009) *Review of the Pilot Flood Protection Grant Scheme in a Recently Flooded Area*. London: Department for Environment, Food and Rural Affairs.

House of Commons (2015) *Defra Performance in 2013–14: Eighth Report of Session 2014–15 (House of Commons Environment, Food and Rural Affairs Committee)*. London: The Stationery Office Limited.

Johnson, C. & Priest, S.J. (2008) Flood risk management in England: A changing landscape of risk responsibility? *International Journal of Water Resources Development*, 24(4), 513–525.

Lamond, J.E., Proverbs, D.G. & Hammond, F.N. (2009) Accessibility of flood risk insurance in the UK: confusion, competition and complacency. *Journal of Risk Research*, 12(6), 825–841.

Local Government Association (2012) Managing flood risk: Roles and responsibilities. http://www.local.gov.uk/topics/civil-emergencies/flooding/local-flood-risk-management/managing-flood-risk-roles-and (Date Accessed: 22nd May 2017).

Kuhlicke, C. & Steinführer, A. (2013) Searching for resilience or building social capacities for flood risks? *Planning Theory & Practice*, 14(1), 114–120.

Masterson, J.H., Peacock, W.G., Van Zandt, S.S., Grover, H., Schwarz, L.F. & Cooper Jr, J.T. (2014) *Planning for Community Resilience: A Handbook for Reducing Vulnerability to Disasters*. Washington, DC: Island Press.

McCarthy, S. & Tunstall, S. (2008) *Risk Communication: Inter-Professional Flood Risk Management*. London: Flood Hazard Research Centre, Middlesex University.

Meijerink, S. & Dicke, W. (2008) Shifts in the public-private divide in flood management. *Water Resources Development*, 24(4), 499–512.

Neill, J.O. & Neill, M.O. (2012). *Social Justice and the Future of Flood Insurance*. York: The Joseph Rowntree Foundation.

NFF internal database (2015) A database containing flood group names and locations in England. Personal communication with the National Flood Forum. Unpublished document, available upon request.

Norris, F.H., Stevens, S.P, Pfefferbaum, B., Wyche, K.F. & Pfefferbaum, R.L. (2008) Community resilience as a metaphor, theory, set of capacities, and strategy for disaster readiness. *American Journal of Community Psychology*, 41(1–2), 127–150.

O'Brien, L., Ambrose-Oji, B., Morris, J., Edwards, D. & Williams, R. (2014) Volunteers' contribution to flood resilience. *Research Report by Forest Research*. UK: Environment Agency.

Parker, D.J. & Handmer J.W. (1998) The role of unofficial flood warning systems. *Journal of Contingencies and Crisis Management*, 6(1), 45–60.

Pitt, M. (2008) *Learning Lessons from the 2007 Floods, an Independent Review by Sir Michael Pitt*. London: Cabinet Office.

Porter, L. & Davoudi, S. (2012) The politics of resilience for planning: A cautionary note. *Planning Theory & Practice*, 13(2), 329–333.

Priestley, S. & Allen, G. (2016) Flood risk management and funding. *House of Commons Library, Briefing Paper, Number CBP07514, 31st March 2016*. http://researchbriefings.parliament.uk/ResearchBriefing/Summary/CBP-7514 (Date Accessed: 9th May 2016).

Restemeyer, B., Woltjer, J. & van den Brink, M. (2015) A strategy-based framework for assessing the flood resilience of cities – the Hamburg case study. *Planning Theory & Practice*, 16(1), 45–62.

Salemink, K. & Strijker, D. (2015) Breedbandcoöperaties op het platteland: Leerscholen voor Next Generation Plattelandsontwikkeling. *Bestuurskunde*, 24(2), 40–50.

Schelfaut, K., Pannemans, B., van der Craats, I., Krywkow, J., Mysiak, J. & Cools, J. (2011) Bringing flood resilience into practice: The FREEMAN project. *Environmental Science & Policy*, 14(7), 825–833.

Scott (2013) Living with flood risk. *Planning Theory & Practice*, 14(1), 103–106.

Scott Wilson Kirkpatrick and Co Ltd, Risk and Policy Analysts Ltd, Jones, P. & Sheate, W. (2003) *Community and Public Participation: Risk Communication and Improving Decision-Making in Flood and Coastal Defence*. London: Defra.

Tapsell, S.M. & Tunstall, S.M. (2008) "I wish I'd never heard of Banbury": The relationship between 'place' and the health impacts from flooding. *Health & Place*, 14, 133–154.

Terluin, I.J. (2003) Differences in economic development in rural regions of advanced countries: An overview and critical analysis of theories. *Journal of Rural Studies*, 19(3), 327–344.

Thaler. T. & Priest, S. (2014) Partnership funding in flood risk management: New localism debate and policy in England. *Area*, 46(4), 418–425.

Thorne, C. (2014) Geographies of UK flooding in 2013/14. *The Geographic Journal*, 180(4), 297–309.

Tierney, K. (2014) *The Social Roots of Risk: Producing Disasters, Promoting Resilience*. Stanford, CA: Stanford University Press.

Twigger-Ross, C., Coates, T., Deeming, H., Orr, P., Ramsden, M., & Stafford, J. (2011) Community resilience research: Evidence review. *Report to the Cabinet Office and Defence Science and Technology Laboratory*. London: Collingwood Environmental Planning.

Twigger-Ross, C., Kashefi, E., Weldon, S., Brooks, K., Deeming, H., Forrest, S., Fielding, J., Gomersall, A., Harries, T., McCarthy, S., Orr, P., Parker, D. & Tapsell, S. (2014) *Flood Resilience Community Pathfinder Evaluation: Rapid Evidence Assessment*. London: Defra.

UK Government (2010) Flood and Water Management Act 2010. www.legislation.gov.uk/ukpga/2010/29/pdfs/ukpga_20100029_en.pdf (Date Accessed: 9th May 2016).

UK NEA (2014) UK National Ecosystem Assessment: The UK National Ecosystem Assessment: Synthesis of the Key Findings. UNEP-WCMC, LWEC, UK. Oxford: Information Press.

Van der Vaart, G., Trell, E.M., Restemeyer, B. & Bakema, M.M. (2015) Resilience: Just do it?! Governing for resilience in vulnerable places, University of Groningen, 9–10 October 2014. *Resilience: International Policies, Practices and Discourses*, 3(2), 160–171.

Waylen, K., Aaltonen, J., Bonaiuto, M., Booth, P., Bradford, R., Carrus, G., Cuthbert, A., Langan, S., O'Sullivan, J., Rotko, P., Twigger-Ross, C. & Watson, D. (2011) *CRUE Final Report: URFlood – Understanding Uncertainty and Risk in Communicating about Floods*, p. 109. www.crue-eranet.net/Calls/URFlood_frp.pdf (Date Accessed: 9th May 2016).

White, I. (2013) The more we know, the more we know we don't know: Reflections on a decade of planning, flood risk management and false precision. *Planning Theory & Practice*, 14(1), 106–114.

Wilson, G.A. (2012) Community resilience, globalization, and transitional pathways of decision-making. *Geoforum*, 43, 1218–1231.

8 Meta-decision-making and the speed and quality of disaster resilience and recovery

Stephen Platt

Introduction

Recovering from a disaster involves different decisions as disaster managers and long-term planners respond to the myriad of cascading problems. What is unique in post-disaster situations is that decisions must be made in a compressed period. Communities must rebuild as quickly as possible to maintain existing social networks and get the economy back on their feet. But they must also be deliberate in trying to maximize the opportunities disasters provide for improvement (Olshansky and Johnson 2010). Disaster decision-making is typically posed as a series of dilemmas, for example: balancing short term and long term needs (Ingram et al. 2006), speed or deliberation (Olshansky 2006) or focusing on restoration or reform (Davis 2006). This chapter envisages these dilemmas as meta-decisions. It defines meta decisions as trade-offs between opposing strategies that need to be made by the authorities in charge of managing recovery. It tests the idea that meta decision-making is a factor in the speed and quality of post-event recovery and contributes to the future resilience of vulnerable places.

The chapter begins by defining resilience, recovery and meta decisions and describing how these terms are used in relation to disasters. It uses comparative data collected by the author from fieldwork after ten major disasters to analyse the meta decisions taken. Finally, it assesses the speed and quality of recovery after each event and relates this to meta decision-making. The aim of studying recovery in this comparative way is to try to identify the underlying causes of speedier and higher quality recovery. The author argues that better (meta) decision-making will result in faster and better quality recovery, which also potentially leads to more disaster resilient places. A key aspect of better decision making, this chapter argues, is that meta decisions are thought through and made before the disaster event. The precise questions the chapter seeks to answer are therefore: (1) Do countries that make meta decisions quickly recover faster? (2) Do countries that achieve a balance of meta decisions build back better?

Resilience and recovery

The word resilience derives from the Latin word *resiliēns* meaning to rebound. In engineering, resilience is defined as a measure of how easily a material returns to its original shape after elastic deformation (Hollnagel et al. 2006; Oxford Dictionary of Construction, Surveying and Civil Engineering 2013). In ecology Holling (1973) and Perrings (2001) defined resilience as the capacity to absorb shock and linked resilience to the idea of systemic stability. In social science, resilience is considered as the complex web of social interactions, characteristics and capacities that enable a community to live with the hazards they face (Porter and Davoudi, 2012). Keck and Sakdapolrak (2013) argue that social resilience consists of three dimensions: coping capacities, adaptive capacities and transformative capacities.

All the above qualities are relevant for places affected by disasters. It is therefore not surprising that the concept of resilience has been used extensively in disaster research (Tierney 1997; Petak 2002; Bruneau et al. 2003). Zhou et al. (2010) define disaster resilience as the capacity to resist loss during disaster and to recover after disaster in a specific area in a given period. Resilience can, therefore, be conceived as both the loss potential and the biophysical/social response. Zolli and Healy (2012, p. 7) define resilience as "the critical ability to anticipate change, heal when damaged, to reorganize ... to maintain core purpose, even under radically changed circumstances".

In the context of disasters, resilience encompasses a society's capacity to bounce back after a disaster, its level of preparedness to confront or deal with a disaster and its ability to recover quickly and successfully (Alexander 2013). The UNISDR (2004, p. 16) in their Global Review of disaster risk reduction define resilience as "the capacity of a system, community or society exposed to hazards to resist, absorb, accommodate to and recover from the effects of a hazard in a timely and efficient manner, including through the preservation and restoration of its essential basic structures and functions".

Societal resilience, the level of preparedness and rapid and successful recovery depend, to a large extent, on good decisions (Coles and Zhuang 2011). This chapter explores what effect, if any, meta decision-making had on earthquake resilience and recovery in ten major disasters. Rose (2004) defines economic resilience as the inherent and adaptive responses to hazards that enable individuals and communities to avoid potential losses. He distinguishes between *static economic resilience* (the ability of a system to maintain function when shocked), and *dynamic economic resilience* (the speed at which an entity or system recovers from a severe shock to achieve the desired state).

Bruneau et al. (2003) define seismic resilience as the ability of a system to reduce the chances of a shock, to absorb such a shock if it occurs and to recover quickly after a shock. They argue that a resilient system is one that shows reduced failure probabilities, reduced consequences from failures, in terms of lives lost, damage, and negative economic and social consequences, and reduced time to recovery (restoration of a specific system or set of systems to their "normal" level of functional performance). Bruneau et al. (2003) define community resilience as the ability of families, organizations and communities to meet hazards, contain the effects of disasters when they occur, and carry out recovery activities in ways that minimize social disruption and mitigate the effects of further earthquakes.

Resilience is, therefore, a multi-dimentional concept encompassing social, economic, physical, technological and natural dimensions. A paper by Tierney and Bruneau (2007) used resilience to measure disaster loss reduction and Chang (2009) made an important advance in elaborating a conceptual resilience framework for physical, financial, human and natural capital.

Recovery is a complex process that starts immediately after a disaster. Recovery is defined in this chapter as "the act or process of returning to a normal state after a period of difficulty" (Merriam-Webster). Most (lay) people think about disaster recovery as a return to normality although this raises the question of what is "normal". The "normal" may not be a return to the status before the event; in fact, this may be undesirable. Quarantelli (1999) suggests that the word recovery implies an attempt to bring the post-disaster situation to some level of acceptability. Bruneau et al. (2003) include restoration of the system to its normal level of performance in their definition of recovery.

Recovery overlaps with the period of immediate response and relief, which depending on the nature of aftershocks and cascading crises, may last from a month to more than six months. It also merges into the long-term development processes that may even be accelerated by the disaster. The UN Office for Disaster Risk Reduction (UNISDR 2015, p. 25) defines disaster recovery as "decisions and actions aimed at restoring or improving livelihoods, health, as well as economic, physical, social, cultural and environmental assets, systems and activities, of a disaster-affected community or society, aligning with the principles of sustainable development, including build back better to avoid or reduce future disaster risk". The Cluster Working Group on Early Recovery (CWGER) of the UN Development Program in their Guidance note on early recovery define the aim of disaster recovery as restoring the capacity of national institutions and communities to recover from a disaster and to "build back better" (UNDP 2008, p. 9).

Kates (1977) addresses the question of the pace of recovery and argues that it is principally related to the magnitude of the damage. However, the resources available for recovery, the prevailing pre-disaster economic and demographic trends and factors such as the quality of leadership, planning and organization, are also important and exceptional performance can reduce recovery time by as much as half (Kates and Pijawka 1977).

Researchers at the University of Buffalo (MCEER 2006) showed how disaster recovery typically follows an s-shaped curve and developed the idea of the "resilience triangle" (Tierney and Bruneau, 2007). Resilience-enhancing measures aim to reduce the size of this triangle by making the society more robust i.e. resistant to the impact of the disaster, and by reducing the time to recover. Chang and Shinozuka (2004) suggest that it is useful to consider robustness and rapidity as distinct ends of resilience-enhancing measures. Chang (2010) went on to apply a framework to measure urban disaster recovery from the 1995 Kobe earthquake.

Figure 8.1 shows a theoretical cumulative frequency graph of one indicator of recovery – Regional GDP. Immediately after a catastrophic event, there is a decline in GDP as local businesses are unable to maintain output. The survival rate, the proportion 'undamaged' and functioning, in this case GDP, is a measure of robustness. In the green scenario, there is a 30% drop in GDP i.e. Robustness R1 is equal to 70%. In the red scenario, there is a 50% drop in GDP i.e. a Robustness level of 50%. Slowly the local economy recovers, perhaps in steps, until the curve flattens and stability returns. Recovery takes five years in the green scenario and twice as long in the red. If GDP remained constant the loss in Regional GDP over ten years would be approximately 7.5% in the green scenario and three times higher at 25% in the red scenario. Resilience in Regional GDP is therefore 92.5% the pre-disaster in the green scenario and 75% in the red.

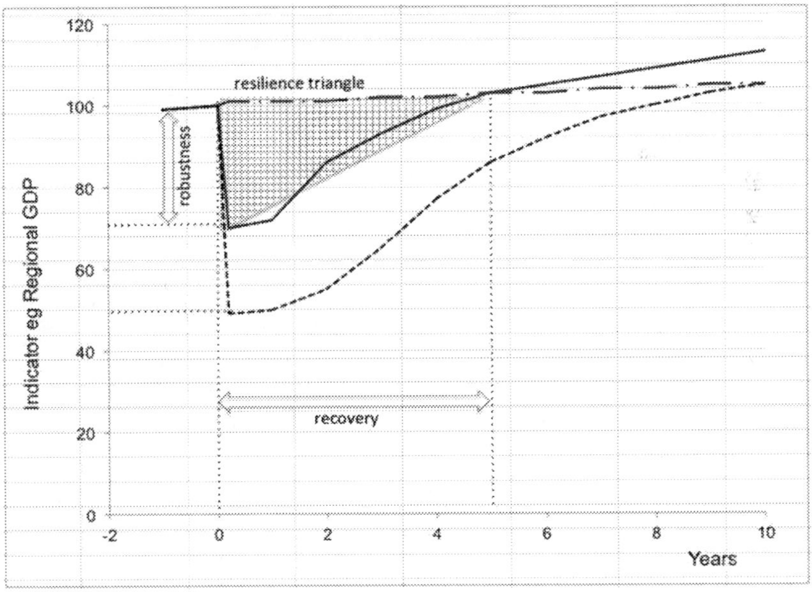

Figure 8.1 Recovery curves: solid line is more 'resilient' than dotted line because recovery wastwice as fast; R1 is more 'robust' than R2 because the loss was 20% less.

Source: Platt et al. (2016).

Meta-decisions

Understanding resilience is important because it helps guide post-disaster decision-making (Tierney 1997; Webb et al. 2000; Rose and Liao 2004). Kottemann (1986) suggests that three different types of disaster decision-making can be distinguished: problem recognition, meta-decision making and primary decision-making. Meta-decision making is the process of deciding how to make decisions i.e. establishing the high-level criteria under which alternative courses of action are taken, for example vesting responsibility for disaster recovery in existing ministries or in a new special authority (Boureau et al. 2015). Meta-decisions are relevant to disaster recovery planning when people are faced by cascading crises and need to think calmly and strategically because they establish a framework for subsequent operational decision-making and because they can save time and mental anguish by eliminating whole areas of indecision (Platt 2015). The importance of meta decisions in strategic thinking has been recognised for at least twenty years (Singer 1996). They are usually the responsibility of the Office of President, Prime Minister or the Cabinet and are generally taken by high-ranking politicians and senior civil servants, and typically made in response to media pressure and reports of failure to take effective action (Davis 2006).

Davis (2014) defined six issues he called disaster decision "dilemmas" (Figure 8.2). A dilemma is defined as a difficult choice between two or more alternatives, especially ones that are equally undesirable (Oxford Dictionaries 2016). The choices Davis (2014) outlined, however, are not necessarily mutually exclusive; a country can opt for a mix of strategies, and in this sense, they are not true dilemmas. In disaster recovery, an optimum or desirable solution might be a balance or mix of alternative approaches. These meta-decisions are akin to a balancing act in which policy makers should weigh trade-offs between contradictory approaches or strategies. For example, in Chile in the coastal settlements devastated by the 2010 Maule earthquake, critical facilities were relocated to higher ground whilst housing and commerce, apart from buildings right next to the coast, were rebuilt on the same sites, albeit in more tsunami proof ways. This planning strategy aimed to increase resilience by achieving a balance between increased safety on the one hand and business continuity and economic recovery on the other.

Figure 8.2 compares the six dilemmas identified by Davis (2014) with the six suggested meta-decisions. Five of them coincide. The dilemma Davis poses of whether resources should go to short-term relief or long-term recovery was omitted since spending on immediate relief is quite separate to recovery and long-term development and no government in the case study countries confounded the two decisions. Governance, whether decision-making should be top down or bottom up, was not considered by Davis but was found to be important in recovery decision-making.

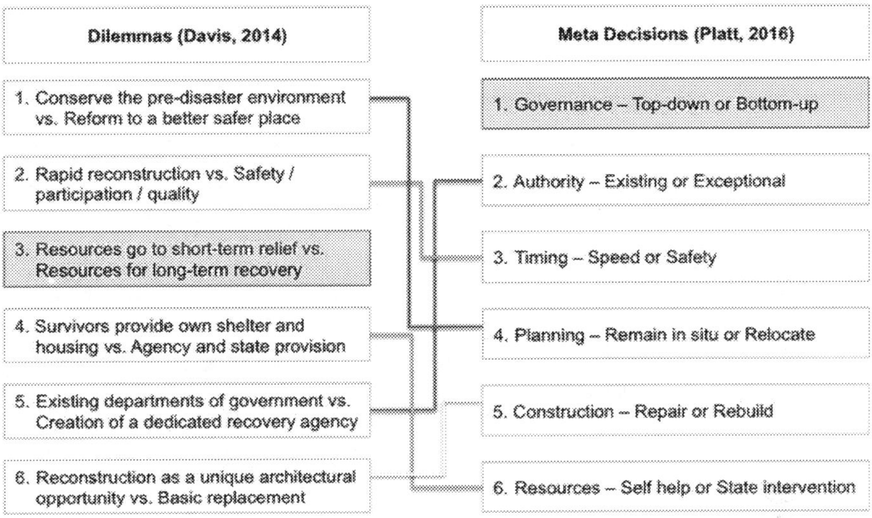

Figure 8.2 Comparison of dilemmas and meta decisions.
Source: Author.

Methodology

The author has studied recovery in ten places affected by earthquakes (see Table 8.1). Insights from these case studies are used to illustrate the relevance of meta decisions for resilience and recovery.

Table 8.1 provides a comparison of the scale of the disaster in different countries. For clarity, this chapter focuses on case studies of six of the most recent of these major earthquakes and tsunami, highlighted above. One can see immediately what a huge disaster the Tohoku earthquake was in Japan both in terms of fatalities and economic loss. Size is measured by the formula: Size = deaths * loss/gdp. (Dacy and Kunreuther 1969; Padli et al. 2010; Barton and Nishenko 2015).

Data collection

Three types of data collection methods were used in a complementary way to provide both quantifiable and qualitative data and to improve the reliability of the evidence. The methodology of measuring recovery and resilience is reported in more detail in Platt et al (2016).

1 *Remote sensing:* Manual and semi-automatic analysis of satellite imagery were used to provide an accurate quantifiable measure of recovery of relatively small sample areas in Pakistan, Thailand, China, and Turkey. Twelve indices of recovery were identified covering transport,

Table 8.1 Data from 10 major earthquakes

Country	*Name*	*Year*	*Date*	*Mw*	*Displaced*	*Deaths*	*Loss US$ bn*	*Size*
USA	Northridge	1994	Jan-17	6.7	125,000	61	44	0.1
Iran	Bam	2003	Dec-26	6.6	75,000	26,271	1.5	82
Thailand	Indian Ocean	2004	Dec-26	9.2	1,690,000	276,025	14	3,979
Pakistan	Kashmir	2005	Oct-08	7.6	3,500,000	100,000	2.3	1,313
China	Wenchuan	2008	May-12	8.0	1,940,000	90,000	75	1,393
Italy	L'Aquila	2009	Apr-06	5.8	67,000	309	16	0.7
Chile	Maule	2010	Feb-27	8.8	800,000	550	30	45
New Zealand	Christchurch	2011	Feb-22	6.3	25,000	185	16	39
Japan	Tohoku	2011	Mar-11	9.0	130,927	18,499	235	5,502
Turkey	Van	2011	Oct-23	7.1	50,000	604	1	0.4

Source: Platt (2015).

housing, shelter, services, environment and livelihoods (Platt et al. 2016). However, the satellite imagery analysis was partial. The analysis covered only part of the affected area for specific snapshots over the first two years of recovery.

2 *Interviews:* Semi-structured interviews and focus groups were conducted with decision-makers, planners, stakeholders and residents. Typically, thirty-key informants were interviewed in each location and about half of them attended a focus group workshop to explore issues in greater detail. Their perceptions and opinions formed the basis of the meta-decision analysis reported below. No specialised software was used but interview quotes were coded into a thematic framework using a standard ethnographic procedure.
3 *Surveys*: Household surveys of a small sample of residents were used in six of the ten disaster locations (Chile, Japan, New Zealand, Pakistan, Thailand and Turkey) to collect data about the timing and quality of recovery plus many other qualitative aspects of the process. Household surveys of fifty households chosen randomly were used to collect data about the timing of recovery. People were asked by what percentage different aspects of society (access, debris clearance, environmental recovery, schooling, healthcare, mains water and livelihoods) had recovered at given intervals after the disaster. Other resilience factors such as governance, leadership, planning, science and construction were derived in part from published sources and in part from the interviews.
4 *Analysis of published material:* As much use as possible was made of reports, statistical data and documents produced by government departments and international agencies. This helped provide base-line data on population, housing and economic activities and was used to validate the extent and timing of various aspects of recovery, for example, school and health provision. There was, however, limited data about rehousing, business continuity, funding recovery and regional GDP was available for some of the case studies. Published sources also provided data about the impact of the disaster in terms of deaths, displaced persons and economic loss, and pre-disaster resilience attributes for example demography, economic product and socio-economic factors such as equity and education. It would have been most helpful to have obtained published data about the timing of recovery, for example about population movements, housing and the local economy, but it was extremely difficult to get any useful information.

Measuring the speed and quality of recovery

Speed of recovery was measured using key informant interviews in every case and satellite imagery analysis in Pakistan, Thailand, Turkey, Italy, China and New Zealand. The timings reported by key informants was compared to that from remote sensing and was found to correlate closely (Platt et al. 2016).

Ten indicators were used to calculate a single measure of the speed of recovery, "return to normality", based on the number of months taken to return and comply with all the conditions listed in Table 8.2.

Recovery quality was assessed using interviews data, field observations and published material. Seven indicators were used (see Table 8.2) to calculate a composite measure of quality of recovery based on the concept of "building back better" (Kim and Olshansky 2015). Each indicator was assessed in terms of whether the recovered state was worse, the same or better than the pre-disaster state and assigned a score (–1, 0, or 1). These scores were summed to give a single composite measure of the quality of recovery in each country.

This was a similar approach to that adopted by Burton (2012) in research that aimed at measuring the multi-dimensional nature of disaster resilience. He asked, "what set of indicators provide the best comparative assessment of disaster resilience and to what extent do these indicators predict ... disaster recovery" (Burton 2012, p. 3).

The balance of meta-decision making was measured using a five-point Likert scale in which the mid-point indicated a balance between the two alternatives, for example between top-down or bottom-up governance structures. This assessment was made principally based on the key informant interviews. It should be stressed that there is no 'right answer'. Higher scores are not better than lower scores and a balanced mix of strategies devised to suit particular circumstances may be the 'best' approach in terms of balancing speed and quality. Finally, a single measure of balance was calculated for each country summing the absolute deviations from the mid value of three using the formula:

$$\text{Balance} = \Sigma_{n}^{1} 12 - (\mathit{Abs\,score} - 3)$$

Table 8.2 Indicators of speed and quality of recovery

Speed indicators		*Quality indicators*	
Access	Fully restored		Worse (–1) same (0) better (1)
Debris	Completely cleared	Safety	–1, 0 or 1
Environment	≥90% restored	Amenity	–1, 0 or 1
Temporary housing	Completely cleared	Environment	–1, 0 or 1
Permanent housing	≥90% displaced rehoused	Infrastructure	–1, 0 or 1
Schooling	≥90% children in school	Housing	–1, 0 or 1
Local admin.	Fully functional	Urban design	–1, 0 or 1
Power	Fully restored	Local economy	–1, 0 or 1
Mains water	Fully restored		
Livelihoods	≥90% back in work		
Return to "normality" = time taken for all above conditions to be met		Recovery quality = sum of indicator scores	

Source: Author.

In the following sections evidence from the remote sensing, interviews, surveys and document analysis is used to illustrate aspects of the six meta-decisions. Of necessity, these examples are in no sense comprehensive but have been chosen to highlight different aspects of meta decision-making.

Governance – top-down or bottom-up

Governance is defined in this chapter as the extent to which control and decisions about recovery are "top-down" and centralised or "bottom-up" and delegated to regional and local authorities with a degree of community consultation and involvement. In five of the ten countries (China, Iran, Pakistan, Thailand and Turkey) there is a top-down governance structure. There are, however, differences of detail.

In Pakistan governance is conducted through military institutions and government departments. Turkey also has a centralised top-down structure with little tradition of community involvement. Van is in the far east, away from the centres of power in Ankara and Istanbul, and local involvement of stakeholders was hampered by political tensions of the Kurdish separatist movement. Decisions about reconstruction were taken by AFAD, the Prime Minister's Office for Disaster Management, and Toki, the Government Housing Agency. Interviews with personnel in AFAD revealed that geologists made planning decisions in Van on the basis of distance from a known fault and whether the land was government-owned; there was no public consultation (Platt and Durmaz Drinkwater 2016). Iran, Thailand and China have similar autocratic top-down governance structures.

In Italy, decision-making was initially top-down, but after the first phase there was a failure of governance and a lack of coordination between regional, provincial and municipal authorities. There was little genuine community involvement and consultation even by local architects, engineers or academics. Governance after the L'Aquila earthquake might be characterised by chaos and failure of government. The many people who spoke at the Forum organised by the OECD (OECD, 2012) and Groningen University (Brezzi and McCann 2012) on recovery in L'Aquila, attended by the author of this chapter, related how the national, regional, provincial and municipal authorities had failed to cooperate effectively, with each accusing the other of being the cause of delay. This judgement is supported by Alexander (2010) and Daziel (2012).

In contrast governance in the USA, Japan, New Zealand and Chile was more balanced with delegation of authority to regional and local government and with stakeholder involvement and community consultation. In Chile, the government appointed a national coordinator to develop a reconstruction plan. The plan was based on the premise that "*the State is unable to reconstruct everything or even control the process of recovery centrally from Santiago. With the support of the state, it is the responsibility of each region, town council and community to develop its own plans*" (MINVU 2010, p. 108; English translation MINVU 2013, p. 2). This meant that authority was delegated to the regional government. The distinctive aspect about recovery in Chile, however, was the quality of the participation process that involved the community in decision-making and kept them informed about progress (See Figure 8.3). The architects heading the three teams master planning recovery in the eighteen coastal settlements, visited their areas at least once a week, briefing resident's groups and business people and walking the streets to monitor progress and meet residents. Maps, sketches and plans were used throughout this process to communicate ideas and get feedback. The main objective was to get business up and running again. So, restaurants and fish processing plants operated in temporary structures while permanent accommodation was planned and built.

Similarly, in Japan after the Tohoku disaster in 2011, the central government took control providing the resources and setting the agenda and the regional and municipal authorities interpreted this policy and implemented plans. There is also a legal obligation in Japan to consult members of the community. But there are cultural differences between Chile and Japan that impacted the speed and quality of recovery. The political structure in Japan is more strongly centralized and the national government maintains a closer oversight over the prefectures, cities and other local government

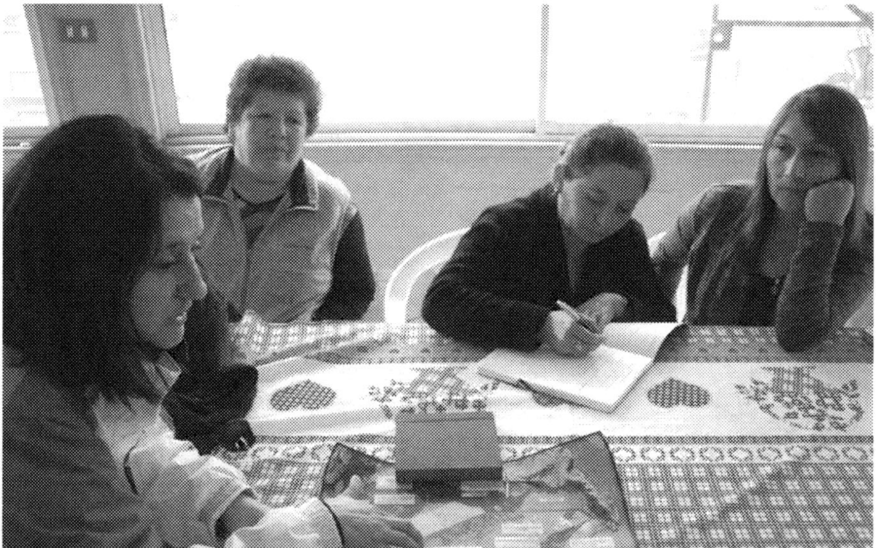

Figure 8.3 Architect Carolina Arriagada showing plans to the residents at a community association meeting in Tubul, Chile, 15 December 2011.

Source: Author.

institutions so there is much less delegation of decision-making (Sorensen 2004). Public consultation in Japan was, therefore, more formalised, less inclusive and gave priority to a smaller section of opinion. One of the interviewees Miura Tomayukin, a residents' association leader, claimed that elderly men dominated decision-making in Tohoku and tended to be conservative and safety conscious.

In New Zealand, the Canterbury Earthquake Authority (CERA) and Christchurch City Council (2011) made efforts to involve citizens in the debate about the future of the city. CERA conducted community workshops and public consultation on the Recovery Strategy for Greater Christchurch (CERA 2011). The City Council planning department's focus was on re-planning the central business district and it ran the *Share an Idea* campaign that involved residents through an interactive website and an exhibition attended by over 10,000 people (Carlton 2013). However, despite these initiatives more power lay with the Minister for Canterbury Earthquake Recovery and CERA than with the city council or local citizens and stakeholders.

Authority – existing or exceptional

There were considerable differences in who had responsibility and authority for decisions in each researched country. Authority is defined as whether existing ministries and local government are in charge or a dedicated body has been constituted and a minister or committee is in control. Typically, creation of a dedicated body may need special legislation. In six of the ten case studies (China, Iran, New Zealand, Pakistan, Thailand and Turkey) authority was vested in a special body.

The Government of Pakistan established the Earthquake Reconstruction and Rehabilitation Authority (ERRA) on October 24,2005, two weeks after the disaster, to control all aspects of relief and recovery. ERRA is a military-led organization comprising armed forces personnel, civil servants and technocrats. ERRA's mission is to "convert adversity into opportunity" by "building back better" (GFDRR 2014, p. 4). In coordinating the many organisations involved in relief and recovery ERRA adopted the UN cluster approach response that grouped humanitarian organisations into specific areas or 'clusters' of responsibility, for example, health and water/sanitation. This cluster approach was developed in 2005, after the Indian Ocean tsunami, when the UN under Secretary General for Humanitarian Affairs, Jan Egeland, commissioned a review of failure in the international response to humanitarian crisis (United Nations 2005). The early performance of clusters in Pakistan was uneven, responsibilities not clearly defined and some clusters struggled until government departments were involved, but it provided a framework for coordination in a chaotic operational environment (Hidalgo and López-Claros 2007).

In New Zealand initially, the local authorities, Christchurch City Council and Waimakakiri District Council, were in charge. The state of emergency was lifted two weeks after the September 2010 earthquake. The Christchurch Mayor said this represented *"a move closer to business as usual"* (BBC News 2010, p. 1). Damaged buildings were evacuated but the centre remained open (Platt 2012a). This changed after the second more devastating earthquake the following February 2011. Two weeks after the February quake the Government passed emergency legislation, the Canterbury Earthquake Recovery Act 2011, by order in Council. The act granted extraordinary powers to the Canterbury Earthquake Recovery Authority (CERA) as a department of government with Foreign Affairs Minister, Gerry Brownlee, to coordinate recovery and to make recommendations to Government. Instead of working to strengthen the City Council, CERA took over its core recovery functions and the City Council was, initially, side-lined. However, despite the tensions, CERA and the municipal authorities managed to cooperate. In January 2015 CERA was downgraded from a department to an agency within the Department of the Prime Minister. Over time the balance of power gradually reverted to the City Council.

After the disaster in Tohoku in 2011, the Japanese government immediately sought to broaden the recovery strategy by setting up an advisory council. Within two months the council issued 'seven principles for the reconstruction framework', that became the basis for the government guidelines that were decided by the National Policy Unit three months after the disaster (Government of Japan 2012). The new governmental Reconstruction Agency, reporting to the Cabinet, was established in February 2012. Its aim was to plan and coordinate all national reconstruction policies and measures and to support the efforts of afflicted local governments by serving as a 'one-stop shop'. The role of the central government was, therefore, to provide guidelines for reconstruction and support in terms of finance, human resources and know-how, but the main administrative actors were the municipalities.

In Chile, the central government recognised it would be unable to reconstruct everything or even control the process and national coordination was limited to defining the scale of the problem and allocating resources. Planning and implementation were the responsibility of regional government and specialist teams of experts. What distinguished recovery in Chile was the community consultation and the desire from the bottom up to rebuild as quickly as possible but also to build back better.

Timing – speed or safety

Decisions about whether the emphasis should be on rapid reconstruction or on increased safety and "building back better" are perhaps the most critical of post-disaster meta-decisions (Kim and Olshansky 2015). The key question facing the authorities is whether they should aim to reinstate livelihoods and rebuild homes as quickly as possible or is the crisis an opportunity to change – to increase safety, to strengthen the economy and to improve the urban environment. Speed of reconstruction was exceptionally fast in two of the studied countries, China and Turkey, where a large proportion of displaced families were rehoused within two years (Miao 2010; Dunford and Li 2011).

In Italy, after the L'Aquila earthquake in 2009, the main issue was the slow recovery of the local economy. Most of the historic buildings were safeguarded with an exoskeleton of scaffolding however it may take years to repair them (see Figure 8.4).

Meanwhile, much of the city centre of L'Aquila was closed and the University, the main economic driver in the region, was operating in temporary rented accommodation. Local architects and engineers devised a master plan for the city. But Central Government rehousing projects were poorly planned, the Regional, Provincial and Municipal authorities refused to collaborate and reconstruction and economic regeneration stalled. The priorities of residents were: repair and reconstruction of their homes, reconstruction of the historic centre and re-establishing employment (OECD 2012), but the centre of L'Aquila city is still not repaired or rebuilt, although the process of rebuilding had begun by 2012 on the outskirts of the town (EEFIT 2013). Instead of repairing existing homes the

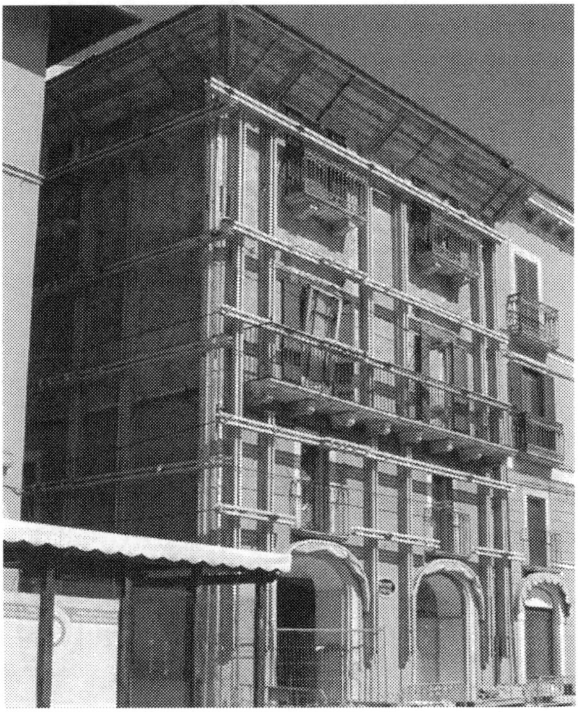

Figure 8.4 Protecting cultural heritage in L'Aquila.
Source: Author.

government built 12,000 new homes in 19 new settlements 15 kilometres from the old city centre (Alexander 2010). These were built in only eight-months and the idea was that they would have a transitional use and as soon as the reconstruction was complete, they would be used as university accommodation.

Chile achieved a better balance of speed and deliberation. There was intense pressure from the residents to rebuild homes, restore facilities and get the economy moving (Comerio 2013). But there was also a desire on the part of the authorities to develop new urban plans that would improve these communities and make them safer. Master Planning of the 18 coastal settlements affected by the disaster was completed within ten months by a team of architects and planners seconded from the University of Bio-Bio. The main thrust of these master plans was to restart business, rehouse residents and to improve safety. This involved relocating critical facilities such as the fire station and moving buildings back from the beach. The sea defences included a setback for buildings of 50–80 metres, a 20–30 meters band of trees and a promenade forming a sea wall. The teams also produced designs for tsunami resistant housing. The houses have a reinforced concrete ground floors and timber-frame second-storey. These were nearing completion when the author visited the area 18 months after the disaster (Platt 2012b).

Japan was traumatised by the unanticipated scale of the 2011 Tohoku earthquake and tsunami. The Japanese government's top priorities were also economic revival and safety. In contrast to Chile, however, these two aims seemed to be at odds and were causing delay in rehousing people and revitalising business. The safety imperative in Japan meant that ways of life and people's relationship to the sea had to change and this was painful and caused dissent. For tsunami protection, up to nine-metres-high levees are being built (see Figure 8.5). Homes were moved to higher ground along the fiord-like Rias Coast and on the Sendai Plain, where there are no natural hills, housing was concentrated on raised platforms (Platt 2013). By law the authorities have to consult people and it is in the nature of Japanese society to try to reach consensus rationally (Heath 1995; Kopp 2012). This takes time, which undermined the possibility of recovery in places that were already in economic and demographic decline.

In Turkey the imperative was speed, particularly to rehouse people in permanent housing. In the days immediately after the earthquake 300,000 people were housed in temporary shelter, mainly tents, and 200,000 out of a population of about one-million left Van and Ergis to stay with relatives (Basburg et al. 2015). Transitional shelter in containers was provided within three months. A total of 35 camps comprising 30,000 containers and 175,000 inhabitants were established in Van and Ergis (Erdik et al. 2012). The 21-metre^2 temporary container houses were smaller than those provided in Japan and housed much bigger families, but people didn't have to stay in them nearly as long as people did in

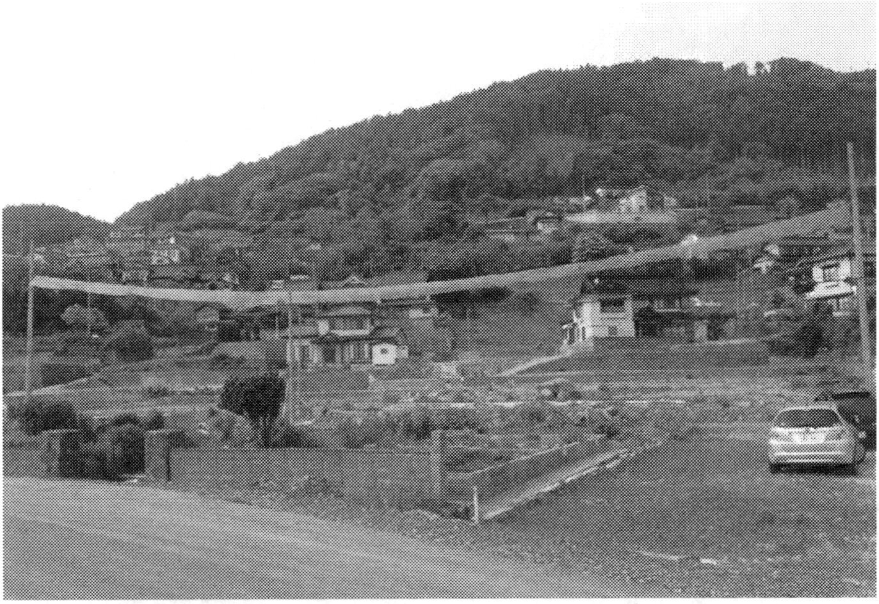

Figure 8.5 Shibitachi, near Kesannuma, Japan 5 June 2013 (The banner indicates the height of the proposed sea wall).
Source: Author.

Japan. The author visited Van ten-months after the earthquake and all the tents had been replaced with containers and the temporary camps were full. They were well policed and contained shops, schools and play facilities. The author visited again 18-months after the disaster and the camps were nearly all empty. Within 15-months, the Ministry Housing Development (TOKI) had built 10,000 dwellings in Van, and 5,000 in Erçis. This rate of reconstruction is unprecedented (Platt and So 2016). The new TOKI housing (Figure 8.6) is more earthquake-proof than previous homes and new hospitals, schools and government buildings were built to code. This was part of a nation-wide policy known as 'urban transformation' aimed at upgrading construction after the 1999 İzmit earthquake (Elincin 2014). All buildings must be inspected before they can be repaired and, in theory, dangerous buildings that cannot be repaired will be demolished.

However, despite aiming to rebuild a better Van, it was almost impossible for the urban planners to produce plans to improve the city centres of Van or Erciş. Senior planners in the Ministry of Environment and Urban Planning in Ankara responsible for planning Van said in an interview that it is difficult to 'expropriate' private land in Turkey and owners don't want to give up land for parks or public space.

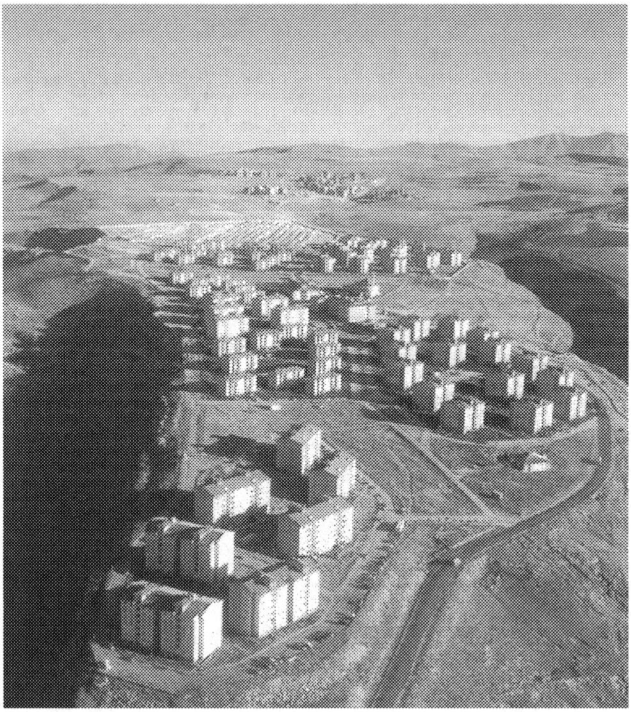

Figure 8.6 New Toki housing in Van, Turkey.
Source: Author.

Planning – remain in situ or relocate

An aspect of the wider question about speed and safety is whether homes and activities should be reconstructed in the same place or relocated to safer areas. Relocation is generally considered as a last resort because of land ownership issues and public opposition (Gonzalez Muzzio 2012). Although the policy decision to relocate is taken at high levels, detailed implementation involves local land-use planning decisions about which built-up land should be abandoned and new green-field or agricultural land be taken into use.

In Christchurch, in neighbourhoods bordering the lower River Avon and along the River Waimakariri in Kaiapoi to the north, there was widespread liquefaction (Quigley et al. 2012; Ballegooya et al. 2014). The water table raised nearer the surface and the crustal thickness was reduced and less able to support the weight of built structures. Severe widespread liquefaction affected many of the Christchurch suburbs, especially Avonside, Avondale, and Bexley, and its central business district. This meant a loss of large areas of the city. Approximately 20,000 houses were seriously affected by liquefaction, out of which between 6,000 and 7,500 were damaged beyond economic repair and were abandoned (Cubrinovski 2012). Buried pipe networks suffered extensive damage and the wastewater system was particularly affected resulting in loss of service to large areas (MacAskill 2016). Extensive areas along the lower River Avon and around the estuary and coastal zones, and in the town of Kaiapoi, were deemed as unsuitable for rebuilding, and the government 'bought' the affected properties, and cleared the land. Complete neighbourhoods and some communities were displaced (Swaffield 2013).

In Pakistan, after the 2005 earthquake, the Government of Pakistan decided to relocate the city of Balakot. In the North-Western Frontier Province (NWFP), Balakot was the area worst hit by the earthquake. Situated on the conjunction of major fault lines, Balakot city was declared a "red zone" and unfit for the reconstruction (Quzai 2010). ERRA instituted a new reconstruction project named "New Balakot City Development Project" at Bakarial, a site 23 kilometres south, where, it was claimed, most of the land was government owned (Ismail 2012). Yet owners of some of the land designated for the new city refused to leave (Shafique and Warren 2015). When the author visited the town nine months after the disaster new inhabitants had already migrated to the town because of its strategically important location and had set up businesses and were building homes. The key issue seems to have been a failure to involve the local community (Asad 2014). Shafique (2016, p. 77) reports that "due to severe clashes between government agencies and local land owners, the work on project was suspended on various occasions and the completion dates revised from 2010 to 2012 and then to 2013. In 2016, the project has achieved less than 15% of its targets".

Construction – repair or rebuild

Unless the decision is to relocate the whole city or settlement, governments and building owners need to decide whether to repair or rebuild after a disaster. Two case study countries – Iran and China-opted for complete rebuilding. The remaining countries opted for a mixed strategy.

In New Zealand, there was a feeling amongst engineers that some decisions to demolish were unjustified and that demolition was driven by the high level of insurance penetration and by a conservative approach to safety (Lynch 2012). The engineers the author interviewed at Canterbury University in Christchurch and GNS Science in Wellington confirmed this. One of the key issues was that few cities hit by recent earthquakes had suffered such a high intensity of aftershocks and this had influenced decisions about reinsuring buildings in Christchurch (Merkin 2012; Watson 2012). Owners had to lodge an application to demolish, but permission seems to have been automatic. It is possible that some buildings were under-insured and were too costly to repair. The most profitable option may have been to demolish and reinvest the insurance pay out, especially since the Christchurch City Council constrained the number of storeys they can rebuild. The main policy outlined in the Christchurch City Council's Central City Plan was for a more compact, low-rise, greener city centre, in which building heights would be strictly controlled (Christchurch City Council 2011). City centre businesses were relocated to the periphery.

The City Council was also engaged in a debate about saving historic buildings, the most heated concerned the Anglican Cathedral (Burdon 2015). Christchurch was unusual for the quality of its Gothic Revival public buildings and the city's Victorian and Edwardian character (Lockhead 2012). A serious architectural loss was the collapse of the Canterbury Provincial Council Chamber (1865), a remarkable colonial example of High Victorian Gothic by the local architect, Benjamin Mountfort (New Zealand Historic Places Trust 2012). This example from New Zealand, an advanced country that values its historic buildings, illustrates the importance of decisions about repair or demolition and how, unless these issues have been debated and decided in advance the is a risk that irreplaceable cultural heritage will be lost in the heat of the moment.

Emergency legislation removed all statutory protection for heritage buildings and over 150 listed heritage buildings were demolished in Christchurch. In contrast in L'Aquila, over 3,000 medieval buildings were damaged, many as badly as those in Christchurch, but were subsequently supported with scaffolding (Comune di L'Aquila 2011). Over half of the city centre was demolished, many historic buildings were lost and extensive areas of residential land were taken out of use. There is clearly a tension between a desire to conserve the familiar and repair damage, usually the preferred option of residents, and the ambition to make safer and 'build back better, often led by government (Contreras et al. 2014). Balancing these competing goals is one of the main aims of meta decision-making.

In Pakistan, after the earthquake in 2005, the federal government directed the Housing Ministry to upgrade building codes to match international standards and in March 2006, the Ministry, in collaboration with National Engineering Services Pakistan Limited (NESPAK) drafted new building codes. But in the years following the release of the codes there was evidence that few people had followed recommended construction practice (Hasseb et al. 2011). The high cost of standard building materials, especially steel and cement, the lack of understanding about sound concrete construction and the lack of adequate site supervision meant that reconstruction was not as safe as supposed. "Owing to the complicated design and high cost of construction material, the victims were forced to abandon ERRA's technical architectural plan, depriving majority of the victims with the third and fourth instalments of compensatory payments" (Sadaqat 2012, p. 2).

Resources – self-help or state intervention

The final meta-decision is about financing business continuity and reconstruction. These are decisions about whether businesses should fend for themselves or receive support, whether individual households or the state should rebuild homes, and whether government should try to control resource allocation and price or leave demand and supply to market forces. In part these decisions depend on sovereign wealth and insurance penetration. Insurance penetration ranged from near 100% in New Zealand to virtually zero in Pakistan. Chile was somewhere between these extremes. Nevertheless, insurance played a major role in Chile in facilitating the financial means for recovery and reconstruction (Franco and Siembieda 2010). Although insurance penetration was low (30% of the residential properties in the Santiago metropolitan area and 10% elsewhere, and about 60% for commercial and industrial properties throughout the country) the insurance system worked well and provided financial coverage for between 20% and 30% of the monetary losses.

All the countries studied, with the possible exception of Iran, prioritised business continuity and some gave significant amounts of assistance to help business continue. In Chile, Japan and New Zealand the local government financed the construction of temporary shops and restaurants and these became local tourist attractions (see Figure 8.7).

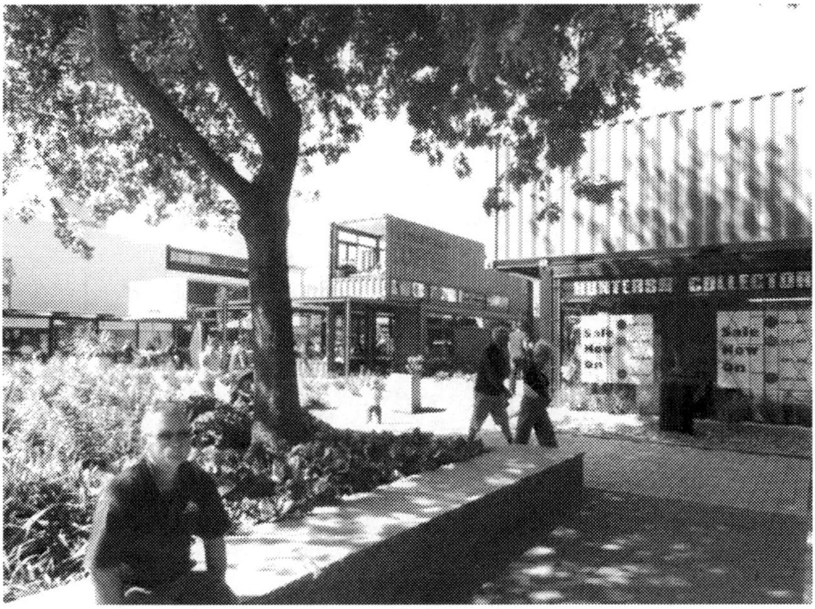

Figure 8.7 Business continuity and temporary retail outlets (ReStart shopping mall, Christchurch New Zealand 9 May 2012).

Source: Author.

In terms of housing reconstruction, most reconstruction in China was done by the state and in Japan and New Zealand funding for reconstruction came from the state or the global insurance industry (OECD 2015). In Turkey and Italy a proportion of new homes were also built by the state but to facilitate construction they were built far from where people would have chosen. In contrast, in Pakistan, to ensure that homes were rebuilt the way people wanted, the policy was for people to self-build on the same plot with government advice about safer construction (Bajwa 2007). It was hoped that this approach would more adequately match people's detailed needs than state rebuilding, but it was only partially successful for two reasons: the financial assistance was insufficient, the technical advice was unclear and people lacked understanding of safe construction practice.

Comparison of meta decisions in 10 countries

Figure 8.8 profiles the ten countries in terms of the six meta decisions. The top of the graph indicates centralised state control and intervention. The bottom of the graph implies people fare for themselves. The middle implies a balanced approach. Of the ten countries, only Chile achieved a completely balanced approach. This is reflected in the graph below where meta-decision making in Chile is shown as a flat light green line. (A failure to take a decision would be represented by a break in the graph line).

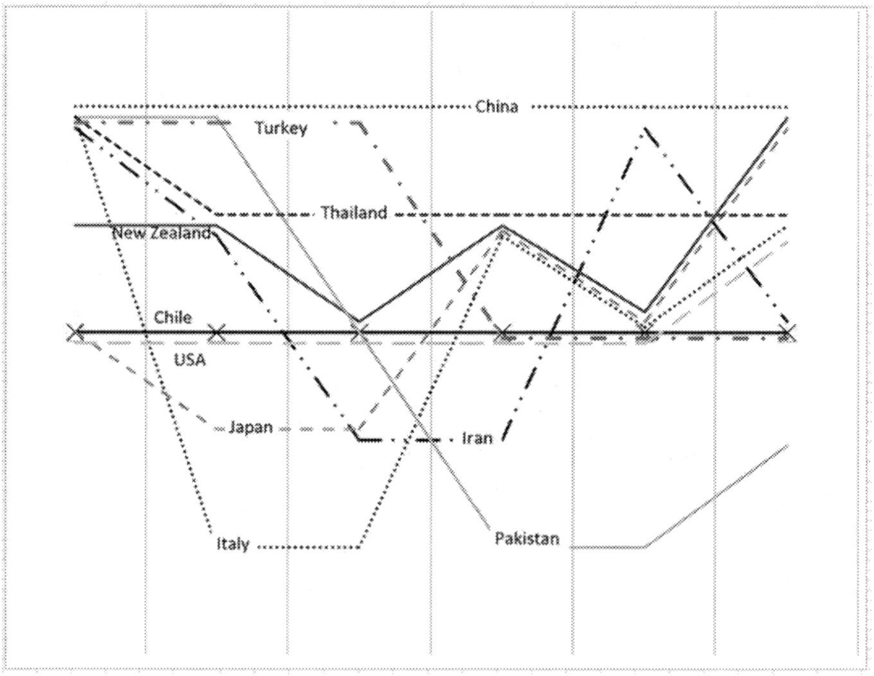

Figure 8.8 Comparison of meta-decision making in 10 countries.
Source: Author.

At first sight there appears to be no pattern; each country has a quite different profile. China's state control is reflected in the flat yellow line at the top of the graph. Thailand is similar but not so extreme. Japan and Italy have a similar shaped profile, but Japan is closer to middle. New Zealand might have been expected to have a similar profile to Japan, but the failures by the city authorities lead to the central government taking more control than might have been expected. Chile and USA have similar balanced profiles and in middle of the graph. Pakistan's profile looks like a ski jump, reflecting the high level of state planning but people still having to largely reconstruct themselves. Turkey is similar to Pakistan but there was more state aid for reconstruction. In Iran, the almost total collapse of mud brick structures in Bam meant that, apart from repairing the Arg of Bam, the government decided on a complete rebuild. This will significantly improve safety and resilience, but the new built form is unsympathetic to the local vernacular or climatic conditions.

As described earlier a single measure of balance of meta decision-making was devised for each country. Figure 8.9 shows that using this subjective measure Chile had the most balanced meta decision-making and China the least. This measure will be used to attempt to answer the questions posed at the beginning of this chapter.

Do countries that can make meta-decisions quickly recover faster?

Logically recovery should be faster if meta decisions are made quickly or in advance of disaster rather than slowly after. For example, Kim and Olshansky (2015) argue that recovery planning is best done before disaster

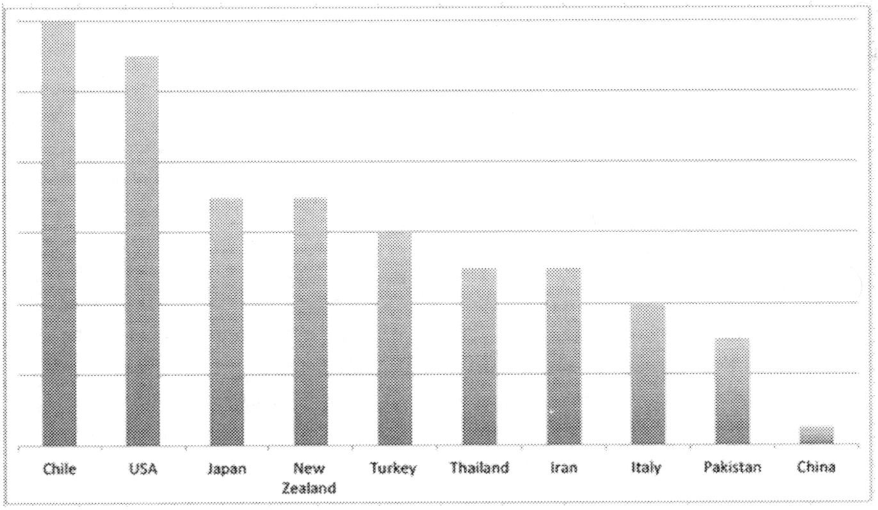

Figure 8.9 Balance of meta-decision making.
Source: Author.

Table 8.3 Speed of meta decision making and speed of recovery

	Quick meta decision making	*Return to normality(years)*
Chile	yes	5
China	yes	5
Thailand	yes	5
Turkey	yes	5
USA	yes	5
New Zealand	no	10
Italy	no	15
Japan	no	15
Pakistan	no	15
Iran	no	25
	Correlation =-0.846	

Source: Author.

strikes and cite as evidence an analysis of 87 local recovery plans in eight US states by Berke et al. (2014). Table 8.3 relates the speed of meta-decision-making to the speed of recovery and shows a strong correlation (–0.846). Half the countries studied Chile, China, Thailand, Turkey and the USA made quick meta decisions and all "returned to normality" in five years. The other half, Iran, Italy, Japan, New Zealand and Pakistan, made meta decisions more slowly and took longer to recover (between 10- and 25-years to "return to normality").

Do countries that achieve a balance of meta decisions build back better?

Figure 8.10 shows there is also a strong correlation (R^2=0.88) between balance and the quality of recovery as measured by determining whether a range of eight factors have been "built back better" or not. However, until there is a more robust measure of quality this finding must be speculative and tentative. It should also be noted that there are large differences in the demography, economies, politics and culture of the ten studied countries and that what is understood by quality of recovery may vary from country to country.

This has implications for our understanding and assessment of resilience. A country like Turkey, Iran or Pakistan, with a young population, a high birth rate, strong family bonds and extended family networks, may be more "socially" resilient than a developed country like the USA, Japan or New Zealand. In contrast developed countries may be more "physically" resilient, in terms of built environment and infrastructure, more "technically" resilient in terms rescue and relief systems and disaster management institutions and more "financially" resilient in terms of sovereign wealth, insurance cover and business continuity.

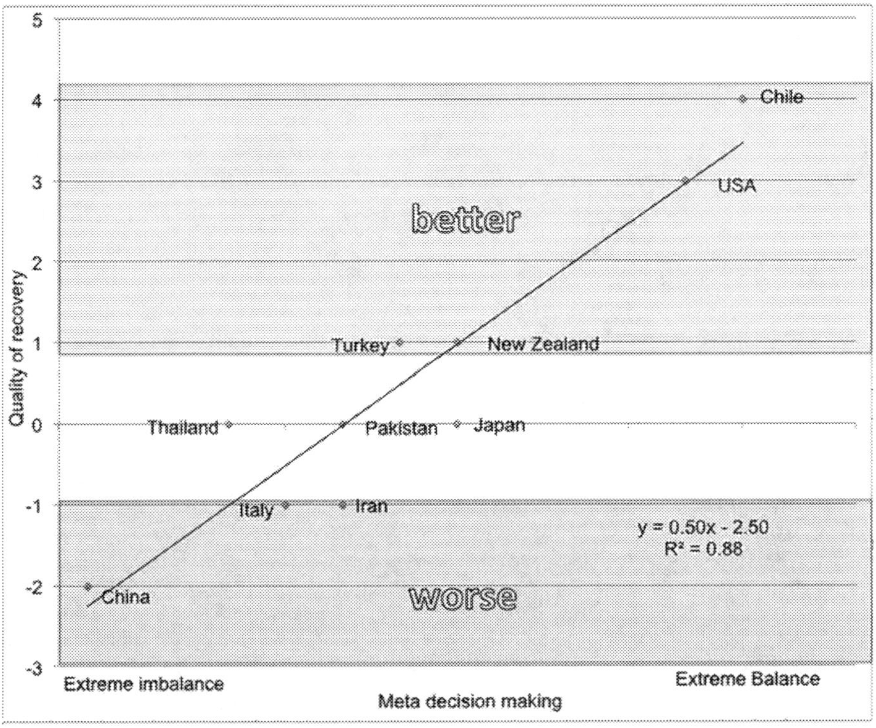

Figure 8.10 Correlation of balance of meta decision making with quality of recovery.

Source: Author.

Conclusions

This chapter defined resilience and recovery as they are currently used in the disaster management field. Resilience was defined as the ability to both resist a hazard and to recover from loss. Recovery was defined as reaching a stable state of "normality. The chapter also discussed six meta decisions or strategic trade-offs and analysed recovery after ten major earthquakes in terms of these decisions. The purpose was to explore whether meta decision-making affects the speed or the quality of recovery.

Two main conclusions can be drawn from the preceding analysis. Firstly, that the combination of pre-existing robustness and post-event response determines recovery outcomes. This means that resilience can be determined by how well a society resists the impact of a disaster and by how quickly it recovers. But the analysis also suggested that speed is not everything and that as well as "returning to normality, " "building back better" is also important in assessing recovery since it increases resilience to future disasters.

The key issue for governments and decision makers should therefore be to explore what factors increase resilience and improve recovery outcomes.

Secondly, the chapter explored the effect of meta-decisions in guiding recovery and suggested that better recovery is achieved by striking a balance between the opposing strategies implied in meta decision-making. For example, recovery seemed to be quicker and better in countries with both strong leadership and citizen involvement. And the quality of recovery outcomes appeared to be better for example in countries that adopted a judicious combination of relocation and in situ rebuilding and repair. Only Chile achieved this balanced strategy on all the six dimensions of meta decision-making and this concurs with the author's observation that recovery in Chile was the most 'successful' of the ten case study countries.

Finally, the chapter attempted to measure the effect of meta decision-making on the speed and quality of recovery. It found evidence that timely decision making did speed up recovery and that balancing meta decisions significantly improved the quality of outcomes in terms of "building back better". However, the speed of recovery was principally influenced by the size of the disaster and pre-existing socio-economic conditions and that a balance of meta-decision making had no effect on the speed of recovery.

References

Alexander, D. (2010) The L'Aquila Earthquake of 6 April 2009 and Italian Government Policy on Disaster Response. *Journal of Natural Resources Policy Research*, 2(4), 325–342.

Alexander, D. (2013) Planning for post-disaster reconstruction. www.grif.umontreal.ca/pages/papers2004/Paper%20-%20Alexander%20D.pdf.

Asad, A. (2014) Disaster, Development, Good Governance and the Time Frame Nexus: A Case Study of Balakot, Hazara, Pakistan. *Journal of Humanities & Social Sciences*, 22(3), 53.

Bajwa, E. (2007) Urban Development: A Strategy for Reconstruction, Rehabilitation and Development of Earthquake Affected Urban Areas. Government of Pakistan.

Ballegooya, S., Malana, P., Lacrossea, V., Jackam, M., Cubrinovski, M., Bray, J., O'Rourke, T., Crawford, S., Cowane, H. (2014) Assessment of Liquefaction-Induced Land Damage for Residential Christchurch. *Geomechanics*, 30(1), 31–55.

Barton, C., Nishenko, S. (2015) Natural Disaster – Forecasting Economic and Life Losses. USGS Fact Sheet. U.S. Geological Survey. http://pubs.usgs.gov/fs/natural-disasters/.

Basbug, B., Karanci, N., Kalaycıoğlu, S., Özden, T., Çalışkan, I., Özakşehir, G. (2015) From Emergency Response to Recovery: Multiple Impacts and Lessons Learned from the 2011 Van Earthquakes. *Earthquake Spectra*, 31(1), 527–540.

BBC News (2010) State of emergency ends in quake-hit Christchurch. 16 September 2010. www.bbc.co.uk/news/world-asia-pacific-11323891 (Accessed 20 September 2016).

Berke, P., Cooper, J., Aminto, M., Grabich, S., Horney, J. (2014) Adaptive Planning for Disaster Recovery and Resiliency: An Evaluation of 87 Local Recovery Plans in Eight States, *Journal of the American Planning Association*, 80(40), 310–323.

Boureau, Y., Sokol-Hessner, P., Daw, N. (2015) Deciding How To Decide: Self-Control and Meta-Decision Making. *Trends in Cognitive Sciences*, 19(11), 700–710.

Brezzi, M., McCann, P. (2012) Building resilient regions after a natural disaster. Abruzzo 2030: On the wings of L'Aquila. Issue paper for the Forum of 17 March 2017. OECD and Groningen University.

Bruneau, M., Chang, S., Eguchi, R., Lee, G., O'Rourke, T., Reinhorn, A., Shinozuka, M., Tierney, K., Wallace, W., von Winterfeldt, D. (2003) A Framework to Quantitatively Assess and Enhance the Seismic Resilience of Communities. *Earthquake Spectra*, 19(4), 733–752.

Burdon, P. (2015) Cathedral demolition simply not an option. *The Press*. www.stuff.co.nz/the-press/opinion/67547535/cathedral-demolition-simply-not-an-option (Accessed 20 September 2016).

Burton, C. (2012) The development of metrics for community resileince to natural disasters. PhD Thesis. University of South Carolina.

Carlton, S. (2013) Share an Idea, Spare a Thought: Community Consultation in Christchurch's Time-Bound Post-Earthquake Rebuild. *Journal Human Rights Commonwealth*, 2, 4–13. sas-space.sas.ac.uk/5219/1/1714-2293-1-SM.pdf.

CERA (2011) Draft Recovery Strategy for Greater Christchurch Canterbury Earthquake Recovery Authority. http://cera.govt.nz/sites/default/files/common/draft-recovery-strategy-for-greater-christchurch.pdf (Accessed 22 May 2017).

Chang, S. (2009) Conceptual Framework of Resilience for Physical, Financial, Human, and Natural Capital. Burnaby, British Columbia: School of Community and Regional Planning, University of British Columbia.

Chang, S. (2010) Urban Disaster Recovery: A Measurement Framework and Its Application to the 1995 Kobe Earthquake. *Disasters*, 34, 303–327.

Chang, S., Shinozuka, M. (2004) Measuring Improvements in the Disaster Resilience of Communities, *Earthquake Spectra*, 23(1), 41–62.

Christchurch City Council (2011) Central City Plan. Draft central city recovery plan for Ministerial approval. https://ccc.govt.nz/assets/Documents/The-Council/Plans-Strategies-Policies-Bylaws/Plans/central-city/CentralCityPlanTechnicalAppendicesP02-S.pdf (Accessed 22 May 2017).

Coles, J., Zhuang, J. (2011) Decisions in Disaster Recovery Operations: A Game Theoretic Perspective on Organization Cooperation. *Journal of Homeland Security and Emergency Management*, 8(1), Article 35.

Comerio, M. (2013) Housing Recovery in Chile: A Qualitative Mid-Program Review. PEER Report 2013/01. Pacific Earthquake Engineering Research Center.

Comune di L'Aquila (2011) Il piano di ricostruzione dei centri storici di L'Aquila e frazioni: Linee di indirizzo strategico. Parts 1–4 Dicembre.

Contreras, D., Blaschkea, T., Kienbergera, S., Zeila, P. (2014) Myths and Realities about the Recovery of L'Aquila after the Earthquake. *International Journal of Disaster Risk Reduction*, 8, 125–142.

Cubrinovski, M., Henderson, D., Bradley, B. (2012) Liquefaction impacts in residential areas in the 2010–2011 Christchurch earthquakes. Tohoku Special Conference Paper 183. http://ir.canterbury.ac.nz/handle/10092/6712.

Dacy, D., Kunreuther, H. (1969) *The Economics of Natural Disasters: Implications for Federal Policy*. The Free Press, New York.

Davis, I. (2006) Learning from Disaster Recovery: Guidance for Decision Makers. International Recovery Platform (IRP), May 2006.

Davis, I. (2014) *The Architecture of Recovery*. Presentation to The Martin Centre Research Seminar Series 21 May 2014. http://talks.cam.ac.uk/talk/index/52206.

Daziel, P. (2012) Quake lessons shared in L'Aquila. *The Press*. Christchurch New Zealand. 9 April. www.stuff.co.nz/the-press/opinion/perspective/6711790/Quake-lessons-shared-in-L-Aquila (Accessed 20 September 2016).

Dunford, M., Li, L. (2011) Earthquake Reconstruction in Wenchuan: Assessing the State Overall Plan and Addressing the 'Forgotten Phase'. *Applied Geography*, 31, 998–1009.

EEFIT (2013) Return mission to the L'Aquila earthquake. A joint evening meeting EEFIT/SECED/ISTRUCTE. Institution of Structural Engineers, 25 March 2013.

Elincin, Y. (2014) Neoliberal transformation of the Turkish City through the Urban Transformation Act. *Habitat International*, 41, 150–155.

Erdik, M., Kamer, Y., Demircioğlu, M., Şeşetyan, K. (2012) 23 October 2011 Van (Turkey) earthquake. *Natural Hazards*, 64, 651–665.

Franco, G., Siembieda, W. (2010) Chile's 2010 M8.8 Earthquake and Tsunami: Initial Observations on Resilience. *Journal of Disaster Research*, 5(5), 577–590.

GFDRR (2014) Pakistan Earthquake 2005: The Case of Centralized Recovery Planning and Decentralized Implementation. Country Case Study Series Disaster Recovery Framework Guide May 2014. www.gfdrr.org/sites/gfdrr/files/documents/docs/Pakistan_April%202014.pdf (Accessed 20 September 2016).

González Muzzio, C. (2012) Planning back better, urgent and important. Salzburg Congress on Urban Planning and Development 45th Annual SCUPAD Congress May 9–12, 2012 Salzburg, Austria. www.scupad.org/web/sites/.../2012_Congressppt_Muzzio_Chile.pdf.

Government of Japan (2012) *Road to recovery*. Reconstruction Agency, Prime Minister's Office. www.kantei.go.jp/foreign/incident/road_to_recovery.html (Accessed 5 September 2013).

Haseeb, M., Xinhailu, A.B. Khan, J., Ahmad, I., Malik, R. (2011) Construction of Earthquake Resistant Buildings and Infrastructure Implementing Seismic Design and Building Code in Northern Pakistan 2005 Earthquake Affected Area. *International Journal of Business and Social Science*, 2(4), 168–177. http://ijbssnet.com/journals/Vol._2_No._4;_March_2011/20.pdf.

Heath, R. (1995) The Kobe Earthquake: Some Realities of Strategic Management of Crises and Disasters. *Disaster Prevention and Management*, 4(5), 11–24.

Hidalgo, S., López-Claros, A. (2007) Humanitarian Response Index 2007: Measuring Commitment to Best Practice. Development Assistance Research Associates (DARA).

Holling, C. (1973) Resiliency and Stability of Ecological Systems. *Annual Review of Ecological Systems*, 4, 1–24.

Hollnagel, E., Woods, D.D., Leveson, N.C. (Eds.) (2006) *Resilience Engineering: Concepts and Precepts*. Aldershot: Ashgate.

Ingram, J., Franco, G., Rumbaitis-del Rio, C., Khazai, B. (2006) Post-Disaster Recovery Dilemmas: Challenges in Balancing Short-Term and Long-Term Needs for Vulnerability Reduction. *Environmental Science & Policy*, 9(7–8), 607–613.

Ismail, M. (2012) Bridging the GAP from Destruction to Rehabilitation for Balakot Town, Pakistan. *Journal of Seismology and Earthquake Engineering*, 14(1), 69.

Kates, W. (1977) Major Insights: A Summary and Recommendations, in *Reconstruction Following Disaster*, edited by J. Eugene Haas, Robert W. Kates, Martyn J. Bowden. Cambridge, MA: MIT Press, pp. 261–294.

Kates, R., Pijawka, D. (1977) From Rubble to Monument: The Pace of Reconstruction, in *Reconstruction Following Disaster*, edited by J. Eugene Haas, Robert W. Kates, Martyn J. Bowden. Cambridge, MA: MIT Press, pp. 1–23.

Keck, M., Sakdapolrak, P. (2013) What is Social Resilience? Lessons Learned and Ways Forward. *Erkinde*, 67(1), 5–19.

Kim, K., Olshansky, R. (2015) The Theory and Practice of Building Back Better. *Journal of the American Planning Association*, 80(4), 289–292.

Kopp, R. (2012) The decision making process in Japan. *Japan Close-Up Magazine*. April 2 www.japanintercultural.com/en/news/default.aspx?newsID=154 (Accessed 13 July 2016).

Kottemann, J. (1986) Some requirements and design aspects for the next generation of decision support systems. *Proceedings of the 19th Annual Hawaii International Conference on Systems Sciences*, pp. 339–343.

Lockhead, I. (2012) An endangered city: Christchurch New Zealand and the earthquakes of 2010 and 2011 Society of Architectural Historians of Great Britain Newsletter No. 105 Winter/Spring 2012.

Lynch, D. (2012) Quake destruction avoidable. *New Civil Engineer*, p. 6.

MacAskill, K. (2016) Post-disaster reconstruction of civil infrastructure networks. Unpublished PhD manuscript, University of Cambridge.

MCEER. 2006. MCEER'S resilience framework. http://mceer.buffalo.edu/research/resilience/ Resilience_10-24-06.pdf (Accessed 15 October 2009).

Merkin, R. (2012) The Christchurch Earthquakes Insurance and Reinsurance Issues. *Canterbury Law Review*, 18, 199–154.

Miao, H. (2010) Wenchuan earthquake 2008: Recovery and reconstruction in Sichuam Province. Recovery Status Report 04. United Nations International Strategy for Disaster Reduction (UNISDR). www.unisdr.org/we/inform/publications/16777.

MINVU (2010) Plan de Reconstrucción "Chile Unido Reconstruye Mejor" Ministerio de Vivienda y Urbanismo. Ministerio de Vivienda y Urbanismo, Gobierno de Chile 3era Edición Octubre 2010.

MINVU (2013) MINVU Reconstruction Plan: A United Chile Rebuilds. Government of Chile. http://documentos.minvu.cl/min_vivienda/paei2013/Documents/02%20CUMPLIMIENTO%20DE%20COMPROMISOS%20GUBERNAMENTALES%20Iniciativa%20de%20mejoramiento%20de%20la%20gestión/1_Chile%20Reconstruction%20Plan%20after%20February%2027th%20Earthquake.pdf.

New Zealand Historic Places Trust (2012) Pouhere Taonga Report for the Canterbury Earthquakes Royal Commission – Heritage Buildings, Earthquake Strengthening and Damage, The Canterbury Earthquakes September 2010–January 2012 Final, 8 March.

OECD (2012) Building resilient regions after a natural disaster "Abruzzo 2030: On the wings of L'Aquila". Issue paper Forum – 17 MARCH 2012 Laboratori Nazionali del Gran Sasso, L'Aquila. www.oecd.org/gov/regional-policy/49866886.pdf (Accessed 20 September 2016).

OECD (2015) *Disaster Risk Financing: A Global Survey of Practices and Challenges*. OECD Publishing, Paris.

Olshansky, L.B. (2006). Planning after hurricane Katrina. *Journal of American Planning Association*, 72(2), 147–153.

Olshansky, L.B. & Johnson, L.A. (2010). *Clear as mud: Planning for the rebuilding of New Orleans*. Chicago, IL: American Planning Association.

Oxford Dictionary of Construction, Surveying and Civil Engineering (2013) Oxford University Press. www.oxfordreference.com/view/10.1093/acref/9780199534463.001.0001/acref-9780199534463-e-5743?rskey=f8DtdK&result=5739.

Oxford Dictionaries (2016). Dilemma. www.oxforddictionaries.com/definition/english/dilemma.

Padli, J., Habibullah, M., Baharom, A. (2010) Economic Impact of Natural Disasters' Fatalities. *International Journal of Social Economics*, 37(6), 429–441.

Perrings, C. (2001). Resilience and Sustainability. In Folmer (ed.) *Frontiers of Environmental Economics*. Cheltenham, UK: Edward Elgar.

Petak, W. (2002) Earthquake Resilience through Mitigation: A System Approach. Paper presented at the International Institute for Applied Systems Analysis, Laxenburg, Austria.

Platt, S. (2012a) *Reconstruction in New Zealand Post 2010–11 Christchurch Earthquakes*. Cambridge: CAR.

Platt, S. (2012b) *Reconstruction in Chile Post 2010 Earthquake*. Cambridge: CAR.

Platt, S. (2013) Urban planning and recovery. In Recovery two years after the 2011 Tohoku Earthquake and Tsunami: A return mission report by EEFIT.

Platt, S. (2015) A decision making model of disaster resilience and recovery. SECED 2015 Conference: Earthquake Risk and Engineering towards a Resilient World 9–10 July, Cambridge.

Platt, S., Durmaz Drinkwater, B. (2016) Measuring Resilience and Recovery. *International Journal of Disaster Risk Reduction*, 17, 220–237.

Platt, S., So, E. (2016) Speed or Deliberation – A Comparison of Post Disaster Recovery in Japan, Turkey and Chile. *Disasters* (Available online). doi:10.1111/disa.12219.

Platt, S., Brown, D., Hughes, M. (2016) Measuring Resilience and Recovery. *International Journal of Disaster Risk Reduction*, 19, 447–460. doi:10.1016/j.ijdrr.2016.05.006.

Porter, L., Davoudi, S. (2012) The Politics of Resilience: A Cautionary Note. *Planning Theory and Practice*, 13(2), 329–333.

Quarantelli, E. (1999) The disaster recovery process – What we know and do not know from research. Preliminary Paper #286. University of Delaware Disaster Research Center.

Quigley, M., Bastin, S., Bradley, B. (2012) Recurrent Liquefaction in Christchurch, New Zealand, During the Canterbury Earthquake Sequence. *Geology*, 41(4), 419–422.

Quzai, U. (2010) Pakistan: Implementing People-Centred Reconstruction in Urban and Rural Areas, in *Building Back Better: Delivering People-Centred Housing Reconstruction at Scale*, edited by M. Lyons, T. Schilderman, C. Boano. London: Practical Action Publishing, pp. 113–134.

Rose, A. (2004) Defining and Measuring Economic Resilience to Earthquakes. *Disaster Prevention and Management: An International Journal*, 13(4), 307–314.

Rose, A. (2007) Economic Resilience to Natural and Man-made Disasters: Multidisciplinary Origins and Contextual Dimensions. *Environmental Hazards*, 7(4), 383–395.

Rose, A., Liao, S. (2005) Modeling Regional Economic Resilience to Disasters: A Computable General Equilibrium Analysis of Water Service Disruptions. *Journal of Regional Science*, 5(1), 75–112.

Sadaqat, M. (2012) Balakot City: A tale of a forgotten town. *The Express Tribune*. http://tribune.com.pk/story/448530/balakot-city-a-tale-of-the-forgotten-town/ (Accessed 20 September 2016).

Shafique, K. (2016) Success of Post-Natural Disaster Reconstruction Projects – Significance of Community Perspective. *International Journal of Business and Management*, 11(9), 69.

Shafique, K., Warren, C. (2015) Significance of community participation in success of post natural disaster reconstruction project – Evidence from developing country. Paper ID: 533. 5th International Conference on Building Resilience. Newcastle, Australia 15–17 July.

Singer, A. (1996) Strategic Thinking without Boundaries: Transitions and Meta-Decisions. *Systemic Practice and Action Research*, 9(5), 531–537.

Sorensen, A. (2004) *The Making of Urban Japan: Cities and Planning from Edo to the Twenty-First Centuries*, Nissan Institute Routledge Japanese Studies Series. New York: Routledge.

Swaffield, S. (2013) Place, Culture and Landscape after the Christchurch Earthquake. *Space Place and Culture*. www.futureleaders.com.au.

Tierney, K. (1997) Impacts of Recent Disasters on Businesses: The 1993 Midwest Floods and the 1994 Northridge Earthquake, in *Economic Consequences of Earthquakes: Preparing for the Unexpected*, edited by B. Jones. New York: National Center for Earthquake Engineering Research, University at Buffalo, pp. 189–222.

Tierney, K., Bruneau, M. (2007) Conceptualizing and Measuring Resilience: A Key to Disaster Loss Reduction, *TR News* 250, May–June.

UNDP (2008) *Inter-Agency Standing Committee (IASC) Guidance Note on Early Recovery*. www.undp.org/content/undp/en/home/librarypage/crisis-prevention-and-recovery/guidance-note-on-early-recovery-cwger-april-2008.html (Accessed 22 May 2017).

UNISDR (2004) *Living with risk: A global review of disaster reduction initiatives*. www.unisdr.org/files/657_lwr1.pdf (Accessed 3 June 2016).

UNISDR (2007) *Disaster risk reduction: Gobal review*. www.unisdr.org/files/1130_GlobalReview2007.pdf (Accessed 3 June 2016).

UNISDR (2015) Proposed Updated Terminology on Disaster Risk Reduction: A Technical Review Background Paper. www.preventionweb.net/files/45462_backgoundpaperonterminologyaugust20.pdf (Accessed 19 September 2016).

United Nations (2005) *What are Clusters?* https://business.un.org/en/documents/249 (Accessed 23 May 2015).

Watson, W. (2012) New Zealand re/insurance industry feels aftershocks of quakes. 6 February http://blog.willis.com/2012/02/new-zealand-reinsurance-industry-feels-aftershocks-of-quakes/ (Accessed 20 September 2016).

Webb, G., Tierney, K., Dahlhamer, J. (2000) Business and Disasters: Empirical Patterns and Unanswered Questions. *Natural Hazards Review*, 1, 83–90.

Zhou, H., Wang, J., Wan, H., Jia, H. (2010) Resilience to Natural Hazards: A Geographic Perspective. *Natural Hazards*, 53(1), 21–41.

Zolli, A., Healy, A. (2012) *Resilience: Why Things Bounce Back*. New York: Free Press.

9 The Resiliency Web – a bottom-linked governance model for resilience and environmental justice in the context of disasters

Kevin Gooley and Melanie M. Bakema

Introduction: how does a natural phenomenon become a disaster?

The powerful forces of nature are ubiquitous elements in the lives of many people, none more so than those residing in the planet's coastal areas. These areas repeatedly face a multitude of natural hazards, including cyclonic storms, flooding, tsunamis, and earthquakes. Historically, humans have settled in these regions because of their fertility and proximity to the open sea for resources and trade opportunities. This trend is even more prevalent today; humans have been migrating to coastal areas at an unprecedented rate over the course of the past century (UN Habitat, 2012). The rapidly increasing population and urbanization of coastal zones, combined with their natural hazard vulnerability, creates a social-environmental relationship through which a disaster can easily be born. When natural forces negatively intersect with the human world and overwhelm our governance systems, infrastructure, and livelihoods, these hazards become dangerous disasters. Moreover, the impacts of disasters can be exacerbated by inappropriate governance responses (Ahrens and Rudolph, 2006; Aldrich, 2012; Pelling et al., 2015). A disaster is consequently generally understood as "a serious disruption of the functioning of a community or a society involving widespread human, material, economic or environmental losses and impacts, which exceeds the ability of the affected community or society to cope using its own resources" (UNISDR, 2016).

This notion of natural-social interdependency was already recognized in the late 1970s when O'Keefe et al. (1976) started to question the 'naturalness of natural disasters'. The argument that disasters are just as much – or perhaps even more – the result of social-economic as/than of natural factors, is the basis for our analysis of environmental injustice hindering resilience in the face of disasters. When a disaster occurs, different sections of society are affected and respond differently based on their geographic location and access to certain socio-economic assets. This disproportion exists between groups of different socio-economic standing, as lower socio-economic groups are more vulnerable, and therefore more negatively affected with higher losses of lives. For example, due to their lack of capacities, resources to recover from disasters and/or inability to freely choose their settlement location, such groups have in general a longer and more difficult recovery time (Adger, 2006; Blaikie et al., 2003; Cannon, 1994; Cutter et al., 2003; Turner et al., 2003). Consequently, environmental injustices are a widely present phenomenon in the context of disasters, and disasters have a cumulative negative effect on the resilience of such poorer communities. In this context, resilience is understood as the ability of a system to absorb a disturbance and retain its essential structures, processes and feedbacks in societies (Adger, 2006).

In this chapter, we explore disasters as the result of a societal system's interaction with the extremes of the natural environment and, moreover, analyse how governance systems can be created for enabling and triggering transitions to more equally resilient societies. We view the disproportionate distribution of negative impacts of disasters on poorer communities and the lack of capacities that such communities must cope through the lens of environmental justice, which is defined as all communities and persons having the same degree of protection from environmental and health hazards (Morse, 2008). The concept of environmental justice gives us the opportunity to better understand the different social, spatial and temporal dynamics of disasters. Environmental justice helps us to highlight that vulnerability is inherent within our social structure, and that poorer communities generally lack the basic protections that would limit the impact of hazards as well as the physical and financial assets that would help them recover from (potential) disasters (e.g. Adger, 2006; Moser, 2008). By focusing on environmental justice, we by extension aim to add to current debates on the concept of resilience and help to foster the academic dialogue about resilience, with an emphasis on the question 'resilience of whom, to what?' (Davoudi, 2012). Furthermore, our aim is to contribute to debates on governance in academia and to governance practice through developing a governance framework to increase resilience of vulnerable communities – termed the '*Resiliency Web*'.

In our analysis, we build upon a 'bottom-linked' governance model (Pradel et al., 2015) to conceptualize resilience through environmental justice. This model attempts to outline ways to establish relationships between actors with the capacity to implement a service or provide a resource with those who need them, i.e. more vulnerable communities (Pradel et al., 2015). Using research on disaster governance, environmental justice, vulnerability and resilience, we construct the Resiliency Web with four 'distribution channels' that we refer to in this chapter as '*RISK Pathways*' (*Resources, Information, Services and Knowledge*). The different elements representing the RISK Pathways were determined through an in-depth literature review and represent the flow of different forms of capital that communities could use to become more resilient to disasters. In addition, a case study was conducted of disaster governance structures in Bangladesh in order to test and apply the Resiliency Web and RISK pathways. By doing so, we aimed to develop the model further to create a better understanding of how to design a governance system that can contribute to strengthening the resilience of communities in the context of disasters.

In the following sections, we explore the theoretical concepts that we used to construct the Resiliency Web. Following the theoretical explanation and the presentation of the Resiliency Web, we apply it to a case-study in the context of Bangladesh, investigating ways in which governance changes can be triggered to enhance the resilience of vulnerable people in disaster-prone places. We chose to explore the linkages between environmental justice and resilience in the context of Bangladesh as this country is known to be extremely vulnerable to disasters. Moreover, a number of specific disaster preparedness programs that are aimed to contribute to resilience have been created for the area. To give recommendations for disaster governance, we will analyse these disaster preparedness programs of Bangladesh. Finally, we draw the main conclusions about the dynamic interrelationships between environmental justice and resilience and propose a governance framework that can contribute to making communities in vulnerable places more resilient to disasters. The framework serves first and foremost as a structuring framework to create and guide governance actions, but also as an analytical tool through which actions of communities in the context of disasters can be better understood.

Linking environmental justice to resilience

How can applying the concept of environmental justice to the context of disasters provide us with a better understanding of resilience, and ultimately be useful for increasing the overall community resilience in vulnerable places? We begin to answer these questions by using the justice-lens of Sen (2009) who points out that "a calamity would be a case of injustice only if it could have been prevented, and particularly if those who could have undertaken preventative action had failed to try" (p. 503). It could be said that providing preventative services – e.g. shelter or early warning systems – to vulnerable communities that do not have access to assets, would, in theory, be a just act. Rectifying injustices that result from the unequal access to and distribution of assets, would entail undertaking actions that allow for communities to mitigate, absorb, recover and evolve from – or: become more resilient to – the impact of hazards such as tropical storms. Nevertheless, whereas the aim to rectify injustices entails the implicit assumption that governments need to undertake action, disaster scholarship argues that relying solely on governmental bodies is not the most efficient and effective way to foster resilience. Instead, establishing relationships across different public, private and community sectors may be a more effective strategy and such strategies are increasingly appearing in the context of disaster management, governance and risk reduction (e.g. Fois and Forino, 2014; Swyngedouw,

2005; Tierney, 2012). Such strategies craft resilience in a unique way that could especially aid in the protection and empowerment of disenfranchised and vulnerable communities (Bakema et al., 2014).

In the following sections, we present the theoretical underpinnings that we use for exploring environmental justice of societies in the face of disasters. We begin with an examination of the idea of environmental justice, and then relate this idea to the concept of vulnerability. From our understanding of the links between these two concepts, we can better explore resilience in the context of disasters, especially in terms of enhancing the resilience of vulnerable communities. This exploration leads to an analysis of different governance approaches used in disaster management and how these approaches often fail in contributing to resilience.

The lens of environmental justice

By incorporating the notion of justice into environmental issues, the goal is to elevate

> "concerns for the distributive and corrective effects of laws and decisions pertaining to health, the environment and natural resources, as well as concerns for the opportunities of those potentially affected to participate in such law-making and decision-making in the first place"
> (Ebbesson, 2009, p. 1).

By looking at this definition one can notice that environmental justice is mainly centred on the idea of fairness, which is a sentiment long-established in justice theory (Sen, 2009). Morse (2008) states that "in the legal realm, the goal of environmental justice is to secure for all communities and persons the same degree of protection from environmental and health hazards, and the same opportunity to influence the decision-making process" (p. 1). Morse's definition is similar to Ebbesson's (2009) contributions to environmental law. Deducing and simplifying the definitions provided by Ebbesson (2009), and Morse (2008), we can determine two goals for fostering environmental justice to which we will refer throughout the remainder of this chapter:

- Goal One: Creating an equal share of environmental benefits and equal protection from environmental hazards among all citizens;
- Goal Two: All citizens having equal opportunities in the decision-making process to determine the distribution of these benefits and hazards.

Building on the notion that a "disaster marks the interface between an extreme physical phenomenon and a vulnerable human population" (O'Keefe et al., 1976, p. 566), environmental justice can serve as a window to understand how a natural phenomenon, like a tropical cyclone, becomes a disaster. Whereas in the past the concept of environmental justice has been mainly applied to cases dealing with the allocation of polluting industries near lower income families (e.g. Morse, 2008), the concept of environmental justice can also be valuable for disaster management, especially for understanding and dealing with the impact of hazards on vulnerable groups. Disasters are wicked problems with both apparent and ambiguous causes and effects (McPhearson, 2013). A single event can simultaneously disrupt and destroy multiple components of a society (Pelling, 2003). The elements generating the disruption and destruction can be technical, socio-economic, ecological, cultural and/or psychological. These elements, crossing multiple disciplines and practices, are difficult to 'fix' with technical solutions. In addition to technical solutions, examining societal systems in an integral way, including different socio-economic processes and the so-called systems thinking, could provide more insight into the resilience building processes and understanding of the ways that the different elements are interrelated. The systems thinking approach entails identifying the social and environmental vulnerabilities of a community and addressing these using as much local capacity as it would allow (Adger, 2006; Becker, 2009; Berkes and Folke, 1998).

Vulnerability in human-environment interactions highlights the susceptibility of communities to environmental stresses. Vulnerability has been used in disaster literature since the 1970s and is promoted with different foci (Gaillard, 2010). O'Keefe et al. (1976) referred to the social construction that causes the fragility of some groups of people, stating that "the necessary concentration on the vulnerability of a population to a future disaster can only be done successfully through an understanding of the marginalization process" (p. 556). More recently, the focus in vulnerability studies shifted to measuring the vulnerability of regions combining quantitative and qualitative indicators (Gaillard, 2010; Haase, 2013). A third focus relates to forecasting potential damage of the built environment using the vulnerability concept (Cutter et al., 2008; Gaillard, 2010). In addition, the concept of capacity – or: entitlement – was promoted in the late 1980s as a contradictory concept to vulnerability. Whereas vulnerabilities were suspect to external factors of a community, capacities were regarded as rooted in the internal characteristics of a community. Capacities could, therefore, be influenced, opening the way for a decrease of vulnerability and increase of resilience (Gaillard, 2010).

A lack of entitlements, meaning "sources of welfare or income that are usually realized or latent" (Adger, 2006, p. 270), is an antecedent to vulnerability. According to Sen (1984), entitlements are a "set of alternative commodity bundles that a person can command in a society using the totality of rights and opportunities that he or she faces" (p. 497). By linking these entitlements with the rights of individuals, their realization is an issue of environmental justice. Whatever form these entitlements take – one specific resource, certain information, a reliable service or useful knowledge – their presence and realization are key to providing equal protection from natural hazards across all social groups. A lack of these entitlements creates sensitivity to stressors from the natural environment and a decline in the capacity to handle hazardous events. When these sensitivities intersect with a natural hazard it could create a disaster situation. Any area that is in an area that is vulnerable to different kinds of disasters would need measures to improve resilience that could help communities to prevent and/or to recover from possible disasters (e.g. Cannon, 1994). However, these measures often fail to reach and to really be effective for poorer communities. Elliot and Pais (2006) point out that disasters supply a rare glimpse into social identity and resource disposal, showing how society consists of "overlapping subsystems cross-cut by social and economic inequalities" (p. 296). For example, lower income housing, especially in developing countries, is frequently placed in former marshlands that have been drained and developed, leaving them extremely susceptible to flooding (Morse, 2008). In addition, because of a lack of political representation, such areas often lack sufficient infrastructures, such as levees or dykes, that would protect them from flooding (Elliot and Pais, 2006; Mohit, 2011).

The level of income is repeatedly referred to as a major factor in determining vulnerability – lower income groups are labelled as the most vulnerable mainly because of a lack of access to financial assets and consequently a disproportionate exposure to hazards (Adger, 2006; Blaikie et al., 2003; Cannon, 1994; Cutter et al., 2003; Turner et al., 2003). Here the interrelationship between socio-economic inequality and environmental injustice is particularly well visible; groups of lower socio-economic status are predominantly the people that have been pushed to settle in more vulnerable areas in both developing and developed countries and are hence more exposed to natural disasters such as floods (e.g. Morse, 2008). The above indicates that by extension also the negative consequences of disasters are disproportionally and environmentally unjustly placed on such groups of people. The above ideas on vulnerabilities and capacities connect directly to our goals for fostering environmental justice. When creating the Resiliency Web below, we therefore explicitly address the 'lack of entitlements' that contribute to vulnerability by proposing a model for distributing the necessary resources, information, services and knowledge. In this way, we attempt to begin building resilience by understanding vulnerabilities and framing them in a justice context.

Resilience: bouncing-forward to justice

How can the environmental justice lens help to transform vulnerable places and communities into more resilient ones? (How) can we use such lenses to enhance resilience for all groups in society, regardless of their socio-economic or political status? In other words, for whom and to what can resilience be created? These are the central questions we focus on in the discussion below.

Originating from ecology and later transferred to engineering, economic and social sciences, the concept of resilience is increasingly used among several different disciplines today. In social and ecological sciences, Adger (2006) states that resilience is the ability of a system to absorb a disturbance and retain its essential structures, processes and feedbacks. This refers to the ability of a community to 'bounce-back' from a disaster and return to a previous state or 'normalcy' (Manyena et al., 2011). However, this return to normalcy could re-create a situation that initially caused the disaster. Such understanding of resilience disregards the fact that disasters have the ability to completely change the physical and social structure of a place, making the concept of bounce-back' not only undesirable but also impossible. Moreover, another problem with such definition of resilience is that it does not embrace the dynamic elements of a social-environmental system. For a society to be resilient, it must embrace change as a necessity (Davoudi, 2012). In this sense, resilience reflects the capacity of societies to either get back to pre-disturbance development pathways or to shift to new development pathways that could increase resilience to future disasters (Van der Vaart et al., 2015). When moving to an understanding of resilience which includes organizational learning and 'bounce-forward' strategies, we may be able to understand and tackle the initial problems that led to the disaster in the first place (Manyena et al., 2011). By 'bounce-forward' we refer to the ability of a society to learn from what occurred in a previous disaster situation, analyse the elements that contributed to the disaster situation, and adjust those elements in order to be more resilient to future hazards. Here the concept of vulnerability becomes relevant; by understanding and rectifying problems that can cause vulnerability we can potentially enhance resilience.

In a resilient human-environment system, the actors involved would in ideal have the capacity to respond to changing conditions and acute disturbance events by adapting to the new characteristics of and threats within their environments. This type of system calls for a strong network and equal distribution of different forms of capital (Mayunga, 2009). Above we argued that vulnerability can be the result of a lack of entitlements (Adger, 2006; Blaikie et al., 2003; Cannon, 1994; Cutter et al., 2003; Turner et al., 2003). We also categorized these entitlements into Resources, Information, Services and Knowledge (RISK). These different entitlements form the basis of our Resiliency Web, a system of governance which is designed to enable and facilitate the distribution of these entitlements to the communities that need them to increase the adaptive capacity of individuals and strengthen their collective resilience.

Bottom-linked governance: forging the network

As Davoudi (2012) and Tierney (2012) point out, for a long period of time, the prevailing focus in disaster studies was on emergency management, disaster preparation and mitigation. Recently, an increasing number of disaster studies are centred on the importance of public engagement in the recovery processes (e.g. Aldrich, 2012; Cox and Perry, 2011), on risk governance (e.g. Renn and Klinke, 2015) as well as vulnerability and resilience (e.g. Berkes, 2007). Furthermore, the importance of the concept of disaster risk reduction is rising, reflecting a shift from 'response and recovery' to 'prevention and preparedness' (e.g. Becker, 2009; Jones et al., 2015; López-Carresi et al., 2013). Linked to these shifts in the focus of disaster studies, disaster management practice has traditionally operated using a top-down structure, relying on technological measures and engineering to reduce risk and large relief organizations to distribute aid with support of (national) governmental agencies. This type of hierarchical management focuses predominantly on overall economic well-being and less on 'people-centred development' (Yamin et al., 2005).

The common critical responses to the rather traditional management of disasters by the (central) state tend to focus on bottom-up strategies. This would imply that disaster management needs to be handled at the local level with little interaction from national governments or international NGOs (e.g. Tierney, 2012). The problem with disaster management at only the local level is that many local actors do not have the capacity or knowledge to create and implement preparedness programs without the help of larger organizations (Gaillard and Mercer, 2012). Instead, a real sharing of governance roles and responsibilities is needed between different state- and non-state actors (Parra, 2010). Sharing governance roles could build resilience of communities as community members could take on responsibilities such as constructing flood control infrastructure or providing medical assistance, normally carried out by relief organizations. It is therefore argued that an adaptive and dynamic governance strategy that facilitates the cooperation of public, private and civil society actors at different horizontal and vertical organizational levels is needed (Folke et al., 2005). This governance strategy is referred to as 'bottom-linked' governance, combining bottom-up initiatives with top-down policies (Pradel et al., 2015).

The aim of this style of governance is the "creation of new mechanisms for the provision of resources" (Pradel et al., 2015, p. 159). However, it is not just resources that this governance strategy could help distribute. Information, services and knowledge, can all be useful for resilience in the context of disasters. Scientific information on the environment, insights into disaster preparedness from experts and flexible technological fixes can all be developed by larger agencies and government bodies and distributed to individuals and communities. In addition, resources, information, services and knowledge, originating from community members or local small businesses could aid in designing broader approaches and applications of disaster management used by various organizations and institutions. Bottom-linked governance opens the disaster management process to non-state actors by giving them more room to intervene in the design and implementation of policies, and to integrate their local (tacit) knowledge in the processes (Gaillard and Mercer, 2012). Such governance structure can help to meet social needs by enabling equal capital distribution, empowering marginalized populations, reducing social exclusion by transforming social and governance mechanisms and, consequently, increase the overall resilience of communities (Pradel et al., 2015).

A bottom-linked governance model is the basis of the Resiliency Web proposed in this chapter. By establishing direct distribution channels between entities with the proper resources, information, services and knowledge, and communities who may be vulnerable to natural hazards, we can begin to construct a stakeholder network of actors and benefactors. The establishment of RISK Pathways between actors with the capacity to act and those in need will help to address the lack of entitlements (Adger, 2006) that as argued above create vulnerabilities for certain societal groups.

The Resiliency Web

The Resiliency Web and RISK Pathways can be best understood as a governance model for enhancing resilience in vulnerable communities. The Resiliency Web is based on the establishment of RISK Pathways, in which RISK stands for Resources, Information, Services and Knowledge, while the Pathways refer to distribution channels. Each of the categories represents different entitlements which are important to possess in order to reduce vulnerability (Adger, 2006). The pathways are conceptualized as a double-loop distribution channel, where Resources, Information, Services and Knowledge, flow back and forth between stakeholders. The establishment of the different distribution pathways with the aim to realize the entitlements that are essential to creating greater resilience to natural hazards adds to realizing the goals related to environmental justice (Ebbesson, 2009; Morse, 2008) and in ideal, to increasing resilience (Mayunga, 2009).

Table 9.1 illustrates the meaning of the different Pathways and gives examples of what each Pathway could consist of Figure 9.1 subsequently displays an example of the Resiliency Web and illustrates what the RISK Pathways would look like when established in a governance model.

Table 9.1 Examples of RISK pathways.

Resources	*Information*	*Services*	*Knowledge*
• Finances and funding • First aid supplies • Protective infrastructure • Labor • Food • Water	• Weather forecasts • Early-warnings • Evacuation routes • First-aid stations • Hospital locations	• Health-related services • Emergency related services • Evacuation services • Rescue services • Mobile-based alert systems	• Proper sanitation practices • Emergency procedures • Flood control measures • First-aid procedures

Source: *Authors.*

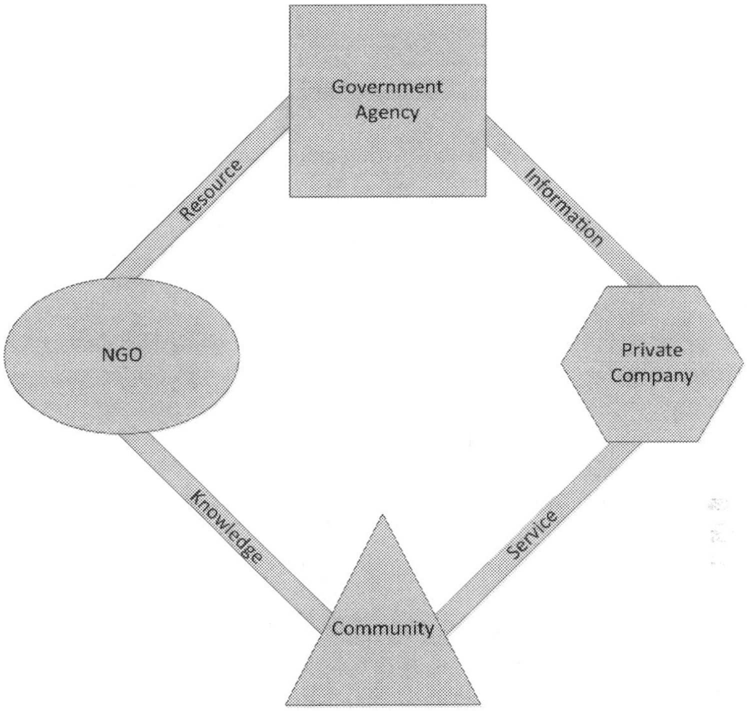

Figure 9.1 The Resiliency Web and RISK pathways.
Source: Authors.

In our model, Resources refer to physical, or tangible, resources that can be used by the community. Financial resources are often the key resources, which could be used to acquire other resources such as first aid supplies and food. Information refers to useful facts that could help a community avoid a disaster situation. Weather forecasts are a good example of information, having accurate information on future weather patterns can allow for a community to prepare for an approaching storm or cyclone. Services refer to any physical or technological assistance that a community could use, such as an evacuation service providing vehicles, to move persons out of areas about to undergo a serious environmental hazard like a cyclone. Knowledge would be anything that can be taught to a community to foster resilience and this knowledge dimension also highlights the relevance of preparedness to a potential disaster. Focusing on a disaster situation, knowledge of good sanitation practices and flood control measures are examples of knowledge as a resource which can help a community mitigate impacts during such potential disaster situations. It is important to differentiate between these different distribution channels of the above resources as it allows for a better understanding of what a community needs to foster resilience at the local level.

The Resiliency Web and RISK Pathways were conceptualized based on a thorough review of theories related to environmental justice and resilience. Each pathway represents a form of entitlement distribution from one actor to another. These entitlements will help address issues of vulnerability in the community, whether it is a lack of knowledge or information, or a specific resource or service. The framework is meant to be a simplified tool to distribute these entitlements, and with its simplification, we open the process of distribution to different kinds of stakeholders, both state and non-state. By simplifying the process and opening disaster governance to many different actors, we aim to address our two main goals of environmental justice and to help transform vulnerable communities into more resilient ones. In the context of disasters, socioeconomic inequalities that lead to environmental injustices make poorer communities highly vulnerable, since the inequalities result in a lack of entitlements among poorer communities that is needed to create resilience. A governance model such as the Resiliency Web can help to facilitate the distribution of those entitlements. The Web itself is a bottom-linked governance model which helps to define relationships and establish distribution channels for building resilience in societies, particularly for disenfranchised communities. In the next section, we apply the Resiliency Web to the case of Bangladesh to illustrate how the governance framework can help to build resilience using environmental justice lenses. Furthermore, we explain how the Resiliency Web could be broadly applied to other scenarios where a vulnerable population could establish RISK Pathways to foster resilience.

Applying the Resiliency Web to the case of Bangladesh

Bangladesh is located in a 'condensed pocket' of geographic and social vulnerability. Its location, topography, geology and climate allow for a myriad of different natural hazards. This susceptibility to nature related hazards coupled with a high rate of poverty and high population density contributes to a high vulnerability to disaster situations (Paul, 2009). To gain a more in-depth understanding of the vulnerability of the area, we first examined academic articles discussing previous cyclones in Bangladesh (e.g. Mohit, 2011; Paul, 2009). Next, to evaluate its usefulness, we applied the Resiliency Web to two disaster management programs in Bangladesh. We examine programs in Bangladesh that focus on ensuring community participation in disaster management efforts because these can shed light on how resilience can be strengthened and by which actors (ISDR, 2005; UNISDR, 2015). To obtain a better understanding of specifically these projects and the underlying associated processes, we conducted three semi-structured interviews in May, June and July 2014 with representatives of Cordaid, Proportion Foundation and the Green Soil Bag Foundation, which are organizations responsible for the projects analysed in this chapter.

Whereas a lot of research has already focused on Bangladesh and its vulnerability to disasters (e.g. Mohit, 2011; Paul, 2009), we use the case of Bangladesh and two examples of disaster management programs to illustrate how the Resiliency Web and RISK Pathways could be used as a framework in strengthening its resilience. The first program we analyse is the Community Managed Disaster Risk Reduction (CMDRR).[1] This program works to empower communities by teaching them disaster risk reduction strategies. We subsequently analyse the Sustainable Dyke Program,[2] which aims to help and prepare communities themselves to implement measures to reduce vulnerability.

Help on the way: Community Managed Disaster Risk Reduction (CMDRR)

The first program we analyse focuses on a remote rural area in Bangladesh. The susceptibility to disasters is especially prevalent in the most remote and rural areas in Bangladesh, referred to as 'the last-mile', meaning the least accessible, mainly residing along the last mile of routes that lead to the Bay of Bengal (interview respondents from Cordaid and Proportion Foundation). These 'last-mile' communities and local governments are usually neglected in national level preparedness programs and lack the resources, information, services and knowledge, to protect their own people effectively. However, the government of Bangladesh – inspired and encouraged by international disaster relief organizations such as the UNISDR (United Nations Office for Disaster Risk Reduction) – has enacted many programs to meet the needs of these communities based on ideas of disaster risk reduction and community empowerment. These ideas are the basis for what is referred to as Community Managed Disaster Risk Reduction (CMDRR). The CMDRR Program tries to address several different aspects of vulnerability, including the use of sub-standard housing, the lack of information regarding early-warning for cyclones and floods, the lack of relief services such as proper healthcare, and the lack of knowledge of disaster preparedness procedures (Costa and Sadeque, 2012; interview respondent from Cordaid). CMDRR has a strong focus on distributing knowledge and services from those with the capacity to those that need it.

Figure 9.2 presents the relationships in the CMDRR Program portrayed in our Resiliency Web. It illustrates the establishment of the particular RISK Pathways and the formation of the Web. The four main entities involved in the program are Cordaid, who operates in a funding role; Caritas, which implements the programs on the ground; the Government of Bangladesh, which cooperates with the organizations and exchanges information and resources; and the communities themselves, who receive the disaster risk reduction programs and strategies. The programs cover a wide variety of pertinent topics. Many involve construction practices that are robust to natural hazards, such as elevating shelters on earthen mounds to protect

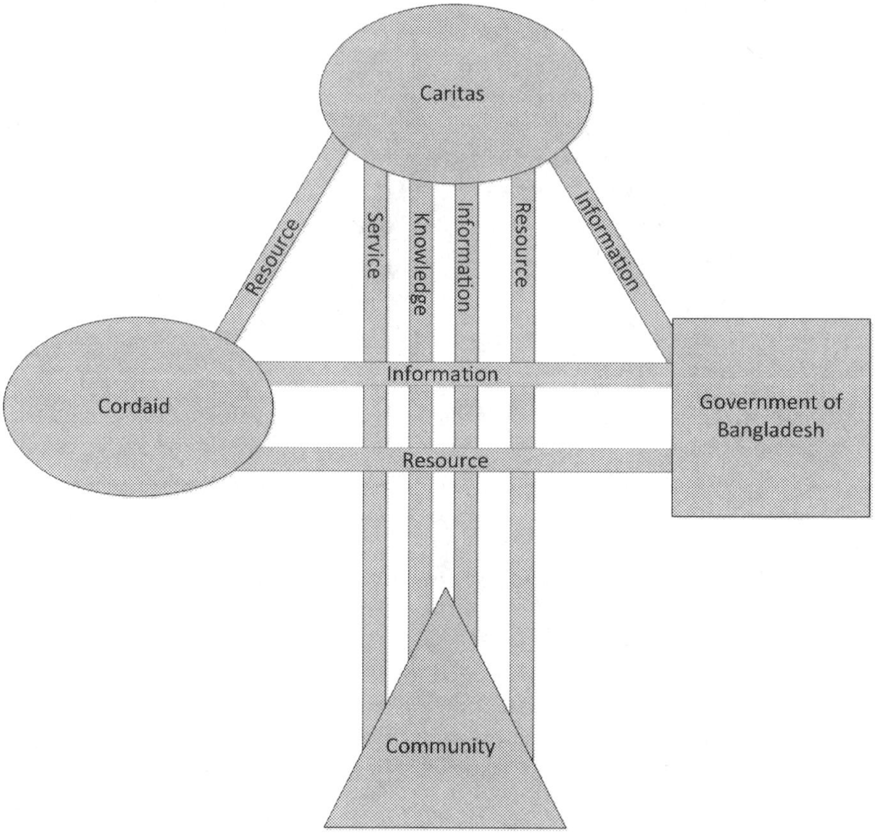

Figure 9.2 CMDRR Resiliency Web.
Source: Authors.

from floodwaters and teaching construction techniques that will withstand strong winds. Others involve preventing water-borne diseases in the aftermath of disasters and include teaching proper sanitation practices and building latrines to prevent the spread of water-borne diseases such as cholera (Costa and Sadeque, 2012; interview respondent from Cordaid).

The RISK Pathways are directly established between the different parties, allowing for easy distribution and feedback. This is in line with the 'bounce-forward' and dynamic resilience strategies of Manyena et al. (2011) and Davoudi (2012). The direct feedback and engagement with community members is an example of 'double-loop learning' where the organizations can learn from their work and improve their efforts in the future. These dynamic feedback channels create a flexible and adaptive resilience strategy that attempts to address some of the antecedent conditions (Adger, 2006) that are present in a community. The CMDRR strategy allows for social learning to occur by engaging the communities to participate in their own resilience-building efforts. Inviting communities into the decision-making and strategy building processes increase their adaptive capacity because it makes them feel part of the (recovery) processes. Moreover, Caritas identifies community leaders who become heavily involved with the programs. These leaders help direct the programs at the local level and fully take on the role of the NGO officials once the official program ends (Costa and Sadeque, 2012). This addresses our second goal of environmental justice; offering the opportunity to participate in the decision-making process (Ebbesson, 2009; Morse, 2008). This process of opening planning processes could then address our first goal of environmental justice, allowing for all citizens to have equal protection from environmental hazards.

So, the CMDRR Program focuses on community empowerment and building resilience at the local level among vulnerable communities in remote areas. However, it still operates in a traditional manner with state actors and large NGO's providing all the resources, information, services and knowledge in a rather top-down manner to the local communities. In addition, the stakeholders of the program do not include non-state business actors. This makes it at this point impossible to judge whether the program meets the first goal of environmental justice of creating an equal share of environmental benefits and equal protection from environmental hazards among all citizens. According to our theory, to build local resilience, other non-state actors should be included and responsibilities distributed evenly (Gaillard and Mercer, 2012; Pradel et al., 2015). In the next section, we will, therefore, look in-depth at a more applied project which better succeeds in illustrating and informing how a successful bottom-linked model can be designed.

The Sustainable Dyke Program

The second program of our study is a flood prevention program which is initialized by the NGO Cordaid. Hard constructions such as dykes and sea walls are a major asset in coastal protection. However, "in Bangladesh nothing is permanent" (interview respondent from Cordaid). Building permanent sea dykes and embankments have been somewhat of a futile effort since the coastline is constantly changing from extreme processes of erosion, storm surges and flooding. The amount of financial capital, resources and manpower needed, to repair destruction of this magnitude is enormous, and once they are repaired they could be easily destroyed again by another cyclone or flood. The Sustainable Dyke Program is trying to remedy this issue by using Green Soil Bags, also known as 'brinkers', that contain a mixture of soil and seeds to repair broken dykes and embankments. The program aims at teaching communities to repair their own river embankments at minimal costs (interview respondents from Cordaid and Green Soil Company). Bags are stacked in areas of the embankment that need repair. Soon thereafter, the seeds sprout and vegetation grows to anchor the bags and stabilize the structure. The repaired embankments are a co-production of international actors – Cordaid, Caritas, Green Soil Bag company and TU Delft – and local community members to improve local flood protection and strengthen both physical and natural capital of the area. Cordaid hired local community members to aid in the construction and because of the cheap cost of the repairs, the Government of Bangladesh is interested in applying the 'brinkers' to multiple broken embankments on the coast (interview respondent from Cordaid).

Figure 9.3 presents the Resiliency Web applied to the Sustainable Dyke Program. State and non-state actors work together to establish RISK Pathways between themselves and with the community, while the community provides services through labor to build the dykes and complete the project. Private business is included, producing a revenue stream which could establish a sustainable and long-lasting business model, meaning that

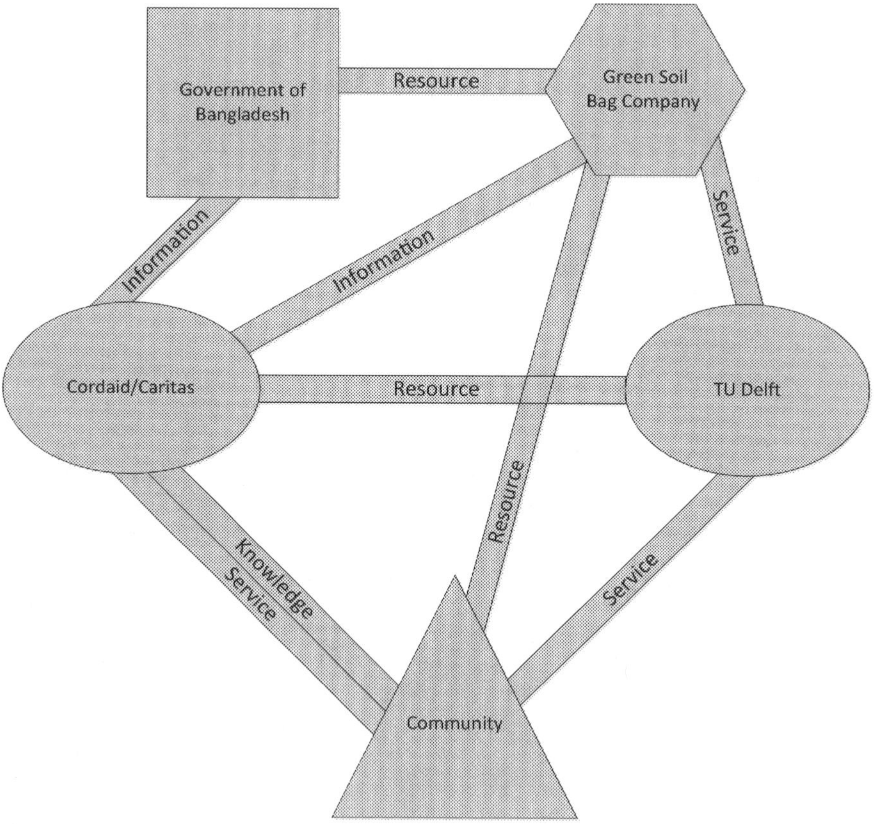

Figure 9.3 Resiliency Web for Sustainable Dyke Program.
Source: Authors.

local actors will have the capacity to take over the project once Cordaid pulls out. Local actors could take over the responsibility of producing the 'brinkers' and strengthening the embankments and their services can be paid for by local community members. Having an established business model allows for financial resources to remain in place. The financial resources give the opportunity for the Sustainable Dyke Project to be maintained by local actors, providing both protection for communities and employment opportunities for community members. Moreover, it keeps financial resources circulating through the community. Increasing financial capital and distributing it among community members is part of our resilience strategy (Manyunga, 2009) and could extend into other resilience-building opportunities. The financial capital could, for instance, go towards improving shelters to withstand hurricanes or paying local farmers to increase their crop yield.

The Sustainable Dyke Program seems promising for meeting both of our goals for fostering environmental justice and stimulating resilience (Ebbesson, 2009; Morse, 2008). Providing the innovative technology to the communities and educating them how to re-create the technology gives them the capacity of determining where the protective measures can be applied and distributed, which relates to our second goal. Giving this power to the communities equalizes the playing field and builds local human and resource capital (Mayunga, 2009), since communities that might not have had the political representation to acquire the resources needed to repair embankments, can now provide these protections themselves without the need to appeal to a relevant authority. Empowering the communities to repair the embankments themselves is important to our resilience strategy. These developments in combination with a wider cultural change in peoples' behaviours and values can make the local communities more self-reliant, flexible and adaptive, and the overall societal system more resilient. This links to our first goal of environmental justice – equal protection from natural hazards – and supports the effectiveness of a bottom-linked governance model.

The application of the Resiliency Web to this program is a better representation of our bottom-linked governance model compared to the CMDRR Program since it promotes the creation of opportunities to increase capital within local capacities using both state and non-state actors. However, there is a risk of governments 'withdrawing' from their responsibilities because of the shared and bottom-linked governance roles. This raises the question if the Resiliency Web based on a bottom-linked governance model would be more effective in creating resilient communities as opposed to more traditional disaster governance approaches. For our strategy to be useful, it must be able to be applied across a wide selection of vulnerable situations and communities. Testing the framework in more cases and analysing it in practice should provide more evidence for its efficiency and adequacy. In the next section, we, therefore, explain how the Resiliency Web could be used as a broader governance framework for building resilience in vulnerable communities and fostering environmental justice.

Discussion: the Resiliency Web as a governance framework for resilience building

Based on the previous explorations of two disaster management programs in Bangladesh, we observed how the establishment of RISK Pathways can help to foster resilience among vulnerable populations. The CMDRR program mainly establishes Information and Knowledge Pathways, while the Sustainable Dyke Program establishes Resource and Service Pathways. To make the ideas of the Resiliency Web and RISK Pathways applicable to any society that is exposed and vulnerable to a possible disaster, the framework needs to be flexible and able to address dynamic differences in places for disaster recovery processes or disaster risk reduction.

The first step in making a general framework – yet considering that this should be flexible to be applicable for different contexts – would be to understand the hazards facing a particular place. To be able to build resilience, communities need to know what they must be resilient to. The next step would be to understand the vulnerabilities to these hazards that are present in the community that resides in a particular place. This would help to guide and direct the future RISK Pathways which need to be established to form a Resiliency Web. Once the vulnerabilities are known, it is important to identify how those vulnerabilities can be addressed and through which RISK Pathway. If a community needs a particular resource, allocating and distributing that resource would add to increasing their resilience. If communities are not well rehearsed in disaster situation procedures, such as evacuation, an information or knowledge pathway would be used for community members to better respond to a disaster situation.

These steps may seem elementary, but what the Resiliency Web provides is a simple framework to understand and potentially put into practice different resilience-building practices or procedures by a multitude of different actors with different roles. This is where the strength of the Resiliency Web comes through; it allows for any individual or group to get involved and contribute to improving resilience. Moreover, in this position, the bottom-linked governance web can respond to questions of resilience of who to what. However, to strengthen resilience among all groups in a society, it is essential to coordinate the distribution of the RISK Pathways throughout a vulnerable place in an adequate manner. In this regard, there is a need to ensure that Resource Pathways do not overlap in areas where resources are scarce to avoid a non-provision of resources at all. As communication technology continues to permeate even in the most remote and vulnerable areas, it would be important to take advantage of these networks in an applied way. An idea could be to build these networks through mobile and web-based applications. By using a mobile or web-based platform there is potential to produce revenue streams, meaning a viable business model to ensure the continuing application and evolution of the Resiliency Web. This will establish the web as a bottom-linked governance model that could be adopted by actors of different capacities and across different social roles at different scales.

In this chapter, we have presented the links between environmental justice, vulnerability and resilience, to illustrate how we can help build resilience strategies through a system of governance that facilitates capital distribution between the relevant state and non-state actors. We believe there is a strong potential for the concept of the Resiliency Web to have a large impact in Bangladesh and other vulnerable areas in both developed and developing countries. An equal distribution of different kinds of capacities and entitlements can form the fertile ground from which communities in interrelation with other state and non-state actors can perform collectives actions which strengthen their resilience. However, it would require a direct application of the model into a resilience building strategy, continuous monitoring and an adequate balance between all actors to analyse its effectiveness. It could empower communities to foster their own resilience, and in turn meet the two goals of environmental justice by allocating and distributing the resources, information, services and knowledge, themselves and help state actors with the facilitation of this.

Conclusion

In this study, we established links between the concepts of environmental justice and resilience to help strengthen vulnerable communities through a governance framework for dealing with disasters. We identified how communities of lower socio-economic standing have a disproportionate share of vulnerabilities to disasters than wealthier communities. We investigated how the concept of resilience could be used to lessen this disproportion and foster environmental justice in the context of disasters. Through the analysis of these concepts, we created a framework called the Resiliency Web, which aims to facilitate the establishment of distribution channels – RISK Pathways – between stakeholders who possess Resources, Information, Services and/or Knowledge and communities and individuals who need them. We applied this governance framework to two case-studies to illustrate how the framework could function in practice.

The Resiliency Web could be valuable as a guide for building resilience in vulnerable places through distributing entitlements as resources, information, services and knowledge, among different actors and coordinating resilience building efforts following a bottom-linked governance model. However, it is not without its own weaknesses. The programs described in this chapter have been financed and managed by international NGOs using their own financial structures. The communities themselves would rarely have the financial or human capital necessary to facilitate these projects. However, the idea of having a framework is that any project can be conceptualized and applied anywhere, considering contextual differences. Some projects might not require a large amount of financial capital and would just need the perseverance of individuals to facilitate the exchange of resources, information, services and knowledge. This is even more evident with the diffusion of mobile communication technologies which could facilitate the establishment of these distribution channels at an extremely low-cost and without a central authority.

Furthermore, by continuing to link environmental justice with governance for disaster management and risk reduction, we can further instil the idea that all people, regardless of income-level or social-standing, are entitled to equal protection from the extremes of nature. Moreover, this protection requires the cooperation and collective efforts of multiple levels of government, private businesses, community leaders and members as well as various organizations. In this way, resilience can go beyond a new buzzword and becomes a goal for which strong and thriving communities continually work towards.

Notes

1 More information about the program can be found at: www.cmdrrforum.org.bd/index.php?option=com_content&view=article&id=2&Itemid=3.
2 More information about the program can be found at: www.cordaid.org/en/projects/sustainable-dykes-for-bangladesh/.

References

Adger, W.N. (2006). Vulnerability. *Global Environmental Change*, 16, 268–281.

Ahrens, J. & Rudolph, P.M. (2006). The importance of governance in risk reduction and disaster management. *Journal of Contingencies and Crisis Management*, 14(4), 207–220.

Aldrich, D.P. (2012). *Building Resilience: Social Capital in Post-Disaster Recovery*. Chicago, IL and London: The University of Chicago Press.

Bakema, M.M., Parra, C., McCann, P., Dalziel, P. & Saunders, C. (2014). Disaster governance for resilience: a post-earthquake Christchurch case-study. Association of European Schools of Planning (AESOP) Annual Congress 2014.

Becker, P. (2009). Grasping the hydra: the need for a holistic and systematic approach to disaster risk reduction. *JAMBA: Journal of Disaster Risk Studies*, 2(1), 1–13.

Berkes, F. (2007). Understanding uncertainty and reducing vulnerability: lessons from resilience thinking. *Natural Hazards*, 41, 283–295.

Berkes, F. & Folke, C. (1998). *Linking Social and Ecological Systems: Management Practices and Social Mechanisms for Building Resilience*. Cambridge: Cambridge University Press.

Blaikie, P., Cannon, T., Davis, I. & Wisner, B. (2003). *At Risk: Natural Hazards, People's Vulnerability and Disasters*. Second edition. New York: Routledge.

Cannon, T. (1994). *Vulnerability Analysis and the Explanation of 'Natural' Disasters. Disasters, Development and Environment*. London: Belhaven Press.

Costa, S.S. & Sadeque, A.Z.M. (2012). CMDRR – A step to change the community. Disaster Management and Development Department. Caritas Bangladesh.

Cox, R.S. & Perry, K.M.E. (2011). Like a fish out of water: reconsidering disaster recovery and the role of place and social capital in community disaster resilience. *American Journal of Community Psychology*, 48, 395–411.

Cutter, S.L., Boruff, B.J. & Shirley, W.L. (2003). Social vulnerability to environmental hazards. *Social Science Quarterly*, 84(2), 242–261.

Cutter, S.L., Barnes, L., Berry, M., Burton, C., Evans, E., Tate, E. & Webb, J. (2008). A place-based model for understanding community resilience to natural disaster. *Global Environmental Change*, 18, 588– 606.

Davoudi, S. (2012). Resilience: a bridging concept or dead end? *Planning Theory & Practice*, 13(2), 299–333.

Ebbesson, J. (2009). Dimensions of Justice in Environmental Law. In J. Ebbesson & P. Okowa (eds.), *Environmental Law and Justice in Context* (pp. 1–36). Cambridge: Cambridge University Press.

Elliot, J.R. & Pais, J. (2006). Race, class and Hurricane Katrina: social differences in human responses to disaster. *Social Science Research*, 35, 295–321.

Fois, F. & Forino, G. (2014). The self-built ecovillage in L'Aquila, Italy: community resilience as a grassroots response o environmental shock. *Disasters*, 38(4), 719–739.

Folke, C., Hahn, T., Olsson, P. & Norberg, J. (2005). Adaptive governance of social-ecological systems. *Annual Review Environmental Resources*, 30, 441–470.

Gaillard, J.C. (2010). Policy Arena. Vulnerability, capacity and resilience: perspectives for climate and development policy. *Journal of International Development*, 22, 218–232.

Gaillard, J.C. & Mercer, J. (2012). From knowledge to action: bridging gaps in disaster risk reduction. *Progress in Human Geography*, 37(1), 93–114.

Haase, D. (2013). Participatory modelling of vulnerability and adaptive capacity in flood risk management. *Natural Hazards*, 67, 77–97.

ISDR (2005). Hyogo Framework for Action 2005–2015: Building the resilience of nations and communities to disasters. *International Strategy for Disaster Reduction*. www.unisdr.org/files/1037_hyogoframeworkforactionenglish.pdf [Accessed on: 25/08/2014].

Jones, S., Manyena, B. & Walsh, S. (2015). Disaster risk governance: evolution and influences. In A.E. Collins, S. Jones, B. Manyena, J. Jayawickrama & J.F. Shroder (eds.), *Hazards, Risks, and Disasters in Society* (pp. 45–61). London: Elsevier.

López-Carresi, A., Fordham, M., Wisner, B., Kelman, I. & Gaillard, Jc. (eds.) (2013). *Disaster Management: International Lessons in Risk Reduction, Response and Recovery*. London and New York: Routledge.

Manyena, S.B., O'Brien, G., O'Keefe, P. & Rose, J. (2011). Disaster resilience: a bounce back or bounce forward ability? *Local Environment: The International Journal of Justice and Sustainability*, 16(5), 417–424.

Mayunga, J.S. (2009). Measuring the measure: a multi-dimensional scale model to measure community disaster resilience in the U.S. Gulf Coast Region. Dissertation Texas A&M University.

McPhearson, T. (2013). Wicked problems, social-ecological systems, and the utility of systems thinking. *The Nature of Cities*. www.thenatureofcities.com/2013/01/20/

wicked-problems-social-ecological-systems-and-the-utility-of-systems-thinking/#respond [Accessed on: 10/08/2015].

Mohit, M.A. (2011). Bastee settlements of Dhaka City, Bangladesh: a review of policy approaches and challenges ahead. *Social and Behavioural Studies*, 36, 611–622.

Morse, R. (2008). Environmental Justice through the eye of Hurricane Katrina. Joint Center for political and Economic Studies, Health Policy Institute.

Moser, C.O.N. (2008). Assets and livelihoods: a framework for asset-based social policy. In C.O.N. Moser & A.A. Dani (eds.), *Assets, Livelihood, and Social Policy*. Washington, DC: The World Bank.

O'Keefe, P., Westgate, K. & Wilsner, B. (1976). Taking the naturalness out of natural disasters. *Nature*, 260, 556–557.

Parra, C. (2010). Sustainability and multi-level governance of territories classified as protected areas in France: the Morvan regional park case. *Journal of Environmental Planning and Management*, 53(4), 491–509.

Paul, B.K. (2009). Why relatively fewer people died? The case of Bangladesh's Cyclone Sidr. *Natural Hazards*, 50, 289–304.

Pelling, M. (2003). *The Vulnerability of Cities. Natural Disasters and Social Resilience*. London and Sterling, VA: Earthscan Publications Ltd.

Pelling, M., O'Brien, K. & Matyas, D. (2015). Adaptations and transformation. *Climate Change*, 133, 113–127.

Pradel, M., Garcia, M. & Eizaguirre, S. (2015). Theorising multi-level governance in social innovation dynamics. In F. Moulaert, D. MacCallum, A. Mehmood & A. Hamdouch (eds.), *The International Handbook on Social Innovation. Collective Action, Social Learning and Transdisciplinary Research* (pp. 155–195). Cheltenham: Edward Elgar.

Renn, O. & Klinke, A. (2015). Risk governance and resilience: new approaches to cope with uncertainty and ambiguity. In U.F. Paleo (ed.), *Risk Governance. The Articulation of Hazard, Politics and Ecology* (pp. 19–41). Dordrecht: Springer.

Sen, A. (1984). *Resources, Values and Development*. Oxford: Blackwell.

Sen, A. (2009). *The Idea of Justice*. Cambridge, MA: The Belknap Press of Harvard University Press.

Swyngedouw, E. (2005). Governance innovation and the citizen: the Janus face of governance-beyond-the-state. *Urban Studies*, 42(11), 1991–2006.

Tierney, K. (2012). Disaster governance: social, political and economic dimensions. *Annual Review of Environmental Resources*, 37, 341–363.

Turner, B.L., Kasperson, R.E., Matsone, P.A., McCarthy, J.J., Corell, R.W., Christensene, L., Eckley, N., Kasperson, J.X., Luers, A., Martello, M.L., Polsky, C., Pulsipher, A. & Schiller, A. (2003). A framework for vulnerability analysis in sustainability science. *PNAS*, 100(14), 8074–8079.

UN Habitat (2012). Sustainably Urbanization. UN System Task Team on the Post-2015 UN Development Agenda. www.un.org/millenniumgoals/pdf/Think%20Pieces/18_urbanization.pdf [Accessed on: 25/08/2014].

UNISDR (2015). GAR. Global Assessment Report on Disaster Risk Reduction. Making Development Sustainable: The Future of Disaster Risk Management. The United Nations Office for Disaster Risk Reduction. www.preventionweb.net/english/hyogo/gar/2015/en/gar-pdf/GAR2015_EN.pdf [Accessed on: 25/08/2015].

UNISDR (The United Nations Office for Disaster Risk Reduction) (2016). 'Terminology'. www.unisdr.org/we/inform/terminology#letter-d [Accessed on: 03/04/2016].

Vaart, G. van der, Trell, E.M., Restemeyer, B. & Bakema, M.M. (2015). Resilience: just do it?! Governing for Resilience in Vulnerable Places, University of Groningen, 9–10 October 2014. *Resilience: International Policies, Practices and Discourses*, 3(22), 160–171.

Yamin, F., Rahman, A. & Huq, S. (2005). Vulnerability, adaptation and climate disasters: a conceptual overview. *IDS Bulletin*, 36(4). Institute for Development Studies.

10 Changing stakes

Resilience, reconstruction, and participatory practices after the 2011 Japan tsunami

Malka Older

Introduction

On 11 March 2011, a 9.0 magnitude earthquake unleashed a tsunami that devastated around 500 kilometres of the north-eastern coast of Japan, primarily across the prefectures of Iwate, Miyagi, and Fukushima. It caused nearly 16,000 confirmed casualties, with more than 2,500 people still missing; over 340,000 people were displaced. Recovery from such an event is both a test of existing resilience and the construction of resilience for the future. Japan is among the most disaster-prepared countries in the world, and quickly rolled out an impressive and well-financed plan for recovery. Four years later, the recovery is behind schedule and struggling. This chapter shows that part of the problem stems from confusion over the goals of the effort. Without a firm and widely understood definition of resilience, attempts to achieve it became confused and counterproductive.

Resilience: from conceptual vagueness to efforts at implementation

The concept of resilience has gained rapid momentum over the past decade, both among theorists and practitioners. Resilience has become a keystone of government (DFID, 2011) and non-governmental (Turnbull et al., 2013) disaster management thinking, as well as being referenced across a wide range of other disciplines (see Pendall et al., 2010). Many scholars have noted, however, that the definition of resilience is "fuzzy" (McEvoy et al., 2013; O'Hare and White, 2013; Pendall et al., 2010). The definitions vary across disciplines: Pendall et al. (2010) catalogue differing approaches from ecology, psychology, engineering, and economics as well as disaster studies. As Davoudi (2012) puts it, "it is not quite clear what resilience means, beyond the simple assumption that it is good to be resilient," and there are concerns that resilience is "in danger of becoming just another buzzword" (p. 299).

This broadness in the concept leads to inevitable difficulties in linking theory and practice; what promotes resilience according to one analysis undermines it for another. For example, McEvoy et al. (2013) note that while an early "underpinning notion was one of an ecosystem 'bouncing back' to a functioning state following an external shock," this can be challenged in some contexts since "a return to the normal functioning of a system, or part thereof, after an extreme event may be an inadequate adaptation response or in some cases may actually constitute maladaptation" (p. 285). Hutter and Kuhlicke (2013) point out that "the different definitions of resilience are understood as rather static and frequently mutually exclusive entities," (p. 295) forcing practitioners and theorists alike to choose among them.

There are consequences to the lack of a consistent or concrete definition. For one, a conceptually fuzzy definition can allow a positively connoted buzzword to distract from what's happening in implementation. Many disaster management actors use the concept of resilience to draw attention to community capacities and focus efforts on building or supporting those capacities. The United Nations Office for Disaster Risk Reduction (UNISDR), in many ways the backbone international organization for disaster risk reduction, defines resilience as "the ability of a system, community or society exposed to hazards to resist, absorb, accommodate to and recover from the effects of a hazard in a timely and efficient manner, including through the preservation and restoration of its essential basic structures and functions," and the explanatory comment offered is decidedly in favor of self-help: "The resilience of a community in respect to potential hazard events is determined by the degree to which the community has the necessary resources and is capable of organizing itself both prior to and during times of need."[1] (p. 285). Turnbull et al. (2013) situate resilience in opposition to vulnerability, locating it in the communities at risk of disaster. This suggests bottom-up, participatory mechanisms and support for local capacities.

However, the rhetoric does not always match the impact. O'Hare and White (2013, p. 276, emphasis in the original) write that:

> "many policy documents referencing the term favour articulations that may be considered less progressive than others, whilst elsewhere, it has been observed that resilience has emerged as a *tool* of governance: an effort to exert control, or at least the sense of control, over the manifold challenges faced by contemporary society, and to counter the complexities of spatial and administrative governance."

The buzzword can be used as a cover, suggesting community involvement and vaguely forward-thinking orientations for initiatives that may have nothing to do with those connotations. Alternatively, as O'Hare and White (2013) suggest, the language of resilience can be used to create top-down, rather than bottom-up, policies; for example, by prioritizing as a goal a certain interpretation of resilience, thereby and invalidating more participatory processes that do not align with the desired result.

Discrepancies and gaps in the definition can also confound even the most well-meaning of policy makers. When different definitions of resilience point at different strategies, planning implementation can become paralyzed. McEvoy et al. (2013) find that "if groups of actors (researchers, government, civil society organizations, households, individuals) persistently lack a shared understanding of what constitutes resilience [...], this will lead to inefficiencies in planning processes" (p. 289). The lack of a common conceptual foundation makes it difficult to agree on, measure, or evaluate resilience efforts; if resilience is a planning goal, then it is difficult to agree on or evaluate plans as well, slowing their implementation. This is particularly noticeable in post-disaster reconstruction, in which a concrete demonstration of disaster preparedness failures coexists with attempts to plan for an unknown future. While the theory around resilience often suggests an attribute that seems to be unitary (a community is resilient or it is not) and somewhat static (resilience may be built or supported, but does not seem to fluctuate), the practical issues of recovering from one disaster while planning for the next bring out divisions in the interpretation of the term.

Japan's reconstruction: a promising plan and problematic implementation

In the case of Japanese reconstruction after the 2011 earthquake and tsunami, the vagueness of the goal for resilient post-disaster reconstruction has caused serious delays and disillusionment, despite a well-funded effort apparently based on international best practices. After the disaster, Japan faced the challenge of rebuilding large swathes of inhabited land that had been shown to be highly vulnerable. The plans and approaches designed in the immediate aftermath of the disaster aimed to both express and build resilience, urging a community-driven process. Despite the high levels of resources and technical capacity that the government applied to the problem of reconstruction, they have found considerable difficulties in implementing it according to their approaches. As different stakeholders in a reconstruction process aim for different results, the entire process becomes complicated and stalled, ultimately undermining gains made possible by the conscious application of resilience principles. This chapter highlights three areas where vague understandings of what resilience means caused confusion and delays in reconstruction.

First, post-disaster reconstruction planning highlights the problematic temporality of resilience. The planning process envisions the resilience of a future community as the current community is still determining its capacity for recovery from the event that has just occurred. The impacts of the disaster offer an unparalleled opportunity for learning about existing vulnerabilities, and rebuilding can be an expression of resilience. However, as this chapter shows, extensive planning for resilience in the future may undermine the immediate efforts for cohesion.

Second, with large-scale hazards or disasters, geographic scope provides another area of dissonance in resilience perceptions. What seems resilient at one jurisdictional level may be a vulnerability at another level. This proves particularly problematic in democratic countries or systems with difficulties managing conflicting interests at different governmental levels. Municipalities, prefectures, and national governments, with their different interests and perspectives, can have divergent resilience plans that, though individually logical and reasonable, are mutually incompatible. As more national governments take on greater responsibilities in disaster response and reconstruction, such conflicts are likely to increase.

Finally, response and reconstruction involve both, financial commitments and, particularly in the case of reconstruction, financial gain. The way that these are allocated among the various actors – different levels of government, private firms, and non-profits – can also affect the perception and implementation of resilience.

This chapter argues that a failure to agree on a definition, scale, timeframe and financial structure for resilience can weaken internal mechanisms for absorbing shocks and lead to greater disruption. The case of Japan shows that financial resources and technical capacity are insufficient without clear, broadly understood goals. Divisions over, for example, whether it is individuals, the community as a whole, or a settlement's physical location that needs to revive can stymie processes, reducing the possibilities for any of those to take place and simultaneously weakening future resilience. While it is not realistic to expect consensus across every affected group and different levels of government, better defining both the capacities and the objectives of resilience in the specific context should smooth the processes required to embody it.

The chapter is based on fieldwork conducted in Japan over seven weeks in early 2013. Interview subjects included officials working at the Reconstruction Agency deployed to local, prefectural, and national levels; a consultant supporting the city planning process in one of the affected cities; and a number of city and town officials in affected areas. Interviews were semi-structured, conducted in Japanese, and recorded; all translations are by the author unless otherwise noted. While some interviews were the result of unscheduled visits to city halls, many drew on contacts the author developed while responding to the disaster with international and Japanese NGOs. The chapter also includes documentary research analysis, such as reconstruction plans and evaluations of the disaster response.

This next section will briefly review the case and the context of Japan, in particular, the characteristics that are most salient in terms of recovery. The subsequent section will examine the recovery approach, legal framework, and plans. The body of the chapter examines why, in this promising context, the recovery has so far failed to live up to the plans and the aspirations they embodied, with an emphasis on the enacting of resilience. In the conclusion, the implications of these findings for other countries are considered, along with suggestions for improving outcomes.

The case: the 2011 earthquake and tsunami and Japan's disaster frameworks

The disaster

The 2011 earthquake and tsunami struck along the northeast coast of Japan's Honshu Island, in a region known as Tohoku, causing severe humanitarian crises in Iwate, Miyagi, and Fukushima prefectures (see Figure 10.1). The immediate humanitarian response to the disaster was massive and included the deployment of the Japanese Self-Defense Forces, the construction of nearly 30,000 temporary houses, and unprecedented distributions of goods. As the Japanese government began to shift into reconstruction mode, new challenges began to arise.

The earthquake and tsunami also triggered a number of technological disasters, the most well-known being the Fukushima Dai-Ichi nuclear power plant meltdowns, which led to further evacuations, a long-term exclusion zone, radiation leakage, and a costly clean-up. While the fears of radiation contributed to stress and quite possibly to the loss of tourism (except disaster tourism) and trade nationwide, it should be noted that in

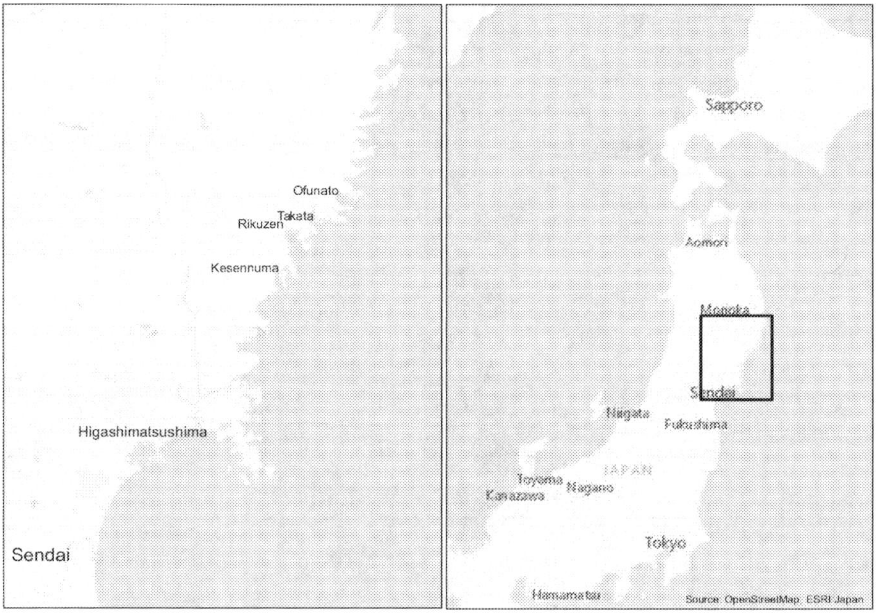

Figure 10.1 The section of Japan's Tohoku (Northeast) coastline discussed in the chapter, including the northern part of Miyagi Prefecture (Higashimatsushima, Kesennuma) and the southern part of Iwate Prefecture (Rikuzen Takata, Ofunato). Created using Mapbox.

Source: Author.

affected areas outside of Fukushima Prefecture, and particularly towards the north of Miyagi and in Iwate, where most of the research for this chapter took place, there were no direct impacts from the nuclear disaster.

Japan has invested heavily in disaster risk reduction (Ranghieri and Ishiwatari, 2014[2]), and this region, where the potential for a tsunami was well known, is no exception. Every municipality was required to have a disaster plan, and drills were frequent. A simulation of a tsunami off the Tohoku coast, where the tsunami hit, had been developed some years before and dramatized in video.[3] Although the simulation underestimated the height of the waves, it was remarkably accurate in terms of some of the cascading effects (for example, fires fed by oil from off-shore facilities that crashed into the cities). The simulation was used as a basis for local disaster risk reduction plans; in particular, the modeling of the wave's reach was used to identify escape routes and evacuation sites. In addition to this "software," many of the cities and towns had seawalls designed to mitigate tsunamis or storm surge. Nearly half of Japan's coastline had some type of seawall in concrete; many also used narrow pine forests as an additional barrier. However, the tsunami of 2011 was far larger than the parameters used for the simulation, overwhelming seawalls and washing away some designated evacuation sites (Interviews, Rikuzentakata City and Kesennuma City, 2013).

The recent history of disaster reconstruction in Japan

The modern legal framework for Japanese government participation in disaster was laid out in the *Basic Act on Disaster Control Measures*, in reaction to the 1959 Ise Bay Typhoon. Oguma (2013) notes four major points in this law: a focus on rebuilding communities, rather than individual property; establishing the local administrative level as the implementers of reconstruction; an emphasis on "hard" disaster risk reduction efforts; and standardization across localities.

This approach was challenged by the difficult and widely criticized reconstruction after the Hanshin-Awaji earthquake in January 1995. Olshansky et al. (2005) describe the recovery as "generally a top-down process" (Olshansky et al., 2005, pp. 6–14) in which "local planning decisions were heavily influenced by the Central government, consistent with Japan's governmental system" (Olshansky et al., 2005, pp. 6–36). As criticism for lack of citizen participation built, however, it was mitigated by "active efforts by Kobe City and Hyogo Prefecture to establish citizen participation organizations to expand local input on rebuilding plans" (Olshansky et al., 2005, pp. 6–36). They began encouraging more widespread engagement through a process known as *machizukuri* (町づくり), literally town-building. However, as Olshansky et al. (2005) note, the impact of these consultative groups post-Kobe was limited: "By the time the *machizukuri* organizations became active, however, major planning decisions for restoration promotion districts had already been made by the City. This reduced the scope of issues considered by participants in the *machizukuri* process" (Olshansky et al., 2005, pp. 6–18; 6–19).

The serious housing crisis following the Hanshin-Awaji disaster also spurred criticism and, eventually, some relatively minor legal changes that offered more funding for individuals who had lost property in disasters, but the amounts remained low and the underlying principle did not change: the national government would support local governments, who would implement recovery projects aimed at rebuilding communities, not replacing individual property. There were cultural changes as well; Chino and Abe (2013) write that in the wake of the disasters of the 1990s and early 2000s, "the importance and necessity of a multi-stakeholder participatory approach that put local citizens at the center when rebuilding from disaster or undertaking disaster prevention urban planning [*machizukuri*] became recognized" (Chino and Abe, 2013, p. 31).[4]

Planning for reconstruction after the 2011 disaster

Machizukuri remained very much in favour after the 2011 tsunami. Based on the concepts of participation and the use of local capacities, *machizukuri* represents principles of resilience, with locals rebuilding their own cities and the ideal that they would be rebuilt in ways more resistant to subsequent disasters. Indeed, *machizukuri* echoes some of the buzzword glow and corresponding concerns over appropriation discussed about the term resilience (Evans, 2002).

Faced with the city- or neighbourhood-wide destruction of cities and towns by the tsunami, the national government rapidly developed an approach for city rebuilding. The *Basic Guidelines for Reconstruction*, released three and a half months after the disaster, espoused a number of resilience principles for recovery, including participation and "putting people at the centre of disaster reduction" (Ranghieri and Ishiwatari, 2014, p. 183). The key structure for the recovery, following in the tradition of the *Basic Act on Disaster Control Measures*, had municipalities as the primary actors in implementing reconstruction.

Although the responsibility of local actors for disaster management was not new, it was unusual for localities to have so much responsibility for large-scale planning and project implementation. In Japan, local governments are largely subservient to the central government, with approximately two-thirds of their budget allocated down from the national level, most of it attached to specific projects (Samuels, 1983). In an interview, a city planner working on the reconstruction of Rikuzentakata, with long experience of non-disaster urban planning, noted that in the past the central government had been much more directive about what was to be done with local development, enumerating exact parameters for projects and closely overseeing them (Interview, Rikuzentakata City, 2013).

Of course, not all the localities had the capacity for large-scale or comprehensive city planning. It would be unusual in any case for a small town with a population in the tens of thousands to have an urban planner on staff, but for most of the municipalities in north-eastern Japan, this was even less likely. As the city planner involved in the reconstruction of Rikuzentakata explained in an interview, population in these cities had been dropping gradually for several decades; while some of the retirement-age staff in the city halls might have had planning experience, anyone younger was unlikely to have seen any growth in the town necessitating new designs (Interview, Rikuzentakata City, 2013).

The weak local capacity would therefore be supplemented by external experts, hired by the central government (this idea had also been tested after the Hanshin-Awaji quake, although in that case the consultants were mainly hired by cities and the prefecture for smaller internal units, such as the *machizukuri* groups; Olshansky et al., 2005). Financially, the localities would be supported by the central government, which had quickly passed supplemental budgets.

To implement the reconstruction, the government also made a structural change in order to subvert one of the persistent bugbears of Japanese bureaucracy: *tatewari* (縦割り), which Samuels calls "the single most important structural feature of Japanese public administration" (Samuels, 1983, p. 81). Samuels goes on to explain that "literally the term means 'vertical administration,' but while the flow from centre to locality is an important component of this 'vertical administration,' of even greater importance are the barriers among the central agencies which the term also implies. 'Sectional centralism' is a more appropriate description of the Japanese administrative apparatus" (Samuels, 1983, p. 81). The system isolates the different functional areas into vertical silos more connected "vertically" up and down the levels of government than "horizontally" within a level; so, for example, a city employee on the Board of Education is likely to have more contact with the prefectural education department than with the city mayor, while the prefectural employee will communicate more with that city employee and with the national ministry of education than with the prefectural governor. This hierarchy is also important to the system; a city employee will communicate with the prefecture, but very rarely directly to the national level. However, as Samuels (1983) notes, the *tatewari* also suggests that the powerful agencies at the central government level are isolated from each other and may compete rather than cooperate.

Despite its centrality to the Japanese system, Samuels (1983) writes that "Japanese observers, both practitioners and scholars, unanimously deplore this" (p. 82), and a new, temporary structure was put in place to reduce the impact of this sectional division on the recovery. A Reconstruction Agency (復興庁) was created and staffed with civil servants from ministries and departments nationwide. The idea was that this new entity would be a "one-stop shop" (a popular buzzword) for localities as they navigated the process of recovery, and particularly recovery funding. Staff from the Reconstruction Agency would be based in the field to support localities; plans, projects and funding requests would be checked by the Reconstruction Agency offices at the prefectural level; and Reconstruction Agency officials in Tokyo would carry out the necessary negotiations with other ministries to secure approvals and funding. In theory, this would allow for cross-cutting programs and the cooperation among different agencies that was normally so elusive while giving local governments a direct advocate at the national level.

Japan seemed to have all the ingredients for a successful recovery. Funding was allocated quickly; procedures were designed to combine local participation with outside expertise; structures were modified to streamline the bureaucracy. Planners were encouraged to combine hard and soft mitigation and use a "people-centred" approach to disaster risk reduction. Yet, three and a half years later, there are delays, divisions, and disillusionment, and many people question whether the recovery is making the places where they live safer and whether their communities will survive. A process that seemed to be both a symptom of current resilience – the quick shift to recovery – and a recipe for improving future resilience – the focus on locally-driven planning – now threatens both.

Putting the plan into practice

Resilience at different levels

What follows below is a short anecdote from the personal experiences of the author that serves to illustrate concretely how different, equally valid perspectives on resilience can work at cross-purposes.

In 2013, as part of the field research used for this article, I spent a few weeks in Kesennuma, a city in Miyagi Prefecture badly affected by the tsunami. The apartment where I stayed was one of four units in a small two-story apartment building. The apartment had hot water, a basic kitchen, a washing machine, and a parking space. What it did not have was a neighbourhood. Our neat, new building stood alone in a flattened landscape.

With almost no housing units available in town, the rents were high, and our own contract had to be paying back some of the investment of building the apartment so quickly after the disaster. However, it was unclear how long the apartment would be able to stay there. After the apartment was built, the city decided that it would be necessary to raise the level of this low-lying area by trucking in soil. Everyone else – assuming there were others who wanted to rebuild – was waiting to see how this would play out before deciding if, where, and how to invest, and the modest apartment building we lived in was likely to be torn down.

This anecdote is indicative, in a microcosm, of some of potential challenges in evaluating resilience. The entrepreneur who rapidly built the apartments and then took advantage of their scarcity could be described as resilient; he or she "bounced back" quickly, restoring limited normalcy (Davoudi, 2012; Pendall et al., 2010). The actor even verges towards those "interpretations of resilience [which] make a discernible effort to treat the potential consequences of risk, not only as threats but also as opportunities that may be capitalized" (O'Hare and White, 2013, p. 275). At the scale of the community, however, that bounce back has not happened; indeed, the window for describing recovery as bouncing back may have already passed. Decision-making failures have slowed the rebuilding and the return to normal function. As Pendall et al. (2010) note, deciding where to draw spatial boundaries around a system can change the meaning of resilience; moreover, "smaller and larger systems affect one another through continual response and adaptation" (p. 78). As that suggests, resilience means different things for the individual who built the apartments and for the community; at the same time, those two definitions interact. The apartments allowed the beginning of rebuilding a settlement in this area, affecting the way the community made decisions about returning; however, when the community (or at least the municipal government) decided that significant physical mitigation was necessary to resettle, the apartment owner's resilience was undermined.

Raising the level of the land is an attempt to make the area safer to live in. The idea is not only to learn from the experience of the tsunami so that a future disaster of the same parameters would not cause the same degree of destruction. The goal is to make the future community at least physically more resilient. This is the ideal of building back better, encapsulated in the tenth proposition of Clinton's (2006) post-Indian Ocean tsunami manifesto: "Good recovery must leave communities safer by reducing risks and building resilience." It is a theme echoed in psychological conceptions of resilience related to getting stronger from trauma, or reaching a "new normal" (Pendall et al., 2010, p. 74).

However, designing and implementing this mitigation project takes a substantial amount of time. In the two years between the disaster and the doubtless polite but difficult negotiations over the lease term of the apartment building, former residents of the neighbourhood were faced with the daily question of how long to wait to rebuild before moving somewhere else. Many were living in temporary housing. They were not necessarily in the same temporary housing complexes as their former neighbours; they would be mourning lost connections or building new ones. The fragmenting of the community reduced day by day the chances that that aspect of the neighbourhood would return to its former state, sapping the capacity for resilience that existed before the disaster.

At the same time, the large rebuilding projects were supplanting pre-disaster livelihoods. A former city crisis management centre employee from the same city, Kesennuma, explained:

> "The main reason people are leaving here is that [rebuilding the fisheries processing industry] is taking too long, because it's taking too long

> working people can't return to their original place of work. By 'can't return' I mean to say, for example, let's say you have a household. Both the husband and the wife work. [...] Now, the fisheries processing industry is starting back up, so there are advertisements asking people to come work in the companies. The thing is, now, because it took too long, that husband and wife are working in recovery construction. It's part time work but [...] the salary is much higher than before the disaster."
>
> (Interview, Kesennuma City, 2013)

The temporary recovery jobs will end, but by the time they do, the fisheries processing companies might have folded for lack of staff. An economy that might have been resilient enough to come back is being adversely affected by the efforts to make the physical location safer; this, in turn, impacts the resilience of the community.

Participatory decision-making

Given that the Japanese government's reconstruction plans prioritize rebuilding communities rather than just physical assets (Ranghieri and Ishiwatari, 2014), mitigation projects that delay or further disrupt community recovery may be counter-productive to the stated national-level goal. Yet it is in part the focus on communities, and specifically on building consensus within the communities, that extends the schedule of large infrastructure projects. A participatory decision-making process that seeks consensus from divided communities for problems without any clear solutions is time-consuming. Certainly, the question of whether to rebuild in the same place or move the entire community farther from the ocean was not an easy one. As one academic involved in the response and reconstruction put it in an interview:

> "Even within one family the father wants to return to the place they used to live, but the children and the wife don't want to or something like that, even within one family there are various opinions, then say the father at first wants to go back to live in the previous house, but doesn't have the means to rebuild the previous house, what should they do? [...] If there are these problems within one household, if there are these problems in local area..."
>
> (Interview, Kobe, 2013)

As this quote suggests, divisions over how to rebuild fragment families and communities. In the dilemma between the desire to stay close to the sea as a source of livelihoods coupled with emotional attachment to the land, and the hope of learning from the disaster to make the community safer for the future, finding a consensus is extremely difficult.

Within this context, the participatory, locally-based planning process touted as both important and, within the Japanese context, new, proved difficult in practice, particularly since local governments were not necessarily qualified to implement it. The World Bank/Government of Japan report *Learning from Megadisasters: Lessons from the Great East Japan Earthquake*, otherwise broadly positive in its assessment, noted that

> "In some cases, even after consultations, community members' views were not properly reflected in recovery plans. This may have been because local governments, which had little experience with community participation and limited staff, had to formulate recovery plans within a limited time span"
>
> (Ranghieri and Ishiwatari, 2014, p. 312).

Chino and Abe (2013) have a similar finding based on their work, research, and observation in Ōfunato, an affected town on the coast of Iwate Prefecture. Despite the town's auspicious early start and its great efforts to include community participation through questionnaires, workshops, and district-level discussion meetings, they find that "the so-called balance of conscientious citizen participation/consensus building and speed is in fact always in confrontation" (Chino and Abe, 2013, p. 40). Like the "hard" measures of raising land and constructing massive seawalls, "soft" mechanisms like participatory decision-making contain the risk of adversely affecting the communities they are supposed to make more resilient in the future, particularly when they are not implemented correctly.

Participation in reconstruction planning is aimed at customizing rebuilding to the needs of each setting. When participatory decision-making seems out of reach, either because it is taking too long or because those in charge of facilitating it don't know how, it becomes harder to tailor plans to individual communities. Hideo Nakazawa, a professor at Chuo University who is closely following the recovery, writes that

> "There are some municipal personnel that feel the temptation to mechanically make budgets flow to models, formats, and standard designs prepared by consultants and general contractors, or more precisely, some believe that this is the only possible way of doing things"
>
> (Nakazawa, 2013).

It is far easier to use existing plans or shoehorn housing needs into large public housing complexes than to contextualize recovery.

In some cases, the difficulty of reaching participatory decisions can be mitigated by tightening the administrative level of the decision. On the Hirota peninsula, a sparsely populated section of Rikuzentakata City in Iwate Prefecture, each tiny hamlet decided the height of its seawall, with variable results. As a city employee and resident of Hirota explained:

> "Here, it's 8.8 meters. The height of the seawall, it's 8.8 meters. Then here, it's 12.5 meters so, this one, the area here, it's better to be able to see the sea so, they don't need a very high one. [...] Being able to

> see the ocean, they are working together with the ocean so, they're better off being able to see the ocean. Here it's the same, here, here also definitely is the same, a place called Nishidake, they don't want it. This Nishidake area also, the current situation of 6.8 meters is fine, they said. In this way, going into each district, listening to the opinions of everyone in the local area, they decide the height so, there are areas with 12.5 meters, there are places with no [seawall], 8.8 meters, 6.3 meters, 8.1 meters, that's how it goes, the heights above sea level vary."
>
> (Interview, Rikuzentakata City, 2013)

While this certainly seems democratic, it raises safety concerns that cross the administrative borders: a high seawall in one location could potentially worsen the impact of the tsunami in a neighbouring location with a lower seawall. The resilience of one community or part of a community, considered in isolation, looks very different when it's considered as part of the larger system. Where the lines are drawn has consequences for how resilience is considered; lack of clarity about the scale of goals and how different administrative units cooperate can lead to counterproductive outputs.

In many places, however, the communities did not have a choice about seawall height. In the main Takata section of the same Rikuzentakata City, the seawall will be built by the prefecture, which therefore decides its height. In skirting the main bay, the seawall also affects the reconstruction of the national highway along the coast, which is conducted by the central government. These jurisdictions are not independent; they interact. According to the planning consultant working with Rikuzentakata, the city originally decided not to undergo the land raising process in the interests of rebuilding more quickly and avoiding some of the problems described above in the context of Kesennuma. However, raising the land would have a big impact on the construction of both the seawall – which, although constructed by the prefecture, would be funded with central government budget – and the national highway, and to facilitate those projects the land raising has been reconsidered (Interview, Rikuzentakata City, 2013).

Just to the south, in Miyagi prefecture, the prefectural government's plans to build high seawalls spurred criticism and protests from residents. Kesennuma was one of the cities with the most effective mobilization against the seawall, going as far as to hold a design competition for an alternative solution. While the winning design – a retractable seawall at the mouth of the harbour, instead of around its curve – was rejected by the prefecture, the activism did eventually win the city a compromise, a somewhat lower wall than that originally planned (from 5.1 meters to 4.1, with additional land raising to compensate). However, this compromise was not reached until early 2014, nearly three years after the disaster. This delay underscored the limits on the freedom of localities to define their own reconstruction, as well as holding up the rest of recovery until the question was settled.

Shifting roles and power

While the idea that local development choices be constrained by the prefecture and the central government could be considered normal in Japan, the disaster response had offered local governments a taste of a different paradigm. During the relief phase, localities had a strong leadership role. According to Samuels (2013, p. 171), "local leaders and analysts claim—and some central officials concede—that localities seized the relief initiative after the central government failed to act decisively." Although the traditional hierarchy normally maintains strict lines of communication, these broke down completely during the catastrophe. City officials in different cities, including a mayor, told me that while they had never directly contacted the central government before, during the response they were on the phone with them frequently – in the mayor's case, twice a day (Interview, Higashimatsushima, 2013).

This shift in role was not limited to government; non-governmental organizations (NGOs) and volunteers working on reconstruction have felt the same shift from open, ad hoc processes to tighter structures. A Tohoku University architecture professor involved with an NGO after the disaster commented that "it is no longer the chaotic time immediately after the disaster, and city halls are thinking as much as possible to return to normal processes to move forward" (Email communication, 11 September 2014).

The role of the reconstruction agency

The Reconstruction Agency was designed in part to balance the roles of local and central government by providing localities with a single pipeline to streamline recovery planning, as well as ideally an advocate. However, in practice, the Reconstruction Agency often seemed to be another layer between localities and the centre of power. As the academic involved in the recovery put it:

> "If you think that the Reconstruction Agency, rather than going to the other ministries, should be there to make decisions itself, then it seems like sort of a superfluous process. So if you ask something to the Reconstruction Agency, and are told, well, we will ask the headquarters, then what are you all...I don't understand, it's really meaningless."
>
> (Interview, Kobe, 2013)

The structure of the Reconstruction Agency's work reflects a built-in tension between supporting local decisions and controlling them. Local plans are created with assistance, or oversight, from Reconstruction Agency staff as well as outside consultants who are also paid by the central government. The plans are then checked at the regional offices of the Reconstruction Agency, even though the staff of the agency, all recent transplants from a wide range of other departments in the bureaucracy, are not necessarily trained in reconstruction planning or qualified to evaluate the plans. Finally, at the national level, the Reconstruction Agency must negotiate with the ministries that hold the funding and can give final approval of the projects.

Moreover, the localities were not given a completely blank slate in designing recovery projects. Rather, the Reconstruction Agency offered them a menu of around forty types of projects to choose from and adapt. While this was framed as a way of making the process easier on the localities, because they would not have to design something from scratch, it was also sometimes described as a means of oversight (Interview, Reconstruction Agency headquarters, Tokyo, 2013). This approach also frames resilience-building in terms of the familiar tension between expert and local knowledge, one aspect of the decentralized-centralized debate so important to Japan's reconstruction.

Financial roles

The thread running through these questions of control and oversight is financial. Since local governments in Tohoku, the area where the disaster was centred, were perceived as unable to pay for recovery themselves, the central government financed projects at one hundred percent, a decision that even some within the Reconstruction Agency did not agree with:

> "It's extremely 'dangerous' I think but, the one hundred percent thing, because 'anything go okay', I think one hundred percent is not good [...] If it's a hundred percent, 'if you buy some food product in a supermarket, they are free, you can get a lot of food.' [...] Because it becomes 'anything okay', I think it's not good. [...] Even now I think that if we had left even one percent it would have been better."
>
> (Interview, Reconstruction Agency headquarters, Tokyo, 2013. Sections in single quotes were in English in the original)

The corollary to the idea that "free" reconstruction will lead to requesting too much is the question of "ownership": if communities have not invested their own budget in a project, will they see it as their own and maintain it appropriately? Often, as in this case, the question of maintenance goes beyond whether communities are committed or not. The lack of surplus budget which is the argument for the complete payment by the central government means that although cities are receiving the projects – often massive pieces of infrastructure – for free, the maintenance could still drive them into debt.

The architecture professor at Tohoku University sees another consequence to this. According to him, because the projects are completely publicly funded, officials are unwilling to make new constructions "too good," worrying that this would be an excessive use of the money they have received (Email communication, 11 September 2014). The large amount of money also attracts large projects, and particularly construction. The massive demand has driven prices up for both material and labour, swelling budgets even further, and further delaying progress.

Japan faces none of the financial or capacity constraints commonly cited as problematic for disaster recovery in developing countries. While Japan's economy had been stagnating before the disaster, the government was nevertheless able to fully fund the prospective reconstruction through a combination of taxes and civil servant salary reduction. Likewise, there have been few allegations of corruption in the use of this money. This is not to suggest that corruption does not exist in Japan (for a discussion see for example Choi, 2007). However, it rarely brought up in comparison to developing countries, and Japan is ranked 18 out of 177 on Transparency International's Corruption Perception Index for 2013.[5]

Ahrens and Rudolph (2006) suggest that "according to empirical evidence, it is especially the poor in developing countries who lack the administrative, organizational, financial, and political capacity to effectively cope with disasters." While this is undoubtedly true, Japan's experiences show that while administrative, organizational, financial, and political capacity, all which Japan has in spades, may somewhat mitigate the impact of disasters, they neither fully protect against them, nor guarantee an effective recovery. Applying the latest theories of resilience – local leadership and participation, rapid start to recovery and transparent, sufficient budgets, integration across ministries – is challenging even under the best of circumstances.

Conclusion

Japan has had many successes, particularly in the response but also in the recovery. If the shine on transitional housing has dulled over the years and particularly because of uncertainty, it is still true that those houses were put up quickly and provided adequate, if cramped, housing for an extraordinary number of displaced people. Substantial efforts were made to maintain communities within the temporary housing, from small community centres to elections of community representatives. The efforts towards bottom-up design and integrated government planning, if imperfectly implemented, still provided more ownership and input from communities than if they had not been done. The rapid allocation of capital provided at least the pathway for quick rebuilding, even if the implementation was later stymied.

However, all these efforts have largely foundered on two difficulties: defining the goal and moving from theories of participation, integration, and rapid reconstruction to practice. As this chapter has shown, lack of consensus on the practical meaning of the broad term "resilience" – what timeframe and geographical scope it refers to – as well as problems putting into practice the admittedly challenging idea of redesigning and building entire towns, have squandered many of the seeming gains of the initial decision-making.

The difficulty that Japan has faced in the ongoing process of managing recovery suggests that disaster recovery, and particularly the building of resilience, is something that goes beyond resources or capital. In fact, having large amounts of money may in some ways be counterproductive for the recovery, as it encourages large and time-consuming infrastructure projects and may delay locally driven recovery. While the consultants on planning that were seconded to local governments seem to have been helpful, additional support for the processes of participation could have helped to smooth the balancing of the need for speed and the desire for consensus. More realism about the challenges of such a large-scale reconstruction particularly carried out from the bottom-up, might help to temper high expectations.

The lack of a common understanding among stakeholders of what "resilience" means, or what the "better" is that we are building back towards, obfuscates the unavoidable choices in rebuilding. Are we rebuilding what was lost, or are we building something adapted to new circumstances and new awareness of threats? What scale of resilience – individual, community, municipality, or nation – should be prioritized?

Perhaps the most difficult problem is the realization that there is no one answer to these questions. Participatory processes, though vitally important, should not be expected to reach a perfect consensus, particularly not in a short period of time. While a 'new normal' will eventually develop, and become accepted, perhaps the key lesson of the Japanese experience is that more than money or technical capacity, the most important constraint on that happening is the belief that it will be easy.

Notes

1 http://www.unisdr.org/we/inform/terminology#letter-r
2 See also Tachi, Kenichiro, "Disaster Risk Expenditure in Japan" http://www.slideshare.net/OECD-GOV/workshop-evidencebasecostsofdisasterstachi
3 One example is available for viewing at http://www.tsunami-museum.com/simulation/sm_001
4 "災害からの復興や防災まちづくりにあたって，地域住民を中心としたマルチステークホルダーが参画することの重要性や必要性が認識されるようになっている" (translated by the author).
5 http://cpi.transparency.org/cpi2013/results/. By contrast, the Netherlands is 8, the United States is 19, and France is 22.

References

Ahrens, J. & Rudolph, P.M. (2006) The Importance of Governance in Risk Reduction and Disaster Management. *Journal of Contingencies and Crisis Management*, 14(4), 207–220.

茅野恒秀、阿部晃士。大船渡市における復興計画の策定過程と住民参加。社会学年報 No. 42（２０１３） 特 集 社会問題としての東日本大震災 [Chino, T. & Abe, K. (2013)

"Ofunato City Disaster Reconstruction Plan Development and Related Community Participation." *The Annual Reports of the Tohoku Sociological Society*, Vol. 42, Special Articles "The Great East Japan Earthquake as Social Problem," 31–42].

Choi, J. (2007) "Governance Structure and Administrative Corruption in Japan: An Organizational Network Approach." *Public Administration Review*, 67(5), 930–947.

Clinton, W.J. (2006) "Lessons Learned from Tsunami Recovery: Key Propositions for Building Back Better." Office of the UN Secretary General's Special Envoy for Tsunami Recovery.

Davoudi, S. (2012) "Resilience: A Bridging Concept or a Dead End?" *Planning Theory & Practice*, 13(2), 299–333.

Department for International Development (2011) "Defining Disaster Resilience: A DFID Approach Paper." www.gov.uk/government/uploads/system/uploads/attachment_data/file/186874/defining-disaster-resilience-approach-paper.pdf.

Evans, N. (2002) "Machi-zukuri as a New Paradigm in Japanese Urban Planning: Reality or Myth?" *Japan Forum*, 14(3), 443–464.

Hutter, G. & Kuhlicke, C. 2013. Resilience, Talk and Action: Exploring the Meanings of Resilience in the Context of Planning and Institutions. *Planning Practice & Research, 28*(3), 294–306.

McEvoy, D., Fünfgeld, H. & Bosomworth, K. (2013) "Resilience and Climate Change Adaptation: The Importance of Framing." *Planning Practice & Research*, 28(3), 280–293.

Nakazawa, H. (2013) "Reconstruction Stuck at the Recovery Level." *The Japan Times by the Yomiuri Shimbun*, 22 July. www.yomiuri.co.jp/adv/chuo/dy/opinion/20130722.html. Accessed on: 21 September 2014.

Oguma, E. (2013) "Nobody Dies in a Ghost Town: Path Dependence in Japan's 3.11 Disaster and Reconstruction." *The Asia-Pacific Journal, 11*(44), 1–34.

O'Hare, P. & White, I. (2013) "Deconstructing Resilience: Lessons from Planning Practice." *Planning Practice & Research*, 28(3), 275–279.

Olshansky, R.B., Johnson, L.A. & Topping, K.C. (2005) *Opportunity in Chaos: Rebuilding after the 1994 Northridge and 1995 Kobe Earthquakes*. Department of Urban and Regional Planning, University of Illinois, Urbana-Champaign, IL; Laurie Johnson Consulting | Research, San Francisco, CA. (Web-published: March 2011).

Pendall, R., Foster, K.A. & Cowell, M. (2010) "Resilience and Regions: Building Understanding of the Metaphor." *Cambridge Journal of Regions, Economy and Society*, 3, 71–84.

Ranghieri, F. and Ishiwatari, M., eds. (2014) *Learning from Megadisasters: Lessons from the Great East Japan Earthquake*. The World Bank.

Samuels, R.J. (1983) *The Politics of Regional Policy in Japan: Localities Incorporated?* Princeton, NJ: Princeton University Press.

Samuels, R.J. (2013) *3.11: Disaster Response and Political Change in Japan*. Ithaca, IL: Cornell University Press.

Turnbull, M., Sterrett, C.L. & Hilleboe, A. (2013) *Toward Resilience: A Guide to Disaster Risk Reduction and Climate Change Adaptation*. Emergency Capacity Building Project. www.ecbproject.org/resource/18341.

11 The value of participatory community arts for community resilience

Gwenda van der Vaart, Bettina van Hoven and Paulus P.P. Huigen

Introduction

Since the early 2000s, the notion of resilience has begun to provide an important conceptual framework for understanding how communities respond and adapt to changes (Wilson, 2012). Resilience is rapidly gaining currency as both a targeted process of societal development and as a research topic in its own right (ibid.). The term, however, has been used to express various meanings by different academic disciplines and these have changed over time (see, for example, Chandler, 2014; McIntosh et al., 2008; Weichselgartner and Kelman, 2014). Beel et al. (2015) noted that "within the resilience literature, due to its founding within ecological studies ... resilience is often framed around the context of how well communities respond to external shocks [such as natural disasters]" (pp. 2–3). Resilient communities are those that bounce back to how they were before a disturbance, dealing with external shocks as they occur. However, as Weichselgartner and Kelman (2014) noted, other authors have extended this ecology-related notion, "aiming to better understand characteristics of vulnerability and resilience of individuals and communities in the face of socio-environmental challenges and changes – that is, how well society could deal with changes and disturbances" (p. 3). Further, Davoudi (2012) observed that a socio-ecological (or evolutionary) view of resilience challenges the idea of returning to an equilibrium after a disturbance. Rather she argued that resilience is about the "the ability of complex socio-ecological systems to change, adapt, and, crucially, *transform* in response to stresses and strains" (p. 302, emphasis added). Weichselgartner and Kelman (2014) noted that these interpretations of resilience "have been moving towards 'anticipation', encompassing 'capacity' and "capability" – and now coming the full way to being suggested as doing better than before by 'bouncing forward'" (p. 4). Here, resilience has become associated with communities having adaptive capacities that give them some level of control over their future direction, rather than being at the mercy of unmanageable external forces (McIntosh et al., 2008). In this chapter, we emphasize that social capital is one resource that communities can draw on to build such adaptive capacities. In line with the extended notion of resilience used in this chapter, we adopt the definition by Magis (2010, p. 402) who argued that community resilience concerns:

> "the existence, development, and engagement of community resources by community members to thrive in an environment characterized by change, uncertainty, unpredictability, and surprise. Members of resilient communities intentionally develop personal and collective capacity that they engage to respond to and influence change, to sustain and renew the community, and to develop new trajectories for the communities' future".

Community resilience can be developed in various ways. Magis (2010) outlined how communities have a variety of internal and external resources (economic, social, cultural, human, political, natural and built) on which they can draw to respond to change. White and O'Hare (2014), however, noted that resilience policy and practice encourages an "equilibrium approach", where resilience is characterized by spatial planning as "a simple return to normality that is more analogous with planning norms, engineered responses, dominant interests, and technomanagerial trends" (p. 934). As a result, policies related to (disaster) resilience often focus on rebuilding the economic and physical infrastructure of a community. However, since resilience is a communitywide and holistic characteristic, other socio-cultural resources also warrant attention.

In this chapter, we look at participatory community arts as a resource and demonstrate their value for building community resilience, thereby giving attention to other socio-cultural resources. The literature suggests that participatory community arts can be of value to community resilience because of their ability to generate community participation and social capital (see, for example, Guetzkow, 2002; Jermyn, 2001; Newman et al., 2003; Williams, 1997). In line with Healy and Côté (2001), Larsen et al. (2004) and Sampson et al. (1997), we argue that social capital is one of the resources that play a role in a community's resilience because it stimulates community members' ability and willingness to work together for a common good and empowers them to protect and pursue their collective interests. This fits with the 'evolutionary approach' to planning for resilience that is attuned to sociocultural conditions and embraces transformability (White and O'Hare, 2014).

To provide a theoretical backdrop for our discussion, the chapter begins by outlining the key aspects of social capital and how these relate to community resilience. We then briefly discuss participatory community arts and their relationship to community development. In building an argument for participatory community arts in building resilience, we examine two international participatory community arts projects. These projects illustrate dimensions of social capital (bonding, bridging and linking) that participatory community arts can generate, and how this contributed to the resilience of the communities where the projects took place.

Social capital and community resilience

In this section, we first introduce the concept of social capital and distinguish three types of social capital: bonding, bridging and linking (see Hawkins and Maurer, 2010; Magis, 2010; Woolcock, 2001). Following this, we elaborate on the link between social capital and community resilience.

Social capital is a widely-debated concept. In the social sciences, Putnam's (1995) view of social capital has been highly influential (Daly, 2005; Hawkins and Maurer, 2010; Woodhouse, 2006; Woolcock, 2001). Putnam defined social capital as "the features of social organization, such as networks, norms, and social trust that facilitate coordination and cooperation to mutual benefit" (1995, p. 67). Social interactions between community members form the basis of social capital. Williams (1997, p. 8), for instance, stated that "the elements which increase social capital are mainly based on interactions ... We need the opportunities to interact with a reasonably broad spread of people, and to build up a level of trust through positive rather than negative experiences". Interaction enhances the formation of social links between community members and, as McCarthy et al. (2004) explained, these social links, or *bonds* and *bridges*, can lead to feelings of trust and expectations of reciprocity and can promote a sense of shared interest or common identity – which are necessary 'ingredients' of social capital.

According to Delfmann et al. (2013), Hawkins and Maurer (2010) and Woolcock (2001), social capital encompasses bonding, bridging and linking capitals. *Bonding* capital refers to the close ties between people in similar situations, these are links that tie individuals together on the basis of homogeneity: around social identity (e.g., professional affiliation), sense of purpose (e.g., membership of a social club) or shared demographics (e.g., socioeconomic or ethnic status) (McCarthy et al., 2004). These ties can build trust, reciprocity and a shared sense of identity and belonging (Delfmann et al., 2013). *Bridging* capital, on the other hand, refers to relationships that are formed between diverse social groups and involves looser ties between people that might otherwise not interact. These looser ties expose people to diversity, enhance people's ability to work with each other and expand the resources available to them (Magis, 2010). Finally, *linking* capital is the extent to which individuals build relationships with individuals and institutions beyond their immediate community that have relative power over them (for instance by providing access to resources or services) (Hawkins and Maurer, 2010). Here, links between people and organizations and governmental bodies are also relevant. Citing Coleman (1988–1989), Magis (2010) argued that this linking social capital is particularly important for "communities poor in resources" as "the more they can link with sources of power and wealth, the greater their access to resources, the more opportunity they will have to make their voices heard, and the better situated they will be to take advantage of opportunities" (p. 407).

Scholars have argued that social capital is beneficial in building resilient communities (Anwar McHenry, 2011; Delfmann et al., 2013; Elstow, 2013; McIntosh et al., 2008; Steiner and Markantoni, 2013; Wilding, 2011). Delfmann et al. (2013), for example, show that the availability and use of social capital by a community determines, at least in part, its ability to cope with stressors and accept changes in a constructive way. In general, social capital is considered to underpin the ability of a community "to act as (and in the interests of) a community, and to identify and work towards community-based outcomes" (Dibden and Cocklin, 2005, p. 5). Revisiting Magis's definition of resilience, social capital thus supports community members in their personal and collective capacities "to respond to and influence change, to sustain and renew the community, and to develop new trajectories for the communities' future" (2010, p. 402).

Focusing on community resilience in the context of emergency management, Elstow (2013) provided some concrete examples of how social capital 'works'. She noted that social capital strengthens group social norms to which community members feel pressure to conform. In the context of an emergency, this is relevant as it could, for example, translate into: "I am going to check on my elderly neighbour in a power cut or share my provisions or I am going to volunteer because I can see that others are doing it too" (Elstow, 2013, p. 10). Elstow (2013) further suggested that social capital increases access to information, as people are better connected to each other and therefore, "will be able to pass on where help and assistance is, and what local risks and hazards are" (p. 10).

A community's social capital can, however, be put under pressure by the economic, social and environmental challenges that it faces. For example, processes such as population decline, economic pressures and austerity can lead to the closure of local facilities or services, such as shops, pubs and churches, that are relevant to maintaining social connections. In their study, Skerratt and Steiner (2013) found that such places not only fulfil their primary functions but also play "an important part in enhancing inter-connectivity of the communities, creating invisible 'glue' which helped communities function well" (p. 332). Such places provide opportunities for socializing and their disappearance may have a negative impact on a community's social capital. In addition to the closure of such key places, population decline can also lead to the departure of key players (such as local entrepreneurs and residents who run the community centre) who play an important role in enhancing the social capital of a community and contribute to its resilience (see Delfmann et al., 2013). The processes described above can subsequently impact on a community's ability to respond to other local threats (Lovell, 2009).

The discussion above highlights two important issues. First, social capital is *one* of the resources that contribute to a community's resilience. As Magis (2010) noted, there are also economic, cultural, human, political, natural and built resources from which communities can draw to respond to change. Stehlik (2003) also reminded us that resilience is "much more than just social capital, for it acknowledges that there is ambivalence about this [social] cohesion, that it may not be successful in every situation" (p. 93). In considering rural communities, McIntosh et al. (2008) noted that it is often not sufficient to possess the necessary social capital to be resilient because the social structures of such communities can be threatened by changes over which they have little or no control, and they could simply lack sufficient scale and critical mass. Second, although social capital was initially thought to be a one-dimensional construct that produced only positive outcomes (see, for example, Larsen et al., 2004), several authors have more recently reassessed the concept and it is generally now acknowledged that there is also a 'dark side' to social capital (Beugelsdijk and Smulders, 2009; Lovell, 2009; McCarthy et al., 2004; McIntosh et al., 2008; Portes, 1998). For example, Lovell (2009) highlighted the 'polarizing effects' of social capital, acknowledging that it can increase inequalities between different groups. Nevertheless, against the backdrop of economic, social and environmental challenges facing communities, social capital is found to have an important role in determining which communities will thrive and which will not (Woodhouse, 2006). Just as social capital can be regarded as the 'social glue' of communities, it can also be regarded as a 'lubricant' that facilitates the development of community resilience.

Participatory community arts in community development

As Bishop (2006, p. 178) noted, there has been a recent surge of artistic interest in "collectivity, collaboration, and direct engagement with specific social constituencies". Such art practices, Bishop (2006) notes, go by a variety of names, such as socially engaged art, community-based art, dialogical art, participatory art and collaborative art. We adopt the term 'participatory community arts' in this chapter, referring to "a collaborative process between a professional practicing artist and a community. It is a collective method of art-making, engaging professional artists and self-defined communities through collaborative artistic expression" (Ontario Arts Council, 1998, p. 7). These artistic activities can take on any art form as long as the community members as well as an artist are involved in the process. Bishop (2006) noted that although the output and objectives of artists engaged in community arts can vary enormously, they are all "linked by a belief in the empowering creativity of collective action and shared ideas" (p. 179). As a result, within the field of participatory community arts, both the resulting artwork and the creative process leading to it are regarded as important, with the process being an essential tool for achieving "collective, collaborative, mutually-beneficial" results (Ontario Arts Council, 1998).

Guetzkow (2002) noted that, in practice, participatory community arts are often initiated in the form of projects that attempt to use 'art' as a tool for human or material development. Projects are designed in the context of a larger goal (such as learning about diverse cultures or improving a neighbourhood) and can involve people who are disadvantaged in some way (such as people in a poor neighbourhood, ethnic minorities or at-risk youth). The idea behind such projects is that the involved community members develop themselves and gather knowledge, skills or insights and that such benefits extend beyond the individual, positively impacting the broader community. Kay (2000) highlighted the role the arts can play in community empowerment and helping communities deal with the challenges they face. Specifically, he stated that "local people ... engage together, develop social and economic skills and assume the power to fashion their future" (p. 415) thus fostering the community's adaptive capacities. More recently, Anwar McHenry (2011) maintained "that the arts can build resilience by providing an avenue for increased social and civic participation" (p. 251), implying that the arts can be a vehicle for building resilience.

The recognized benefits noted by Anwar McHenry (2009, 2011), Guetzkow (2002) and Kay (2000) are more broadly supported by a literature review by Newman et al. (2003) that specifically highlighted the social gains achieved through the adoption of community-based arts projects. Based on their review, Newman et al. (2003) identified four social gains: (1) *personal changes* such as being happier, more creative and confident, making new friends, taking up training; (2) *social changes* such as improved organizational skills and greater cross-cultural community understanding; (3) *economic changes* with an improved community image helping inward investment and impacting on the number of new jobs and people finding work; and (4) *educational changes* such as improved school performance. The personal, social and economic changes reflect the development of the necessary 'ingredients' for building social capital (see also Anwar McHenry, 2011; Guetzkow, 2002; Jermyn, 2001; Kingma, 2001; Williams, 1997). Newman et al. (2003) noted that only a few unintended negative consequences of the community-based arts projects (such as tiredness after the event) were ever mentioned in the reviewed literature, but observed that there were some reservations expressed as "to what extent all sections of a community are reached" (p. 12) by the projects.

It is important to note that despite the consensus on the contribution of participatory community arts to community capacity building, relatively few scholars associate this explicitly with the concepts of social capital and/or resilience (see, for example, Azmier, 2002; Matarasso, 1997). This is not surprising given Hutter and Kuhlicke's (2013) claim that, in general, there has been little research "that connects the concept of resilience to existing assumptions, theories and concepts of social science and planning research" (p. 295). This chapter aims to establish this link.

Having discussed both social capital and participatory community arts, the remainder of this chapter explores in greater depth how participatory community arts projects can generate various forms of social capital (bonding, bridging and linking) using two well-documented participatory arts projects as examples: *Closer* and *Connecting Places: Connected Lives*. It is important to note that our aim is not to present an exhaustive analysis of all participatory community arts projects but rather highlight important aspects in such projects that may contribute to, enrich even, communities' resilience. In our exploration of these two projects, we relied on secondary data, comprising academic articles, project reports, websites and a handbook on the role of the arts in building sustainable communities. We studied the available material and analysed how these projects had contributed to the social capital and resilience of the communities in which they took place.

Two participatory community arts projects

The first project we discuss is a participatory community arts project that was initiated by a housing organization to revitalize two neighbourhoods and create a thriving community. It demonstrates the potential of participatory community arts to engage community members in regeneration activities and yield benefits for the community. The second project was chosen because, in addition to illustrating the ability of participatory community arts to generate bridging capital, it highlights a specific benefit of an arts-based activity by addressing the role of material aspects in building social relationships. This project also engaged the larger community and was seen by the coordinator of the involved refugee-led community organization as far more successful than more formal activities that were also aimed at bringing the local communities together (Askins and Pain, 2011). These two projects were selected because, in contrast to many participatory community arts projects, they are relatively well documented (see also Daly, 2005; Jermyn, 2001; Reeves, 2002). This is essential for our discussion as we want to illustrate the various dimensions of social capital that participatory community arts can generate (i.e. bonding, bridging and linking), to understand the potential of participatory community arts in building community resilience. Furthermore, whereas *Closer* provides an example of a participatory community arts project that was open to the entire community and built social capital in two geographically separated neighbourhoods, *Connecting Places: Connected Lives* presents an example of a project that built social capital in an ethnically separated neighbourhood, with participants being selected based on their age and ethnicity.

In our discussions of the two projects, we first provide information on the communities where the projects took place, including the challenges they faced. We then describe the aim and process of each participatory community arts project. In our discussion, we draw out how the project addressed social capital and contributed to building resilience in the community by helping community members deal with the challenges they faced. After discussing the two projects, we briefly reflect on three critical issues that came to the fore: the importance of sustaining the impacts of participatory community arts projects, the potential downsides of projects, and difficulties in getting funding and support for participatory community arts projects.

'*Closer*'

Closer is a community-based arts project that took place in 2001 in two Liverpool neighbourhoods (Speke and Garston) that are home to a total of around 25,000 people (Beedham and Wade, 2005; Carey and Sutton, 2002, 2004). The Liverpool History Society's (LHS) website (2016) describes the neighbourhoods as the 'lost villages' of Liverpool. They are areas of significant deprivation and disadvantage, with statistics indicating a high incidence of poverty and unemployment, low skills and poor educational achievement. From the LHS website, it is apparent that Speke and Garston have been neglected for decades, being low on the regeneration priority scale, resulting in "a community suffering from appallingly decayed housing stock, significant social problems, and a high crime rate" (p. 1). The website also mentions that there has been a lack of adequate social and community facilities and that the inhabitants felt that they were often regarded as 'outsiders', an indication of low levels of social capital. This environment of neglect and desperation led to "disillusionment, distrust and disenchantment with authority" as Carey and Sutton (2002, p. 12) noted. They stated that, over the years, the communities in these neighbourhoods had been subjected to many unsuccessful 'regenerative' activities. Participation in these initiatives has always been low and tended to attract the same small group of committed community members. This is particularly indicative of a low level of linking social capital which, as explained above, is particularly important for 'communities poor in resources' as it gives them more opportunities to make their voices heard and greater access to resources (see Magis, 2010).

Closer was initiated by South Liverpool Housing (SLH, the largest social landlord in the area) in partnership with Arts in Regeneration (AiR, a locally based community arts organization). The project was an expression of SLH's mission "not just to revitalize the houses and the physical environment, but to work with all the people of Speke and Garston to create a vibrant, thriving community where people are proud to live and work" (Carey and Sutton, 2002, p. 6). Although the authors did not use the terminology, this project's mission implies that the activities were targeted at capacity building and aiming to contribute to Speke and Garston's resilience – so that the neighbourhoods would 'bounce forward'.

Closer set out to develop and deliver six arts and culture projects, each involving a professional artist collaborating with local people, in six different locations throughout Speke and Garston. Activities conducted in the context of *Closer* included two environmental arts projects that focused on the development of children's play areas, a video documentary following the redevelopment of the area in which residents were actively involved in the production and content, and an internet radio station that worked with residents from local sheltered accommodation in setting up the station (see Carey and Sutton, 2002, pp. 4–5, 2004, p. 125). In adopting a participatory approach, *Closer* aimed to create a framework for participation that would yield several benefits for the community including training and support for residents in order to increase their participation and self-reliance, and continued skills development after the completion of *Closer* by joining in other regeneration initiatives (Beedham and Wade, 2005). Such benefits contribute to a community's adaptive capacities and make it more resilient by providing the community with some level of control over its future direction (McIntosh et al., 2008).

Beedham and Wade's (2005) handbook on the role of the arts in building sustainable communities cited *Closer* as a successful and exemplary project, largely because of its ability to "bring the community together". In line with this, Carey and Sutton (2002) concluded, in their evaluation report on *Closer*, that the project met its aim of increasing participation. They found that many people were involved in the project as well as in their community. In a later publication, they noted that there was now "a greater sense of solidarity and commitment to the community from people who live and work in the area" (2004, p. 133), which they viewed as an important long-term legacy of the project. In terms of McCarthy et al.'s definition cited above, this suggests that *bonding capital* had been developed within Speke and Garston. Carey and Sutton (2002) argued that it was the project's arts focus that encouraged people to become involved. They cited (p. 25) a resident who said: "people are wary of authority, whereas with this being art it's been less formal and friendly". Participation in the *Closer* project also resulted in the development of a range of individual skills and qualities that Beedham and Wade (2005) and Carey and Sutton (2002) summarized as including: IT and broadcasting skills; organisational, budgeting, intercommunicative and social skills; increased self-confidence and assertiveness. It is noteworthy that at least some residents intended to expand these skills by "opting to attend personal capacity building courses to maximize their input into the area" (Carey and Sutton, 2004, p. 132).

Benefits of the *Closer* projects extended beyond the boundaries of the individual neighbourhoods. First, Carey and Sutton (2002) emphasized that *Closer* helped to bring the people from the two distinct areas together: prior to the project "it [was] evident that residents from both Speke and Garston view[ed] each other with a certain degree of suspicion and distrust – *'them and us'*. This project has gone some way to healing this rift" (p. 24, original emphasis). They argued that the project's arts focus had "encouraged inclusion through getting different groups of people to work together" (p. 25). The ability to collaborate, and thus expand the resources available to the community, demonstrates the building up of *bridging capital* (see Magis, 2010). Second, evidence was noted of stronger links with key agencies both within and beyond Speke and Garston (Carey and Sutton, 2004). Beedham and Wade (2005) noted that *Closer* raised the profile of SLH and changed residents' perceptions of it. They cited the project leader (the New Business Initiatives Manager from SLH), who said: "it [*Closer*] brought the community together so it was no longer a struggle to get people involved – now people trust us" (p. 45). Such relationships between individuals and institutions beyond their immediate community who have relative power over them are associated with *linking capital* (Hawkins and Maurer, 2010). As outlined earlier, and especially for disadvantaged and rundown neighbourhoods such as Speke and Garston, such linking capital is significant in expanding access to resources and opportunities (see Magis, 2010). In addition, Carey and Sutton (2002) noted that *Closer* positively changed people's perceptions of the value of art as a tool for participation and regeneration, and maintained that the dialogue between the community members and the artists greatly contributed to this. To illustrate this, they quoted a resident who stated: "because the artists came out and listened to people and explained what art can be... that was the thing, that got things going" (p. 26).

To summarize, we can conclude that *Closer* contributed to the development of bonding, bridging and linking capitals in Speke and Garston and, in this way, contributed to the resilience of the neighbourhoods by increasing the capacity of the community members "to respond to and influence change, to sustain and renew the community, and to develop new trajectories for the communities' future" (Magis, 2010, p. 402).

'Connecting places: connected lives'

Connecting Places: Connected Lives was a participatory community arts project that was conducted in Newcastle upon Tyne in the UK in 2006–2007. It involved children from African refugee and from white British backgrounds. As Askins and Pain (2011) noted, separation and hostility between existing and newly arrived groups were key current social and political issues of concern in the UK (and elsewhere). Connected to this, the notion of 'community cohesion' had become a central theme for social policy in the UK, with an "acceleration of efforts to bring different communities together" (Askins and Pain, 2011, p. 804) and the UK government placing a "high priority on the promotion of integration and development of resilient communities through the Cohesion Delivery Framework and Guidance on Meaningful Interaction" (ibid., p. 805). Askins and Pain (2011) explained that community cohesion is outlined as an attempt to build communities with four key characteristics: "a common vision and a sense of belonging for all; the valuing of diversity; similar life opportunities for all; and strong and positive relationships between people from different backgrounds and circumstances in the workplace, in schools, and within neighbourhoods" (ibid., p. 804). What resonates in this is the need to build *bridging capital* which, as explained above, exposes people to diversity, enhances their ability to work with each other and expands the resources available to them (Magis, 2010). This contributes to a community's resilience as it creates the 'glue' that helps communities to function well and deal with the challenges they face.

In fact, it was the researchers Askins and Pain themselves who initiated *Connecting Places: Connected Lives*, which "set out to use participatory art to explore emotional topographies, everyday exclusions, and notions of belonging" (Askins and Pain, 2011, p. 803; see also Durham University, 2016; Pain et al., 2007). The project was conducted in collaboration with African Community Advice North East (ACANE), a refugee-led community organization that aims to

> "support the settlement of asylum seekers and refugees from the African continent, who have been dispersed to the North-East region and Tyneside in particular, and to actively promote their integration with the host community so that they can lead full and active lives, and participate in and contribute to the community on an equal basis".
> (quoted from Involve NorthEast, 2016)

Askins and Pain (2011) explained that although "interaction was part of the collaborative framing of what the project was about", and that ACANE's manager hoped that there would also be benefits in terms of interaction from the project's process itself, that "the research was not specially designed to facilitate it" (p. 808).

Connecting Places: Connected Lives involved twenty-one children, aged five to sixteen, who met at ACANE's community centre with the researchers. They discussed and expressed their feelings about bullying and commonly held negative images of African countries, using diagrams, cartoons and sketches. Their ideas were then developed into images using acrylic paints. First, the participants focused on African countries, then on Newcastle. Subsequently, the connections between these places were discussed. The paintings were an attempt to promote positive images of African countries and of Newcastle and highlight some of the connections between them (see Askins and Pain, 2011; Durham University, 2016).

Connecting Places: Connected Lives contributed to the community in Newcastle upon Tyne by providing a meeting place for African and British children. It stimulated the building of *bridging capital* and, in this way, contributed to the community's resilience. The project engaged the local community, which Askins and Pain (2011) regarded as crucial for success in a community cohesion initiative. They noted that, for ACANE's coordinator, the project was part of a series of efforts to bring the local communities together, and was far more successful than more formal activities (which are not further specified). A quote from ACANE's coordinator illustrates this:

> "I'm happy because they [the two groups] can now even meet, because it used to be that black and white kids were not mixing very much. But

> I'm happy because we start to have those activities where they can come together and let the community know about the things that are important to them – to try to break this ice between those communities".
>
> (ibid., p. 817)

Pain et al. (2007) further reported that the participatory art techniques used in the project helped in this process of breaking down barriers between the children in the group. In addition, they were "useful for expressing feelings, ideas and images of places which are sometimes difficult to put into words" (ibid, p. 2). Not only the paintings themselves, but also the processes and discussion that went into producing them, "began to identify points of similarity between the young people from different backgrounds" (Askins and Pain, 2011, p. 809).

Reflecting on the project, Askins and Pain (2011) noted that, initially, there were negative interactions between the young participants and that "dominant social groupings and power relations were played out through the use/control of objects [that were used in the creative process]" (p. 813). In this sense, the divisive social relationships that the participants encountered in their everyday lives were also present on the site of the project. However, they noted that this changed as the project progressed and interactions between the ethnic groups increased. They stated, for example, that "as young people began to explore *shared* themes about their separate lives in the neighbourhood, unexpected new alliances began to form" (ibid., p. 811, original emphasis) and that "the young people began to interact with us [the researchers] and each other to develop the key themes and produce artwork around them" (ibid., p. 811). As such, bridges were constructed between the research participants, across the two ethnic groups, thereby generating *bridging capital.*

In their article, Askins and Pain (2011) highlighted "the materiality of art (the tools) within participatory practices (the doing of it) in contributing to a space where interactions might take place" (p. 803). They highlighted the important role played by the materials with which the participants worked: "through engaging with materials, then, interaction among the young people increased *and changed* – subtly, but there was a tangible shift in individuals' behaviours with each other" (p. 814, original emphasis). The authors explained that the materials that were used in the project (e.g. pens, tubes of paint) "appeared to suggest interactions, demand communications, and enable conversations across and between the research participants, and researchers and participants – they were *part of* our contact" (p. 813, original emphasis). For example, the participants had to share the materials around within the overall group, asked each other questions regarding the use of the materials, and used the materials in 'non-art' ways (such as using paintbrushes as swords in mock sword fights). Askins and Pain concluded that new social relationships could be prompted or enabled by the physical and embodied experiences of making art and using art-related materials.

In their *Connecting Places: Connected Lives* project, they saw how race-based divides began to break down and new relationships were formed (which were also visible beyond the project), specifically by using the 'stuff' of the art project.

Connecting Places: Connected Lives demonstrates the ability of participatory community arts to generate *bridging capital* – between ethnic groups – that can stimulate community cohesion and help in developing community resources that are beneficial in terms of increasing community resilience.

Critical reflections

Before turning to our conclusions on the value of participatory community arts in building community resilience, it is important to note three critical issues that emerged from the discussed projects.

First, in the literature on both projects, the authors identified the importance of sustaining the impacts of the participatory community arts projects. As such a long-term perspective is highly relevant considering community resilience, which requires communities that can "thrive in an environment characterized by change, uncertainty, unpredictability, and surprise" (Magis, 2010, p. 402). Although a single participatory community arts event has the potential to facilitate new social relationships, Askins and Pain (2011) argued that "policy should recognize the need for repeated activities ... if any transformative changes in relations between people are to become routinized and a new norm" (p. 818). On a similar note, Carey and Sutton (2004) stated that the real value of community development is only achieved if participatory community arts projects are sustainable. They argued that a 'long-term legacy' should be an important outcome of projects and that, ideally, "projects should not 'finish', but should evolve to meet the expanding capacity and aspirations of the community, as well as building on success" (p. 133). In considering *Closer,* they commented that there was a concern among the residents that involvement would be undermined if the successes of the project were not built upon, and that a failure to do so would undermine residents' sense of achievement and belonging.

Second, it is important to bear in mind that participatory community arts projects can also have downsides. Matarasso (1997) noted that arts projects can be poorly planned or executed, or produce negative outcomes such as damaged personal or community confidence. Further, projects could provide unequal opportunities for participation and, in this way, contribute to the exclusion of certain groups in the community (see, for example, Mattern, 2001). Some of the literature tends to ignore these negative aspects, and failed participatory community arts projects are often not documented at all (Belfiore, 2006; Guetzkow, 2002). In contrast, when reflecting on *Connecting Places: Connected Lives*, Askins and Pain (2011) quite extensively reflected on a second, in their eyes less successful, part of the project.

This second part involved a local professional artist and was intended to produce a display at an established public art site. Whereas the first part of the project was hands on, this second part was distinctly less participatory, with the artist doing all the work while the young people watched. Askins and Pain noted how this had a negative impact on relationships among the young people: "relations between young people that had previously begun to shift from avoidance to interaction to positive encounters seemed to be reverting back to longer held and enacted exclusions" (ibid., p. 812). Also, when it came to reflecting on *Closer*, Carey and Sutton (2004) provided some more critical reflections on the participatory community arts project. They reflected on some frustrations that were present in the process of planning and managing *Closer* (including in the fundraising process and in the relationships between the artists and managers involved), and noted that the short timescale of *Closer* indirectly led to some residents feeling excluded and disappointed. They explained that, because of the project's short timescale (six months), several of the micro-projects were unfinished by the time of the grand finale (a party to showcase the work that had been achieved through the project) and that this created negative feelings among some of the residents who were involved in the unfinished micro-projects.

Third, from Carey and Sutton's (2004) reflections, it becomes clear that it can be difficult to obtain the necessary funding and support for a participatory community arts project. They commented that accessing funds for *Closer* took considerable effort and was 'extremely time-consuming'. Moreover, they observed that "some fund-holders' regulations mitigate against project sustainability by ruling out bids from already existing projects" (ibid., p. 128), which they saw as a possible threat to any future development.

Conclusions

In this chapter, we argue that participatory community arts should be considered in community development processes as a means for building community resilience. Resilience policy and practice have, to date, often focused on rebuilding the economic and physical infrastructure of a community (White and O'Hare, 2014). However, as Boon et al. (2012) observed, community events that support social networks and build a sense of place deserve similar emphasis. Together with other resilience-building initiatives, they can assist communities in developing the capacity and resources to deal with the challenges they face and to flourish.

An evolutionary approach to planning for resilience, i.e. one which is more attuned to sociocultural conditions and embraces transformability (White and O'Hare, 2014), offers a suitable framework for including participatory community arts in community development processes. Participatory community arts projects can positively contribute to 'resilience-in-process' (see Davoudi, 2012) because they offer the potential to generate various forms of social capital that contribute to a community's adaptive capacity "to thrive in an environment characterized by change, uncertainty, unpredictability, and surprise" (Magis, 2010, p. 402). Generally speaking, because of the build-up of social capital, community members can become more connected to each other and to their community. Subsequently, they are more willing to contribute to their community and its development (Brennen et al., 2009; Derrett, 2003). This is important for community resilience, as resilience requires (pro-)active communities that can help themselves (Steiner and Markantoni, 2013), with community members intentionally developing "personal and collective capacity that they engage in responding to and influence change, to sustain and renew the community, and to develop new trajectories for the communities' future" (Magis, 2010, p. 402).

As discussed above, various studies have shown how participatory community arts provide a context for social interaction between various and often very different community members, bringing people together, stimulating direct social interaction and, thus, providing opportunities for building bonds (see, for example, Anwar McHenry, 2011; Guetzkow, 2002; Jermyn, 2001; Kingma, 2001; Newman et al., 2003; Williams, 1997). In the two projects we explored in depth, the arts were specifically credited with helping to involve people and to facilitate interactions. *Closer* targeted community members from two geographically separated neighbourhoods, whereas *Connecting Places, Connected Lives* involved participants from within an ethnically separated neighbourhood. Both projects illustrate the ability of participatory community arts to generate various types of social capital. By supporting social networks and building a sense of place, they are excellent examples of the kind of community events that Boon et al. (2012) urged be included in resilience-building initiatives. It is important to note that the successful projects we discussed both took place in a UK context. Other spatial contexts, as well as processes or events that put pressure on local communities (such as those discussed in other chapters of this book), may require different forms of participatory community arts projects.

Participatory community arts projects often take their cues from the everyday, lived experiences of communities and use these to formulate goals for human development (see, for example, Askins and Pain, 2011; Derrett, 2003). In doing so, they can offer interesting tools as part of a resilience policy that "is being directed towards smaller spatial scales and everyday practices" rather than "a command and control approach from central government" (Coaffee, 2013, p. 333). Coaffee (2013) further noted that such "*letting go*" by institutions and organizations is needed to "creat[e] the necessary framework for action" (p. 333, original emphasis). He regarded "this integration of a range of resiliency approaches at the *local* level" as representing "the latest generation of resilience practices that planners are increasingly being asked to adopt" (p. 325, original emphasis).

However, Christopherson et al. (2010, p. 9) emphasized that "we should avoid assuming that the same drivers of change are at work everywhere and if we just pull the right levers, the appropriate drivers will respond and deliver the required outcomes". We would, therefore, like to stress the need to take the specific socio-spatial context in which a participatory community arts project is planned into account when planning for resilience, as each community will have its own characteristics and needs.

In addition, one should be aware of the importance of sustaining the impacts of participatory community arts projects, of the potential downsides of projects, and of the difficulties in obtaining funding and support for projects – critical issues that came to the fore in the two cases we investigated. Mattern (2001) provided a good example of the dividing potential of the arts, showing that they can also act more as a 'social solvent', dividing two groups, than as a 'social glue'. Moreover, when discussing the value of participatory community arts in building community resilience, it is important to note, as Burnell (2012) argued, that they cannot alone resolve the complex socioeconomic issues that many communities face. Nevertheless, Burnell (2012) promoted culture as "an essential resource for change" (p. 138), arguing that the arts and cultural resources "provide a wide range of diverse opportunities aimed at unlocking intangible assets and social capital – opportunities that can lead to an increase in tangible assets being accumulated with the aim of reducing vulnerability and building more resilient and sustainable communities" (p. 147). A view which our findings support.

References

Anwar McHenry, J. (2009). A place for the arts in rural revitalization and the well-being of Australian rural communities. *Rural Society*, 19(1), pp. 60–70.

Anwar McHenry, J. (2011). Rural empowerment through the arts: The role of the arts in civic and social participation in the Mid West region of Western Australia. *Journal of Rural Studies*, 27, pp. 245–253.

Askins, K. & Pain, R. (2011). Contact zones: Participation, materiality, and the messiness of interaction. *Environment and Planning D: Society and Space*, 29, pp. 803–821.

Azmier, J.J. (2002). *Culture and Economic Competitiveness: An Emerging Role for the Arts in Canada*. A Western Cities Project Discussion Paper, Canada West Foundation.

Beedham, G. & Wade, A. (2005). *Creative Neighbourhoods: The Role of the Arts in Building Sustainable Communities*. Chingford: Aston Housing Consultancy.

Beel, D.E., Wallace, C.D., Webster, G., Nguyen, H., Tait, E., Macleod, M. & Mellish, C. (2015). Cultural resilience: The production of rural community heritage, digital archives and the role of volunteers. *Journal of Rural Studies*, pp. 1–10. http://dx.doi.org/10.1016/j.jrurstud.2015.05.002.

Belfiore, E. (2006). The social impacts of the arts – Myth or reality? In: M. Mirza (Ed.). *Culture Vultures: Is UK Arts Policy Damaging the Arts?* (pp. 20–37). London: Policy Exchange Limited.

Beugelsdijk, S. & Smulders, S. (2009). Bonding and bridging social capital and economic growth. *CentER Discussion Paper*, No. 2009–27.

Bishop, C. (2006). The social turn: Collaboration and its discontents. *Artforum*, 44(6), pp. 178–183.

Boon, H.J., Millar, J., Lake, D., Cottrell, A. & King, D. (2012). *Recovery from Disaster: Resilience, Adaptability and Perceptions of Climate Change. Its Effect on Perceptions of Climate Change Risk and on Adaptive Behaviours to Prevent, Prepare, and Respond to Future Climate Contingencies*. Gold Coast: National Climate Change Adaptation Research Facility.

Brennen, M.A., Flint, C.G. & Luloff, A.E. (2009). Bringing together local culture and rural development: Findings from Ireland, Pennsylvania and Alaska. *Sociologica Ruralis*, 49(1), pp. 97–112.

Burnell, J. (2012). Small change: Understanding cultural action as a resource for unlocking assets and building resilience in communities. *Community Development Journal*, 48(1), pp. 134–150.

Carey, P. & Sutton, S. (2002). *Closer: An Evaluation of a Community Arts and Regeneration Initiative*. Liverpool: John Moores University.

Carey, P. & Sutton, S. (2004). Community development through participatory arts: Lessons learned from a community arts and regeneration project in South Liverpool. *Community Development Journal*, 39(2), pp. 123–134.

Chandler, D. (2014). *Resilience. The Governance of Complexity*. Abingdon: Routledge.

Christopherson, S., Michie, J. & Tyler, P. (2010). Regional resilience: Theoretical and empirical perspectives. *Cambridge Journal of Regions, Economy and Society*, 3(1), pp. 3–10.

Coaffee, J. (2013). Towards new-generation urban resilience in planning practice: From securitization to integrated place making. *Planning Practice & Research*, 28(3), pp. 323–339.

Daly, S. (2005). *Social Capital and the Cultural Sector*. London: Centre for Civil Society.

Davoudi, S. (2012). Resilience: A bridging concept or a dead end? *Planning Theory and Practice*, 13(2), pp. 299–307.

Delfmann, H., Markantoni, M. & van Hoven, B. (2013). The role of side activities in building rural resilience: The case study of Kiel-Windeweer (the Netherlands). In: J. Revilla Diez & C. Tamasy (Eds.), *Regional Resilience, Economy and Society* (pp. 251–268). Farnham, UK: Ashgate Publishing.

Derrett, R. (2003). Making sense of how festivals demonstrate a community's sense of place. *Event Management*, 8(1), pp. 49–58.

Dibden, J. & Cocklin, C. (2005). Introduction. In: C. Cocklin & J. Dibden (Eds.), *Sustainability and Change in Rural Australia* (pp. 1–18). Sydney: University of New South Wales Press Ltd.

Durham University (2016). *Art project with ACANE*. www.dur.ac.uk/beacon/socialjustice/researchprojects/acane/ [Accessed on 07/04/2016].

Elstow, L. (2013). *Beyond Z-Cards and Grab Bags: Community Resilience in Urban Communities*. Final Report for Winston Churchill Memorial Trust. www.wcmt.org.uk/sites/default/files/migrated-reports/1121_1.pdf [Accessed on 07/04/2016].

Guetzkow, J. (2002). *How the Arts Impact Communities: An Introduction to the Literature on Arts Impact Studies*. Working Paper Series, 20, Princeton University, Center for Arts and Cultural Policy Studies.

Hawkins, R.L. & Maurer, K. (2010). Bonding, bridging and linking: How social capital operated in New Orleans following hurricane Katrina. *British Journal of Social Work*, 40, pp. 1777–1793.

Healy, T. & Côté, S. (2001). *The Well-being of Nations. The Role of Human and Social Capital.* Report of the Centre for Educational Research and Innovation at the OECD.

Hutter, G. & Kuhlicke, C. (2013). Resilience, talk and action: Exploring the meanings of resilience in the context of planning and institutions. *Planning, Practice & Research*, 28(3), pp. 294–306.

Involve NorthEast (2016). *ACANE – African Community Advice North East.* www.healthsignpostdirectory.org.uk/organisation.asp?org=322 [Accessed on 07/04/2016].

Jermyn, H. (2001). *The Arts and Social Exclusion: A Review Prepared for the Arts Council of England.* London: Arts Council of England.

Kay, A. (2000). Art and community development: The role the arts have in regenerating communities. *Community Development Journal*, 35(4), pp. 414–424.

Kingma, O. (2001). *Enabling Communities through the Arts: Case Studies from the Community Cultural Development Fund of the Australia Council.* Sydney: Australia Council.

Larsen, L., Harlan, S.L., Bolin, B., Hackett, E.J., Hope, D., Kirby, A., Nelson, A., Rex, T.R. & Wolf, S. (2004). Bonding and bridging. Understanding the relationship between social capital and civic action. *Journal of Planning Education and Research*, 24(64), pp. 64–77.

Liverpool History Society (2016). *The 'Lost Villages' of Garston & Speke.* www.liverpoolhistorysociety.org.uk/garston-speke/ [Accessed on 07/04/2016].

Lovell, S.A. (2009). Social capital: The Panacea for community? *Geography Compass*, 3(2), pp. 781–796.

Magis, K. (2010). Community resilience: An indicator of social sustainability. *Society & Natural Resources. An International Journal*, 23(5), pp. 401–416.

Matarasso, F. (1997). *Use or Ornament? The Social Impact of Participation in the Arts.* Stroud: Comedia.

Mattern, M. (2001). Art and community development in Santa Ana, California: The promise and the reality. *The Journal of Arts Management, Law and Society*, 30(4), pp. 301–315.

McCarthy, K., Ondaatje, E., Zakaras, L. & Brooks, A. (2004). *Gifts of the Muse: Reframing the Debate About the Benefits of the Arts.* Santa Monica: RAND Corporation.

McIntosh, A., Stayner, R., Carrington, K., Rolley, F., Scott, J. & Sorensen, T. (2008). *Resilience in Rural Communities: Literature Review.* Armidale: University of New England.

Newman, T., Curtis, K. & Stephens, J. (2003). Do community-based arts projects result in social gains? A review of the literature. *Community Development Journal*, 38(4), pp. 310–322.

Ontario Arts Council (1998). *Community Arts Workbook.* Toronto: Ontario Arts Council.

Pain, R., Askins, K. & Kitoko, G. (2007). *Connecting Places, Connected Lives. An Anti-bullying art Project.* Durham, NC: Durham University.

Portes, A. (1998). Social capital: Its origins and applications in modern sociology. *Annual Review of Sociology*, 24, pp. 1–24.

Putnam, R.D. (1995). Bowling alone: America's declining social capital. *Journal of Democracy*, 6(1), pp. 65–78.

Reeves, M. (2002). *Measuring the Economic and Social Impact of the Arts: A Review*. London: Arts Council of England.

Sampson, R.J., Raudenbush, S.W. & Earls, F. (1997). Neighborhoods and violent crime: A multilevel study of collective efficacy. *Science*, 227, pp. 918–924.

Skerratt, S. & Steiner, A. (2013). Working with communities-of-place: Complexities of empowerment. *Local Economy*, 28(3), pp. 320–338.

Stehlik, D. (2003). Australian drought as lived experience: Social and community impacts. In: L.C. Botterill & M. Fisher (Eds.), *Beyond Drought: People, Policy and Perspectives* (pp. 87–108). Melbourne: CSIRO Publishing.

Steiner, A. & Markantoni, M. (2013). Unpacking community resilience through capacity for change. *Community Development Journal*, 48(3), pp. 1–19.

Weichselgartner, J. & Kelman, I. (2014). Geographies of resilience: Challenges and opportunities of a descriptive concept. *Progress in Human Geography*, 39(3), pp. 1–19.

White, I. & O'Hare, P. (2014). From rhetoric to reality: Which resilience, why resilience, and whose resilience in spatial planning? *Environment and Planning C: Government and Policy*, 32(5), pp. 834–950.

Wilding, N. (2011). *Exploring Community Resilience in Times of Rapid Change*. Dunfermline: Fiery Spirits Community of Practice.

Williams, D. (1997). *The Social Impact of Arts Programs. How The Arts Measure Up: Australian Research into the Social Impact*. Working Paper 8, Stroud: Comedia.

Wilson, G.A. (2012). Community resilience, globalization, and transitional pathways of decision-making. *Geoforum*, 43, pp. 1218–1231.

Woodhouse, A. (2006). Social capital and economic development in regional Australia. A case study. *Journal of Rural Studies*, 22, pp. 83–94.

Woolcock, M. (2001). The place of social capital in understanding social and economic outcomes. *Canadian Journal of Policy Research*, 2(1), pp. 11–17.

12 "If we are not united, our lives will be very difficult"[1]

Resilience from the perspective of slum dwellers in Pedda Jalaripeta (India)

Deepika Andavarapu and Mahyar Arefi

Introduction

Roughly a billion people in developing countries live in slums, and this number is slated to double by 2030 (World Bank, 2013). Large-scale urbanization coupled with unaffordable housing is a reason for the mushrooming of slums (UN-Habitat, 2010). Given their worldwide prevalence, slums are attracting attention from planning professionals and academics. Journals such as Planning Theory and Practice (2011), Built Environment (2011), City (2011), and International Development Planning Review (2012), or Habitat International have had special issues dedicated to slums. It is important to note, that the word 'slum' is loose and considered deprecatory; it has many connotations and meanings, and some of the more sensitive, politically correct lexicons ban the term (Gilbert, 2007). Despite these limitations, we refer to 'slum' in this chapter for two key reasons. First, studies we draw from such as UN-Habitat's State of the World Cities (2010), the World Bank's Global Monitoring Report (2013), or Greater Visakhapatnam Slum Household Survey (GVMC, 2009) refer to these settlements as slums. Second, in countries like India and Thailand, an official slum notification[2] is a prerequisite to qualify for several government aid programmes (i.e., lower water fees, reduced electricity bills, and low-interest housing loans). In these countries, poor communities embrace the term slum and use their political leverage to become identified as one (Naidu, 2006).

Slum resilience literature focuses on disasters such as flooding (Chatterjee, 2010; Wilhelm, 2011; Ajibade et al., 2013), or food (in)security (Keck and Etzold, 2013), which residents have endured, but does not explicitly address 'why' or 'how' residents with modest resources fight for rebuilding or protecting their community. In this chapter, drawing on the concept of social capital, we explore these questions in the Pedda Jalaripeta slum of Visakhapatnam, India. This study expands the resilience scholarship by highlighting lived experiences of community members and their active engagement in developing and enhancing community resilience despite their vulnerable social and spatial position. The chapter is structured as follows.

First, we briefly discuss our theoretical framework for discussing 'slum resilience'. We then discuss the outcomes of our research focussing on two examples that emerged from the data, i.e. (1) recovery and developing resilience after a major fire, and (2) adaptation and enhancing resilience in anticipation of threats imposed by tourism development and gentrification.

Slum resilience

After its introduction in ecological thinking by Holling in 1973, resilience gained traction and prominence across a wide array of discourses from disaster and crisis management to climate change and urban planning. Resilience thinking, although ubiquitous, is far from being accepted as a normative urban planning theory. The multiple meanings and interpretations of resilience created a rich interdisciplinary scholarship in urban planning literature (Patulny and Svendsen, 2007; Dovey, 2012; Davoudi et al., 2013; Desouza and Flanery, 2013; Andavarapu and Arefi, 2015).

In light of our focus on slum resilience, yet without providing an exhaustive list, we highlight six interpretations of resilience which have gained popularity among urban planners and policymakers. Engineers dealing with post-disaster recovery from disasters are interested in devising systems that aim to return to pre-disaster conditions (Campanella, 2006; Haigh and Amaratunga, 2012). Community activists and policy analysts seem to care more about the *equilibrium resilience* or a preferred alternative rather than moving towards the original state (Pickett et al., 2004; Arefi, 2011). *Evolutionary resilience* challenges the existence of an equilibrium and suggests that it is inherent to any system to evolve and change with or without external disturbances (Davoudi et al., 2013). The *adaptive cycles* theory posits that socio-ecological systems go through four phases of development in their life cycle: growth/exploitation, conservation, release/creative destruction, and reorganization (Gunderson and Holling, 2002; Dovey, 2012). *Community resilience* subsequently refers to the development of personal and collective capacities of communities to respond and influence change to sustain and renew the community (Magis, 2010). *Social resilience* finally is quite like this but focuses on three specified capacities, i.e. coping, adapting and transforming (Keck and Sakdapolrak, 2013; Chelleri et al., 2015). Of the six interpretations outlined here, *social resilience* is the most commonly used definition to study how slums and slum residents respond to disasters (Jabeen et al., 2010; Chatterjee, 2011; Wilhelm, 2011; Jabareen, 2013; Keck and Etzold, 2013). In relation to our case study, the identified capacities are interesting as they incorporate both the long-term (gentrification or eviction threats) and short-term and more immediate (flooding, fires, or cyclones) challenges that slum dwellers face. While in former cases, the goal is to seek long-term stability, the latter exemplifies extraordinary conditions of finding immediate shelter and safety. The activities and processes within the three capacities are characterised by the utilisation of different forms of social capital. Since we draw on the concepts of social resilience as well as social capital in the discussion of our case study below, we briefly elaborate on the three capacities and provide a definition of social capital in the following section.

The first capacity, '*coping capacity*', describes the slum dwellers' immediate post-disaster actions. These include activities such as friends and neighbours searching for missing people, rescuing young and elderly, sharing food and comfort when those resources are dwindling (Jabeen et al., 2010; Chatterjee, 2011; Wilhelm, 2011; Keck and Sakdapolrak, 2013). In most countries, institutional relief of goods and other forms of government or private assistance are typically not widely available or accessible to slum dwellers. In those cases, the slum dwellers rely on their own networks in the village (Chatterjee, 2010; Braun and Aßheuer, 2011).

Adaptation differs from coping by referring to the process of adjustment following unpredictable sudden shocks whereby communities learn how to prepare for disasters and its long-term impacts. The second capacity '*adaptive capacity*' in the context of slum dwellers, refers to their proactive practices before disasters strike (fire, flood or eviction) (Chatterjee, 2010; Jabeen et al., 2010). These practices are often low-cost, crude techniques that would help the community to regain normalcy after the disaster. For example, slum residents work together to widen and cover the drains, establish security systems to prevent looting (Jabeen et al., 2010; Wilhelm, 2011). They pool their resources, so the residents have access to food and water during and immediately after the disaster (Wilhelm, 2011) and maintain close relations with the local grocer to access food at credit (Keck and Etzold, 2013). In Jakarta, Indonesia, residents in slums that are prone to flooding created an informal warning system by networking with floodgate operators and relatives and friends living upstream (Wilhelm, 2011).

Third, '*transformative capacity*' represents the slum's transition to a more prosperous mode. Physical transformation refers to redevelopment efforts where services such as roads, water, sewer and electricity, are extended into needy communities, and permanent houses are constructed. It must be noted that the physical transformation of slums or slum redevelopments can be controversial since they are often poorly built, and if constructed well, they are prone to gentrification leading to the eviction of original dwellers and loss of livelihood (Peattie, 1982; Andavarapu and Edelman, 2013; Patel, 2013). The social transformation of slums entails educating and empowering people, which is possible if initiated or facilitated by government or non-government agencies (see, for example, Aldrich, 2011; Islam and Walkerden, 2014). Unlike coping and adapting, the transformation of slums needs significant capital and/or knowledge from external sources.

The previous discussion of the three capacities implies that social resilience relies, at least to some extent, on the development and mobilisation of bonding, bridging and linking social capital. Bonding and bridging capitals represent the internal horizontal linkages within the community (Putnam,

2001; Pelling and High, 2005; Islam and Walkerden, 2014). *'Bonding capital'* is shared among individuals who have similar ethnic and religious identities. These horizontal linkages provide critical services in the immediate aftermath of a disaster. These networks typically represent relationships between immediate family members and relatives. *'Bridging capital'*, on the other hand, are social relationships of exchange between people with common interests but contrasting social identity (Islam and Walkerden, 2014). Several scholars suggest that the slum dwellers' bonding and bridging capital plays a significant role in coping and adapting with disasters, since regardless of the disaster's magnitude, mutual help and support are dominant features in times of crises (Pelling and High, 2005; Chatterjee, 2010; Jabeen et al., 2010; Braun and Aßheuer, 2011; Wilhelm, 2011; Ajibade et al., 2013; Keck and Etzold, 2013; Islam and Walkerden, 2014). Nevertheless, Elliot et al. (2010) assert that even when communities are willing to combat disasters, their efforts often fail. For example, many poor urban neighbourhoods in New Orleans failed to revive after the Katrina, and only those communities with linking capital to external agencies survived Katrina. *'Linking capital'* refers to vertical cross-group boundaries between residents and government or non-government organizations (Putnam, 2001; Pelling and High, 2005; Islam and Walkerden, 2014). These networks can provide political, economic, or knowledge-based support to residents, and often provide the residents with much-needed resources not just to recover and bounce back, but also to transform to a better physical state.

Introducing Pedda Jalaripeta

Visakhapatnam (Figure 12.1) is the largest city in the State of Andhra Pradesh with a population of 1.7 million people. It has the highest percentage of residents living in slums; 44.1% of the city residents live in the 654-slums in the city (Indian Census, 2011).

Pedda Jalaripeta is the largest and oldest slum in the city, it has a little over 7,000 people living on roughly 32-acres. Interestingly, three of the top tourist destinations in Visakhapatnam are in close proximity of the Pedda Jalaripeta slum and Five-star hotels and high-rise buildings surround the slum.

Pedda Jalaripeta, which literally translates as 'large fishing village', could be characterised as a low-income fishing village where 75% of the adults still depend on fishing as their livelihood (Central Marine Fisheries Research Institute, 2005; Immanuell and Rao, 2012). More than 90% of the residents earn less than $1.25 per day, which is below the international poverty line (GVMC, 2009). Nearly 88.5% of Pedda Jalaripeta residents are Hindus and belong to the Jalari caste (GVMC, 2009).

An important feature of Pedda Jalaripeta is its beach: The section of Visakhapatnam beach along Pedda Jalaripeta slum mainly functions as a fishing beach. The fishing beach is an ecological and economic resource (Immanuell and Rao, 2012), and also acts as the social gathering space for

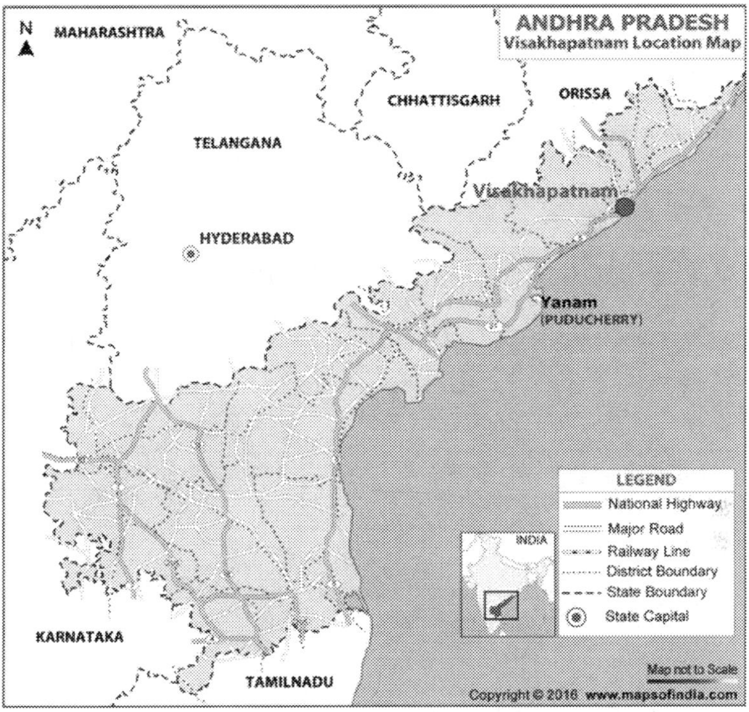

Figure 12.1 Location map of City of Visakhapatnam.
Source: Mapsofindia.com.

men. This is where men store their boats, prepare to go fishing and repair their nets but also where they rest and come to consume (large volumes of) alcohol (Figure 12.2).

With regards to its social organisation, we also wish to highlight the importance of the Grama-Sabha for the slum. Grama-Sabhas are ancient forms of village assemblies in India. These organizations strengthen the communities' bonding and bridging capital through dispute resolution and managing religious events (Aldrich, 2011). Pedda Jalaripeta's Grama-Sabha has existed since before the community was designated as a slum in 1969, and continues to be active to date. For example, it organizes ten – twelve religious festivals such as Poleramma-Jatara, Nookalamma-Jatara, Sri Rama Navami (each of these festivals is aimed at appeasing a Goddess (Poleramma or Nookalamma) or God (Ram)) year-round. As we will discuss below, recently it has taken on an important role in the redevelopment of the slum following a major fire.

Ceremonies and construction activities impose economic burdens, but residents are typically willing to bear them if they help them build their internal and external social networks. The resulting bonding capital is

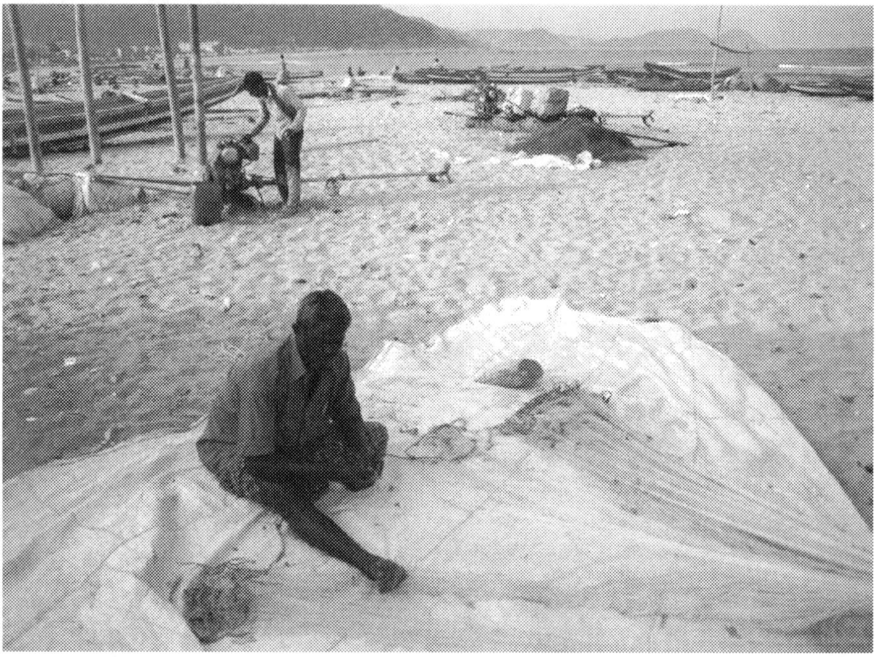

Figure 12.2 Fishermen mending the nets.
Source: Authors.

critical for Pedda Jalaripeta, since, during the off-shore fishing ventures, fishermen rely on friends and family in the nearby boats for first-aid and emergency evacuation. These networks built on the ground save lives on the sea (Focus group, 30 March 2014). One of our respondents commented:

> If we are not united our lives will be very difficult. If we are united here, then when we go in to the sea we help each other out and save each other. So that is the reason for our unity. If someone falls in to the sea, the other person who is fishing far away needs to feel the need to go and save this person. Unity is our strength otherwise we cannot survive. That's why we build temples and conduct festivals. Our safety on the sea is dependent on our unity on the ground.
>
> *(Informal Interview with Retired Senior Fisherman on 22 March 2015)*

In 2006, Grama-Sabha organized a donation campaign for building the Ramalayam temple (Figure 12.3). The slum residents donated three days

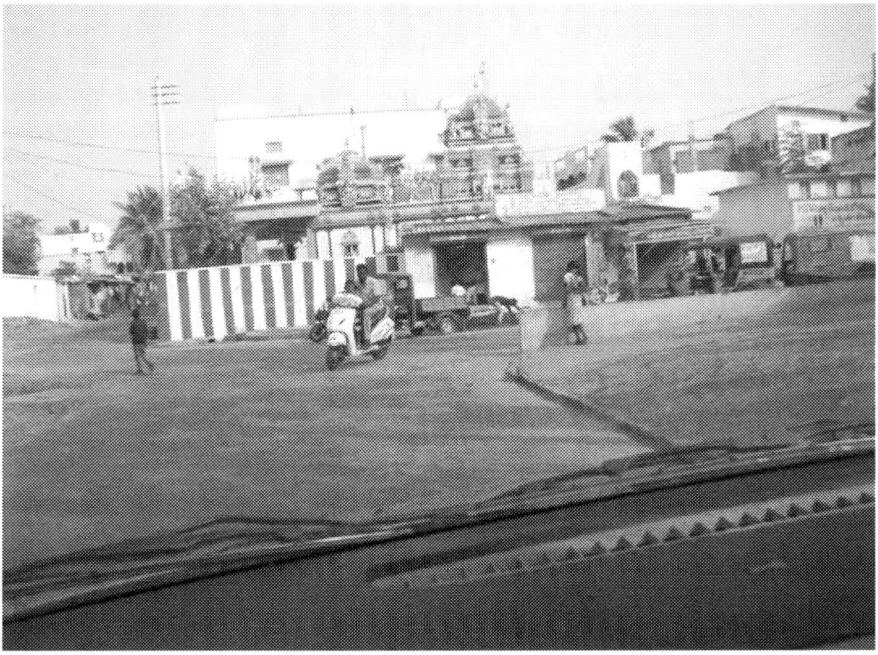

Figure 12.3 Ramalayam temple.
Source: Authors.

of fishing catch equivalent to 1,500,000[3] Indian rupees. The residents continue to donate 1% of their income voluntarily for the temple upkeep and maintenance. Below is an excerpt from the Grama-Sabha president about this effort:

AUTHOR: do you think everyone donates (1% of their income)?
GRAMA SABHA PRESIDENT: In June/July and January/December we (the temple) get donations around 32,000 or 35,000 rupees. The other months we get anywhere from 15,000–20,000 rupees. Those four months are the season for getting fish so our donations in temple are higher in those 4 months. So, yes, I believe that the fishermen donate 1% of their income for the temple upkeep

Over the past forty years, despite multiple challenges, the slum of Pedda Jalaripeta retained its social, cultural and economic identity as a fishing village. It avoided alternative undesirable states, including loss of local control, loss of fishing, gentrification and eviction. In the sections below, we further elaborate on these challenges and how the community has dealt with them.

Methods: data sources and collection

From March to July 2014, Andavarapu, a co-author of this study, spent 15 hours a week in Pedda Jalaripeta to observe and collect data. Andavarapu is a native of the region and is fluent (spoken and written) in the local language (Telugu) both of which are critical for this qualitative ethnographic study.

Fieldwork comprised four sets of activities: (1) observations in popular parts of the slum such as streets, temples and the Pedda Jalaripeta beach; (2) structured interviews with government officials and NGO representatives; (3) casual conversation and informal interviews with slum residents (both fishermen and non-fishermen) in their homes, streets and on the beach; and (4) three focus group meetings with senior fishermen, younger fishermen, and women. Due to the high number of residents who are are fishermen, their experiences and perspectives on developments in Pedda Jalaripeta were crucial in this project.

Observations

The aim of the observations is to gain a deeper understanding of and study the social and cultural bonds within the community. The observations of, for example, the spatial layout of the community, use of public/private space, participation in religious festivals (polaramma jatara), and the feasts on streets were recorded. Andavarapu attended several community affairs including public information meetings organized by the Department of Fisheries, marine cooperative society elections, women's micro-savings group meeting, and the executive board meetings of the Fishermen Youth Welfare Association (FYWA). The researcher entered these observations in a research journal on a daily basis.

Formal interviews

The formal interviews focused on understanding Pedda Jalaripeta's temporal and historical growth, its social capital, and spatial resources. Specifically, our questions were focused on the evolution and history of Pedda Jalaripeta slum, the government funds and projects in the region over the past forty years. We also aimed to obtain a better understanding of the interaction, or lack thereof, between the government agencies and the slum residents. We conducted ten formal interviews with officials from the Department of Fisheries and the Greater Visakhapatnam Municipal Corporation[4]. The interviews lasted on average 45-minutes and several officials were interviewed multiple times.

In addition to government officials, Pedda Jalaripeta community leaders were interviewed[5]. The purpose of these interviews was to understand the history of the slum, the challenges it faced and how it survived them. These interviews took one hour on average.

Informal interviews

The aim of the informal interviews was to understand the day to day challenges of Pedda Jalaripeta slum residents. The purpose of the formal interviews was to learn how the community transformed and the informal interviews revealed what those changes mean to the community members. The informal interviews were conversational but were designed to gain an understanding of resilience and social capital within the community.

All the interviews with the residents were conducted in Telugu (local language) but were translated and transcribed into English for the purpose of data analysis. Key informants were recruited to facilitate conducting the interviews. The key informants introduced the slum residents to Andavarapu and assisted in cultural interpretation. These informants helped to break the ice when the researcher initially met and interacted with the community residents. The three key informants (Past President of Marine Co-operative Society, President of Fishermen Youth Welfare Association and President of FYWA's Women's Co-operative Unit) represent the three primary cohorts within the community (senior fishermen, young fishermen, and women). In addition to these three cohorts, other non-fishermen members of the community were interviewed.

Focus groups

Three focus groups were organized with respectively a group of women, young fishermen, and senior fishermen to explore shared experiences and meanings regarding Pedda Jalaripeta community's resilience, the challenges that the community faced over the past 40-years, the measures they took to survive those challenges, and why the residents fought for their community.

The subsequent section will discuss three key findings that emerged from the analysis of the data, i.e (1) The Pedda Jalaripeta community survived two major disasters over the past thirty years (fire and gentrification/eviction); (2) Retaining access to the beach and coastline and the streets and public space of the Pedda Jalaripeta community motivates the residents to fight for their community and invest time and money, and (3) Despite socio-economic and structural disadvantages, the community proved resourceful and creative in the recovery from a disaster and threat by drawing on different forms of social capital.

"Now we have a better life"[6] – building resilience in Pedda Jalaripeta slum

As noted before, Pedda Jalaripeta faced several disasters and threats of both natural and human origin. In this research, the fire of 1983, as well as recent tourism developments, emerged as central themes. Drawing on our empirical research, we briefly describe both themes in the following part. We then address how the village recovered and developed both in terms of its social and built context.

The fire of 1983

In the middle of the night on 17 December 1983, an election banner hanging near the huts caught fire, and the fire spread throughout the settlement. Our interviews with Government Officials, slum residents and key informants, revealed that 600 of the 800 huts in the slum were burned to the ground. Below are some excerpts from our interviews regarding the incident. The residents whose houses were burned lost everything.

> *When our houses burned down, we ran towards the sea. Since it was winter, we were holding on to blankets and we were shivering. (Respondent in a senior citizen focus group interview on 22 May 2014).*
>
> *My wife was pregnant at that time so my mother took her away from the crowd. I was helping the rest of the residents and could not accompany them. After the rescue work, I started looking for them but it was so chaotic I could not find them. I finally found them away from the crowd sitting in the dark, I was very relieved to find them. My wife gave birth to our son three days after the fire. (President of the Grama-Sabha on 3 April 2014).*
>
> *After the fire we had nowhere to live, some of us lived with our friends and relatives while other built new temporary shacks closer to the beach. (Marine Co-operative president on 22 March2014).*

These quotes suggest that residents had to rescue themselves and had nowhere to go after the fire broke out. In the immediate aftermath of the fire, residents drew on their networks of friends and family to help with the provision of food and shelter.

As part of the recovery and redevelopment of the village, the regional government aimed to deliver support through the Slum Improvement Programme (SIP). The programme was an attempt to improve the living conditions, health and incomes of 190,000 people living in 170 slums across the city of Visakhapatnam. Specifically, the SIP programme included infrastructure improvements (roads, drainage, water pipes, street lights and others), health programmes (primary health centres, nutrition camps, and others) and socio-economic programmes (pre-school education centres, non-formal education centres, adult education centres, reading rooms and others) (Abelson, 1996; Amis and Kumar, 2000; GVMC, 2012). Respondents to this research recall that government officials wanted the slum dwellers to leave their houses to start the redevelopment under the SIP programme. However, residents did not trust the government officials, rejected the redevelopment proposal, and refused to abandon their homes.

An important turning point was the mediation between government and village residents by a local official who understood and successfully conveyed the need for involving trusted, place-based leaders in the redevelopment process. The elected representative of the Pedda Jalaripeta community at the time (Member of Legislative Assembly, MLA) convinced the residents that he would oversee the redevelopment efforts. The MLA at that time was a Jalari born and raised in Pedda Jalaripeta. The residents trusted him and vacated their homes (Personal interviews with Grama Sabha President on 3 April 2014; Marine Co-operative Society Past President on 22 March 2014; and Grama Sabha Secretary on 22 March 2014). The MLA convinced the municipal officers in charge of the redevelopment to appoint the community's Grama-Sabha village assembly as the Neighbourhood Committee in charge of the redevelopment. A key advantage of acknowledging the authority of the Grama-Sabha village assembly was that residents were already familiar with their model of communal investment, for example, in the case of maintaining the temple (see also introduction of Pedda Jalaripeta above).

The way in which the SIP programme was realised in Pedda Jalaripeta was based on John Turner's idea of 'self-help housing' (Turner, 1976). Under this policy, the government lays out the infrastructure (water, sewer, and roads) without constructing the homes. The idea of self-help housing is that the urban poor could mobilize their assets to improve their living conditions (Turner, 1976). The assumption here is that slum residents will strategically upgrade their housing and living facilities while weighing their changing priorities throughout the course of their lives (Nakamura, 2014). Following the Turner model, the Greater Visakhapatnam Municipal Corporation allotted land parcels, building material and limited funding to residents who lost their houses in the fire. The Grama-Sabha monitored the redevelopment and allotted the redeveloped subdivisions to the rightful owners. The redevelopment in Pedda Jalaripeta involved two phases: 432 lots were assigned in the first phase (1984–85), and 50 lots in the second phase (1990–91). Since the residents were responsible for design and construction, homes were personalized per individual taste, and the construction remains still intact after multiple generations (GVMC, 2012).

The following is an excerpt from a senior fisherman in Pedda Jalaripeta who witnessed the redevelopment:

> *In 1984, the government gave us a 60-gajas of land (540 sq.feet). They gave us some rods, cement, gave us Rs. 30,000 ($500) worth of building material. So, we added another Rs. 60,000 and built these houses for a total of Rs. 90,000. But not all of us got the scheme* (Serviced lots were only allotted to the residents who lost their houses in the fire). *I did not get the scheme I built my house by myself. (Marine Cooperative Society Past President on* 15 March 2014*).*

In the context of discussing the development of resilient slums, it is interesting to note that the Turner model was applied in recovery processes in countries like Chile, Pakistan, Iraq, Colombia and Turkey, but many of these programmes failed either due to poor quality construction, infrastructure failures or gentrification after the redevelopment (Peattie, 1982). Pedda Jalaripeta's redevelopment after the fire, however, is narrated by respondents to this research as a success story. This success is largely due to the mobilisation of bonding and bridging capital within the village as well as linking capital facilitated by a key local politician (the MLA).

The comprehensive slum improvement programme resulted in an overall improvement in the health and education of Pedda Jalaripeta community residents. According to the municipal household survey, health, education, birth control, and quality-of-life have significantly improved after redevelopment (GVMC, 2009). In the interviews, these issues frequently came up as well. The residents, especially the older citizens, observed some of the changes in the community within just one generation:

> *Our ancestors used to go fishing with just a loin-cloth. Today, the fishermen are wearing pants while fishing, so we don't know if it's a fisherman or a student. Civilization has increased and has come into our village. (Retired Senior Fisherman on* 22 March 2014*).*
>
> *...civilization has increased, the style has increased. People are also buying new stuff, new clothes, new appliances (TV, fridge). Now people have more money, everybody is working back then we used to have 4 or 5 kids. Now days it is only one or two kids and then operations (family planning). So now they have a better life. They are also educating their kids. (Senior Fisherwoman on 1 April 2014).*

The above excerpts illustrate some differences in the fishermen's lives that were attributed to redevelopment. During the interviews, the residents used the word 'nagarikata' which translates into civilization. The older generation comments on the speed at which younger residents adapted to an 'urban way of life'. They name characteristics typically associated with the city such as education, birth control, and even the use of household appliances (TV, fridge, gas stove, et etera.) which were not part of Pedda Jalaripeta's lifestyle before the redevelopment. It is important to note here, that despite the observed infrastructural and lifestyle changes, the residents we interviewed felt their shared cultural identity as low-income fishing village had been retained.

The threat of gentrification

After the fire in 1983, Pedda Jalaripeta faced a process which can be considered as a second disaster. In early 2000, the slum witnessed a multitude of tourist development projects in and around the community, which not only threatened to gentrify but also challenged the community's livelihood (Equations, 2008; Philipose, 2013). Although gentrification may not immediately be associated with disaster, especially in comparison to potentially deadly consequences of a tsunami or a fire, respondents to this research highlighted tourism developments and gentrification as a key threat to the village. In addition, this example elicited an important process of building community strength and resilience and it shows a different way of 'bouncing forward' not by drawing on the old, established structures of leadership as in the case or the fire and development after that, but instead by drawing on skills, knowledge and motivation of the younger generation.

Previous research has shown that tourism oriented development along the fishing beaches has a detrimental effect on fishermen (Derman and Ferguson, 1995; Benansio et al., 2016). Fishermen lose access to fishing grounds and their fishing gear is often destroyed due to tourist activities such as diving, snorkelling, boat riding and others. Employment in the tourism sector is rarely an option for these fishermen because of their low education background (Derman and Ferguson, 1995; Benansio et al., 2016). As noted above, nearly three quarters of residents of the Pedda Jalaripeta community have limited education and would struggle to find employment in tourism sector (GVMC, 2009). In addition to the loss of fishing resources, any gentrification or redevelopment would result in evicting nearly 65% of Pedda Jalaripeta slum residents. Only about 35% of the households in Pedda Jalaripeta community have possession certificates or some form of rights or documents to their houses (GVMC, 2009). The other 65% of the residents are living on encroached government or private land. Pedda Jalaripeta community residents who do not possess the legal rights are not eligible for any form of compensation in case of gentrification or redevelopment.

In the remainder of this paragraph, we discuss one specific incident within the process of tourism development that illustrates the utility of linking capital to the development of resilience. i.e. a proposal to widen the Beach Road, which is Pedda Jalaripeta primary access road from Visakhapatnam to Bheemunipatnam. This project aimed to attract developments such as beach resorts, hotels, restaurants, yacht clubs, movie theaters and other tourist-oriented developments into the whole region (Equations, 2008; Philipose, 2013). Had this happened, the resort owners would have claimed Pedda Jalaripeta community beach for the tourist activities resulting in the loss of fishing grounds to the local community. The widened road would also make Pedda Jalaripeta attractive for further development resulting in the eviction of most the slum residents. The following is an excerpt from the Fishermen Youth Welfare Association's (FYWA) treasurer regarding the case.

> *It was a Coastal Regulation Zone (CRZ) violation. Firstly, the road would fall under CRZ 1, where construction is not allowed. Second, a lot of fishermen used that area for drying fish and it is a source of income*

> *for us. Third, there is no need for a four-lane road way from Bhimli to here (Visakhapatnam), there is not enough traffic to warrant the demolition of a hill and disturbing the CRZ. (FYWA treasurer on 10 May 14).*

Pedda Jalaripeta residents resisted tourism-oriented projects near their community. In doing so, they utilised their linking capital evident by the presence of Action Aid, an international aid organization. Action Aid started its work in Pedda Jalaripeta in the 1990s. The agency organized fellowship programmes to educate youth in the slum and other fishing communities around Visakhapatnam city. The fellowship programmes trained youth about federal and state regulations such as the Marine Fisheries Regulation Act (MFRA)[7], Coastal Regulation Zone (CRZ), Right to Information Act[8] as well as the judicial process for filing legal petitions against projects that were infringing on the rights of the fishermen and fishing communities. The youth from Pedda Jalaripeta slum, who graduated from the fellowship programme, registered an NGO Fishermen Youth Welfare Association (FYWA) in 2001 (Philipose, 2013).

In 2003, the Fishermen Youth Welfare Association, along with other target communities, filed a lawsuit in the State of Andhra Pradesh High Court against the Visakhapatnam Urban Development Authority (VUDA), arguing that road widening violated the Coastal Regulation Zone (CRZ)[9] notification. The court case halted the project for three years. VUDA was forced to make some modifications to its original plan and eventually, the road widening project was shelved (Equations, 2008; Philipose, 2013).

Thus, fishermen strongly opposed the road widening. The government and other private developers were shocked that 'ordinary fisher folk' had resources to mount a legal battle against a government project (interview with FYWA President 20 April 2014). Between 2000 and 2014, the FYWA filed 13 court cases against the government and private agencies for violating the CRZ guidelines. Over these years, FYWA has perfected a step-by-step approach to fighting or protesting developments that encroach on the coastal protection zone or development that are near Pedda Jalaripeta slum.

This collaboration between the fishermen and an international aid organization transformed Pedda Jalaripeta socially through knowledge and empowerment. Unlike the 1983 fire that ravished Pedda Jalaripeta slum within a few minutes, tourist-oriented development is a slow-moving threat. Just like the fire ushered a new era of development, the tourist-oriented development is triggering a new era of political thinking in the community. The older leaders in Pedda Jalaripeta slum are illiterate and not knowledgeable about laws and legal procedures. These leaders trust the elected representative or depend on the government bureaucrats to assist them with welfare schemes (Senior citizen focus group on 22 May 2014). However, the youth leaders at the FYWA use the media and do not hesitate to take legal action and fight with powerful opposition for their human rights, community rights or their fishermen rights. This drastic change in the community's interaction with the bureaucratic agencies over one generation speaks volumes about the role of education and empowerment.

Conclusions

Academic and policy debates on slums can be placed on a continuum. At one end of the spectrum, slums exhibit signs of underdevelopment and embody a series of problems evident in mega cities (UN-Habitat, 2003). At the other end, they portray creativity, ecological superiority, romanticized entrepreneurialism and adaptability (De Soto, 2000; Appadurai, 2001; Boonyabancha, 2009). The case of Pedda Jalaripeta suggests that, at least to some extent, a slum can transition from one end of the spectrum (underdeveloped) to the other.

Sharing professional and cultural practices using the same key places and spaces in Pedda Jalaripeta has been important in building bonding and bridging capital. The social capital that the residents further built through mutual economic investment in the community (temples) and cultural/religious activities (religious ceremonies) has generated a sense of trust among them and strengthened their commitment to maintaining the community. Pedda Jalaripeta's bonding and bridging capital has been critical for fishermen's safety on the sea and maintaining the community's cultural heritage. However, as other scholars have observed, bonding and bridging capitals, while critical to coping, does not sufficiently help residents to transform and successfully adapt to disasters in the long run (Putnam, 2001; Elliott et al., 2010; Aldrich, 2011; Islam and Walkerden, 2014). Indeed, even though the practices mentioned above, as well as a strong presence of the Grama Sabha, had been in place for generations, and aided the coping capacity of the community, they did not seem to put in motion a process of transformation. As was similarly observed by Elliot et al. (2010), the community's transformative capacity enticed mobilising linking capital with politicians and external agencies. Specifically, linking networks, first with the MLA during the 1980's fire and then with Action Aid starting in 1990's.

The link between slum residents and the government improved Pedda Jalaripeta's physical infrastructure. Those physical transformations, in turn, provided the space and scope for human enrichment, preserved the residents' access to the fishing beach, and retained the social capital within the community. Action Aid provided knowledge and resources to educate and empower youth in the community to fight for their human rights, cultural rights and community rights (Equations, 2008; Philipose, 2013). These types of rights along with the physical upgrading help shield the community against unexpected future threats including gentrification, displacement, or demolition.

Nevertheless, it is important to note that as the city of Visakhapatnam continues to grow, the Pedda Jalaripeta community will continue to face redevelopment and gentrification threats. 'Bouncing forward' relied strongly on political formal leadership. However, with the demise of the previously influential MLA, the community also lost a key link to the regional government. Currently, the strength of the community is related, to an important extent, to the strength of the youth leadership supported by an external partner. It is yet to be seen if the community can withstand the test of time.

Notes

1 Quote from VS on 22 March 2015.
2 A tenure formalization policy, where the state officially recognizes settlements as slums and protects the occupancy rights of the residents (Nakamura 2014).
3 $24,105 at a conversion rate of $1 = Rs. 62.22.
4 Respondents for formal interviews held for his study from the *Department of Fisheries:* Joint Director; Director; Field Development Officer; Field Development Officer; and from *Greater Visakhapatnam Municipal Corporation (GVMC):* Capacity Building Training Coordinator; Urban Community Development Officer; Anganwadi Teacher; Assistant City Planner; City Planner; Zonal Engineer.
5 Respondents from the community: *Grama-Sabha (Village Assembly)*: Secretary, President; *Marine Cooperative Society*: Past President, Current president; *Fishermen Youth Welfare Association (FYWA)*: President, Women's Cooperative president, Treasurer, Secretary.
6 Quote from NM on 1 April 2014.
7 MFRA is a 1994 Indian federal law, which created an exclusive fishing zone within eight kilometers (4.9 miles) from the shoreline for traditional fishermen.
8 A 2005 federal law under which, any citizen may request information from a "public authority" (a body of Government or "instrumentality of State") which is required to reply expeditiously or within thirty days.
9 Coastal Regulation Zone (CRZ) order under the Government of India's Environment Protection Act, became law in 1991. The law aimed to protect and conserve the environment of the coastal regions.

References

Abelson, P. (1996). Evaluation of slum improvements: Case study in Visakhapatnam, India. *Cities*, 13(2), 97–108.

Ajibade, I., McBean, G., & Bezner-Kerr, R. (2013). Urban flooding in Lagos, Nigeria: Patterns of vulnerability and resilience among women. *Global Environmental Change*, 23(6), 1714–1725.

Aldrich, D.P. (2011). The externalities of strong social capital: Post-Tsunami recovery in Southeast India. *Journal of Civil Society*, 7(1), 81–99.

Amis, P., & Kumar, S. (2000). Urban economic growth, infrastructure and poverty in India: Lessons from Visakhapatnam. *Environment and Urbanization*, 12(1), 185–196.

Andavarapu, D., & Arefi, M. (2015). Resilient slums: Role of social capital. *Tekton*, 2(1), 38–54.

Andavarapu, D., & Edelman, D.J. (2013). Evolution of slum redevelopment policy. *Current Urban Studies*, 1(1), 185.

Appadurai, A. (2001). Deep democracy: Urban governmentality and the horizon of politics. *Environment and Urbanization*, 13(2), 21–47.

Arefi, M. (2011). Design for resilient cities: Reflections from a studio. In T. Banerjee & A. Loukaitou Sideris (Eds.), *Companion to Urban Design* (pp. 674–686). London: Taylor & Francis Group.

Benansio, J.S., Wolff, M., Breckwoldt, A., & Jiddawi, N. (2016). Have the fishing communities of Zanzibar Island benefited from increasing tourism development? *Journal of Development and Agricultural Economics*, 8(5), 95–107.

Boonyabancha, S. (2009). Land for housing the poor – by the poor: Experiences from the Baan Mankong nationwide slum upgrading programme in Thailand. *Environment and Urbanization*, 21(2), 309–329.

Braun, B., & Aßheuer, T. (2011). Floods in megacity environments: Vulnerability and coping strategies of slum dwellers in Dhaka/Bangladesh. *Natural Hazards*, 58(2), 771–787.

Campanella, T.J. (2006). Urban resilience and the recovery of New Orleans. *Journal of the American Planning Association*, 72(2), 141–146.

censusura, S. (2014). Impact of slum formalisation on self-help housing construction: A case of slum notification in India. *Urban Studies* 51(16), 3420–3444.

Central Marine Fisheries Research Institute (2005). *Marine Fisheries Census, Andhra Pradesh*. Government of India.

Chatterjee, M. (2010). Slum dwellers response to flooding events in the megacities of India. *Mitigation and Adaptation Strategies for Global Change*, 15(4), 337–353.

Chatterjee, M. (2011). Flood loss redistribution in a third world megacity: The case of Mumbai. In H.G. Brauch, Ú. Oswald Spring, C. Mesjasz, J. Grin, P. Kameri-Mbote, B. Chourou, P. Dunay & J. Birkmann (Eds.), *Coping with Global Environmental Change, Disasters and Security* (pp. 603–612). Berlin and Heidelberg: Springer.

Chelleri, L., Waters, J.J., Olazabal, M., & Minucci, G. (2015). Resilience trade-offs: Addressing multiple scales and temporal aspects of urban resilience. *Environment and Urbanization*, 27(1), 181–198.

Davoudi, S., Brooks, E., & Mehmood, A. (2013). Evolutionary resilience and strategies for climate adaptation. *Planning Practice and Research*, 28(3), 307–322.

Derman, B., & Ferguson, A. (1995). Human rights, environment, and development: The dispossession of fishing communities on Lake Malawi. *Human Ecology*, 23(2), 125–142.

De Soto, H. (2000). *The Mystery of Capital: Why Capitalism Triumphs in the West and Fails Everywhere Else*. New York: Basic Books.

Desouza, K., & Flanery, T. (2013). Designing, planning, and managing resilient cities: A conceptual framework. *Cities*, 35(4), 89–99.

Dovey, K. (2012). Informal urbanism & complex adaptive assemblage. *International Development Planning Review*, 34(4), 349–368.

Elliot, J.R., Haney, T.J., & Sams-Abiodun, P. (2010). Limits to social capital: Comparing network assistance in two New Orleans neighbourhoods devastated by Hurricane Katrina. *Sociological Quarterly*, 51(4), 624–648.

Equations: Equitable Tourism Options (2008). *Right to Information and Tourism*. Bangalore: Equations: Equitable Tourism Options.

Gilbert, A. (2007). The return of the slum: Does language matter? *International Journal of Urban and Regional Research*, 31(4), 697–713.

GVMC (2009). *Survey of Households in Greater Visakhapatnam Municipal Corporation*. Accessed on 24 November 2014: www.apmepma.Gov.In/HHPS/Hh_Rep_Slum.Php?Ulbid=109.

GVMC (2012). *City Development Plan-Greater Visakhapatnam* Cities Alliance Project Output. Accessed on 24 November 2014: www-wds.worldbank.org/external/default/WDSContentServer/WDSP/IB/2012/10/16/000356161_20121016033041/Rendered/PDF/732240WP0P09510reater0Visakhapatnam.pdf.

Gunderson, L.H., & Holling, C.S. (Eds.) (2002) *Panarchy: Understanding Transformations in Human and Natural Systems*. Washington, DC: Island Press.

Haigh, R., & Amaratunga, R. (2012). Making cities resilient: From awareness to implementation. *International Journal of Disaster Resilience in the Built Environment*, 4(1), 5–8.

Holling, C.S. (1973). Resilience and stability of ecological systems. *Annual Review of Ecology and Systematics*, 4(1), 1–23.

Immanuell, S., & Rao, G.S. (2012). Social status of hook and line fishermen in Visakhapatnam. *Fishery Technology*, 49(2), 204–209.

Indian Census (2011). Presentation on Slums. Accessed on 2 August 2013: www.censusindia.gov.

Islam, R., & Walkerden, G. (2014). How bonding and bridging networks contribute to disaster resilience and recovery on the Bangladeshi coast. *International Journal of Disaster Risk Reduction*, 10, 281–291.

Jabeen, H., Johnson, C., & Allen, A. (2010). Built-in resilience: Learning from grassroots coping strategies for climate variability. *Environment and Urbanization*, 22(2), 415–431.

Keck, M., & Etzold, B. (2013). Resilience refused. Wasted potentials for improving food security in Dhaka. *Erdkunde*, 67(1), 75–91.

Keck, M., & Sakdapolrak, P. (2013). What is social resilience? Lessons learned and ways forward. *Erdkunde*, 67(1), 5–19.

Magis, K. (2010). Community resilience: An indicator of social sustainability. *Society and Natural Resources*, 23(5), 401–416.

Naidu, R. (2006). Dilapidation and slum formation. In S. Patel & K. Deb (Eds.), *Urban Studies*. New Delhi: Oxford University Press.

Patel, S. (2013). Upgrade, rehouse or resettle? An assessment of the Indian government's Basic Services for the Urban Poor (BSUP) programme. *Environment and Urbanization*, 25(1), 177–188.

Patulny, R.V., & Svendsen, G.L.H. (2007). Exploring the social capital grid: Bonding, bridging, qualitative, quantitative. *International Journal of Sociology and Social Policy*, 27(1/2), 32–51.

Peattie, L.R. (1982). Some second thoughts on sites-and-services. *Habat International*, 6(2), 131–139.

Pelling, M., & High, C. (2005). Understanding adaptation: What can social capital offer assessments of adaptive capacity? *Global Environmental Change*, 15(4), 308–319.

Philipose, B.P. (2013). *Critical Stories of Change*. Action Aid. Accessed on 15 August 2013: www.actionaidusa.org/india/publications/critical-stories-1-sea-our-life-coast-our-right-visakhapatnam.

Pickett, S.T.A., Cadenasso, M.L., & Grove, J.M. (2004). Resilient cities: Meaning, models, and metaphor for integrating the ecological, socio-economic, and planning realms. *Landscape and Urban Planning*, 69(4), 369–384.

Putnam, R.D. (2001). *Bowling Alone: The Collapse and Revival of American Community*. New York: Simon and Schuster.

Turner, J.F (1976). *Housing by People: Towards Autonomy in Building Environments*. London: Marion Boyars.

UN-Habitat (2003). *The Challenge of Slums*. Sterling, VA.

UN-Habitat (2010). *State of the World's Cities 2010/2009*. Sterling, VA.

Wilhelm, M. (2011). Resilient cities. In K. Otto-Zimmermann (Ed.), *Resilient Cities: Cities and Adaptation to Climate Change* (pp. 45–53). Dordrecht: Springer Netherlands.

World Bank & International Monetary Fund (2013). Global Monitoring Report 2013: Rural-Urban Dynamics & Millenium Development Goals. Accessed on 27 May 2013: http://econ.worldbank.org/wbsite/external/extdec/extdecprospects/0,,contentmdk:23391146~pagepk:64165401~pipk:64165026~thesitepk:476883,00.html.

13 Riding the tide

Socially-engaged art and resilience in an uncertain future

Sage Brice and Seila Fernández Arconada

Introduction

This chapter asks how theoretical and practical approaches developed in the field of socially-engaged art can extend current discourse around resilience and community engagement in the social sciences.[1] We address this question as practising artists, drawing on our experience working collaboratively with different communities – including both academic partners and geographically defined groups – and specifically with flood-affected communities, where resilience is a prominent concern. Our approach is informed by the belief that focusing on relational process rather than output opens space for generative encounters and implies a transformative reading of resilience, in contrast with more directly instrumental approaches. We highlight the central role of uncertainty in the creative processes of art-making and ask how artistic strategies for working productively with uncertainty can contribute – both to understandings of resilience in other disciplines and to promoting community resilience.

This practice-based reflection is further informed by examples from the work of artists and theorists who actively engage with particular social contexts, and with the various challenges faced by different communities. To typify this work we choose the term 'socially-engaged' out of a number of competing terms for what is not an artistic movement but a more-or-less distinct field of practice – one which emphasises dialogue and embeddedness within a broader social arena. Following Kester (2000) we, therefore, define socially-engaged art for present purposes as that in which – firstly – human relations constitute the primary artistic medium, and – secondly – the dialogical process of artist and participant leads the evolution of the work.

Current writing on resilience and the arts tends to revolve around one of two questions – either the effectiveness of art as a tool for social change, or the correct place of instrumental considerations in the evaluation of contemporary art (Belfiore, 2002, p. 9; Matarasso, 2013, pp. 9–10). In this chapter, we seek to extend this conversation by asking instead whether the accumulated critical and practical insights of socially-engaged art might offer new ways of thinking about both resilience and community, beyond the frameworks familiar to social and environmental science, policy and planning.

The word resilience admits multiple interpretations. In the next section of this chapter, we clarify our treatment of some of the key concepts at stake. We discuss briefly how resilience is defined in relation to a perceived climate of uncertainty, and review the implications of habitual discourse around concepts such as community and engagement, as well as the challenges facing co-productive approaches to both research and artistic practice. In the third section, we sketch out the historical development of contemporary socially-engaged art practice and review some of the ethical, aesthetic and political considerations that have shaped its critical evolution. To summarise, we propose four dimensions of socially-engaged art practice we believe have a bearing on how we think about resilience: *New ways of working*, *Embracing Uncertainty*, *Expanded frames of reference*, and *Creative language*. Finally, we review these ideas in relation to a brief case study of our own joint work and discuss some of the practical considerations when putting them into practice.

Critical context: uncertainty, resilience, and the 'social turn'

The current interest in social resilience (Adger, 2000; Brose, 2015; Elms, 2015) arises in the context of an era of perceived uncertainty about global futures – marked by violent conflict, environmental degradation, economic and political crisis, displacement, and the prospect of traumatic climate change. While this state of perceived crisis may or may not be historically exceptional, increasingly extreme weather events, in particular, present the global community with challenges experienced globally at an unprecedented scale. As these events become a frequent feature of everyday life for populations around the globe, the question of resilience and how we achieve it has thus become a matter of significance at societal and community levels. From a government and institutional perspective, promoting the resilience of specific communities is a pragmatic means to mitigate the destabilising impacts of rapid change – in other words, to maintain the function of existing systems in the face of external impact. Top-down implementations of resilience planning, however, raise questions of how resilience objectives are identified and achieved, and by what methods these initiatives can be kept relevant to specific places and specific communities.

Resilience and the paradigm of endemic risk

Models of resilience vary between resilience as the capacity of a system to return to a former state, and as the capacity of a system to produce new adaptations, treating stability as a conservative or progressive concept, respectively. Both readings, however, define resilience in relation to external impacts – leading critics to point out that resilience discourse can obscure structural barriers to the thriving of communities, within existing social systems (Whittle et al., 2010). That the rise of resilience discourse has prompted significant critical concern is reflected in recent literature

(Adger, 2000; Evans and Reid, 2014; McEwen and Jones, 2012), and likewise in the rationale of the conference for which a version of this chapter was originally produced. It is important to bear in mind the different possible implications of current resilience discourse when contextualised, for example, within neoliberal paradigms of serial welfare reform (Macpherson et al., 2014, p. 30).

Brad Evans and Julian Reid, in their recent book *Resilient Life* (2014), point to a problematic conflation of resilience with resistance, or the ability of a system to withstand the negative impact of catastrophic events – effectively reducing the nature of the political to a question of bare survivability. This becomes particularly alarming in the context of a neoliberal order underpinned by the ideology of endemic risk, in which catastrophic events play a politically definitive role (Massumi, 2009). Framing external hazards as the primary threat to society presupposes the existence of an implicitly universal and desirable *status quo*, and in so doing also obscures the links between socio-economic privilege (or lack of it) and vulnerability to extreme events – as evidenced for example by the long history of flood management and differential impacts in New Orleans (McEwen et al., 2012; Smith, 2006). It is a logic which, write Evans and Reid (2014, p. 22), denies the possibility of 'an affirmative thinking', capable of imagining or demanding a different world.

We see cultivating resilience – conceived as the autonomous capacity of communities to thrive despite adverse experience (Macpherson et al., 2012, p. 3) – as a critical part of socially-engaged practice. Unless we are content to maintain things as they are, however, we believe it necessary to think of resilience in transformative terms. Since those most vulnerable to – for example – extreme weather events are often also those most disadvantaged within existing social structures, resilience for these communities may be at least as dependent on the ability to change the *status quo*, as upon the ability to withstand external hazards (Whittle et al., 2010, pp. 11–12). This last point is of particular relevance to our concern here, since socially-engaged art frequently aspires both to initiate transformative processes and to propose radically different frames of reference for imagining and creating social spaces and relations.

Co-production and community engagement

This heightened attention to resilience coincides with a shift in concerns and ways of working within the social sciences and other related disciplines, including a renewed emphasis on co-production of research. Socially-engaged art practice has to some extent co-evolved with participatory research, and both are informed also by activist and social considerations. The increasing focus in both spheres on engaging and working more inclusively, and specifically on engaging with communities identified as 'vulnerable' or 'at risk', reinforces the need for effective ways of working across disciplinary and societal divides. In this context, it becomes necessary to examine the relations of power within a co-productive association. It cannot be taken for granted that co-productive relationships – in either art or academic research – will not replicate or obscure underlying imbalances of power, both within participant groups, and more broadly in society (Askins and Pain, 2011, p. 815; Gaventa and Cornwall, 2006; Macpherson et al., 2014, p. 28). This has implications for any claims of authenticity or appropriateness predicated upon the collaborative nature of the research process. The search for appropriate methodologies to work with and around these difficulties remains an active preoccupation of both artists and researchers attempting to develop exchange-based models for knowledge generation (Flowerdew and Martin, 2005, p. 144).

'Community' in perspective

Community, too, is a concept which often goes unexamined in public and political discourse. Despite its obvious appeal, however, the concept is problematic in many ways and has largely passed out of sociological analysis (Brint, 2001). A given community is defined by specific characteristics held in common – at various registers, from the biological to the metaphysical. Communities are not, however, discrete and homogeneous units – instead community boundaries overlap, clash and disrupt one another. Uncritical treatment of 'community' as a singular entity obscures internal differences, as well as the necessary exclusion implicit in any act of categorisation. In addition, the idealised community can become a vehicle for projected values and assumptions, or as a source of instant validation. Finally, communities are not necessarily comparable across cultures and geographical contexts – a point attested by the lack of truly equivalent terms in different languages.[2] All these considerations must be borne in mind when considering the definition of community resilience, as well as when developing an approach to promoting it in practice.

Art in social context

From formal aesthetics to dialogic practice

The emergence of socially-engaged art is part of a spatial expansion in contemporary art over the past century, from designated art spaces to the public realm. This move beyond the gallery has it roots in the twentieth-century Avant-garde and is perhaps an inevitable consequence of its association with social critique and experimentation. As Bruguera (2011, n.p.) states: "we do not have to enter the Louvre or the castles, we have to enter people's houses, people's lives, this is where useful art is." One of the first and most influential artists to explore this line was Joseph Beuys, whose concept of social sculpture laid the ground for a new generation of practitioners who saw society at large as the medium, rather than the consumers, of artistic practice.

The Artist Placement Group (APG), formed in London in the mid-1960s, developed a new model for artistic practice based on this principle (Rasmussen, 2009; Tate, n.d.). The group negotiated residencies in which artists worked directly in non-art spaces such as government departments and commercial companies. The APG introduced the maxim that 'the context is half the work' – a significant departure from the classic white cube of the gallery, which traditionally treats the artwork as a discrete and self-contained object. They made the case for the relevance of art as an integrated part of contemporary life and production – not as a creative means to improve efficiency or delivery of desired objectives, but as an open-ended, critical, and uncertain mode of production which makes its own necessary and relevant contribution to the social sphere.

Where APG primarily focused on industry and government as spheres of operation, others such as the 'community arts' movement placed an emphasis on working with people in less institutional settings. Later artists drew on both, to inform their models of socially-engaged practice. '*Up in the Air*', a seminal project initiated by artist Neville Gabie and based in a condemned high-rise housing estate in Liverpool, implemented the principles of APG's manifesto in a new setting. By inviting a selection of artists to carry out long-term residencies in empty apartments on the site, the project opened space for exploratory creative processes and relationships to emerge through a dialogic encounter between artists and residents. As the field evolved, artists found diverse ways of working within the new relational dynamics in which they found themselves:

> "These cultural practices indicate the new social order – ways of life that emphasise participation, challenge power, and expand disciplines ranging from urban planning and community work to theatre and the visual arts."
>
> (Thompson, 2012, p. 19)

This attention to the role of art in the social sphere (and concomitantly, the role of the social sphere in art), has presented a complex entanglement of ethical, aesthetic and political considerations. The resulting debate is typified (in the UK) by the critical dispute between Claire Bishop and Grant Kester, which broadly contrast two points of view on the effective sphere of disruptive politics (Bishop, 2005, 2006; Kester, 2006). Where Bishop criticises indiscriminate, conciliatory tendencies in socially-engaged practice, Kester rejects traditional aesthetic parameters as inextricably rooted in cultural dynamics of power and privilege. What both critics have in common is an interest in the inextricably political role of art, and the simplistic inadequacy of models that treat art as a form of social 'improvement'.

The authors of this chapter share Bishop's concern at the instrumentalisation of this kind of work in European cultural policy as it develops in tandem with the dismantling of the welfare state. However, Bishop fails to recognise the potential of dialogic practice for generating politically transformative encounters. The sensibilities and challenges of socially-engaged practice demand a new approach to understanding 'quality' in art (Belfiore, 2002). Traditional frameworks are not merely inadequate in this context; they tend to reinforce the stratifications and perceived boundaries which such practice aims to disrupt. The aesthetic paradigms of modernism and postmodernism, for example, rest heavily on formal innovation as a meter of success, tending to omit or to downplay attention to the subjective and culturally constructed nature of aesthetic parameters (Kester, 2000). Socially-engaged artists instead attempt to find new ways of making meaningful work, or making work meaningful:

> 'In socially-engaged practice, artists attempt to extend the parameters beyond aesthetics to operate in a broader social context: it is not about the next new thing in art, it is about a change that reaches far outside of an art discourse'
>
> (Reyes, 2014, n.p.)

To this effect, artists have moved towards developing new frameworks, such as the functional parameters of Tania Bruguera's *Arte Útil* (Useful Art), which assigns to art a generative and problem-solving role:

> '*Useful Art* is a way of working with aesthetic experiences that focus on the implementation of art in society where art's function is no longer to be a space for 'signalling' problems, but the place from which to create the proposal and implementation of possible solutions. We should go back to the times when art was not something to look at in awe, but something to generate from. If it is political art, it deals with the consequences, if it deals with the consequences, I think it has to be useful art.'
>
> (Bruguera, 2011, n.p.)

Dangers of instrumentalisation

In becoming 'useful', however, artists risk subjecting their practice to instrumentalisation through the implicit and explicit agendas of commissioning and funding bodies (Bishop, 2012). It is important to note, in Bruguera's case, that art is proposed as a generative tool – a way to create space from which to make collaborative solutions that emerge as part of the artistic process. Arts advocates sail close to the wind when they find themselves justifying arts spending by promoting, for example, art's capacity to engage 'hard-to-reach' groups or stimulate economic growth and urban 'renewal'

(Belfiore, 2002, p. 104). Once art is discussed in terms of usefulness it becomes necessary to ask whose interests are served, and how. Caught between aesthetics on the one hand and utility on the other, socially-engaged artists are left to ask what kind of practice most closely reflects both the interests of participants and the aspirations of artistic practice, as opposed to social provision, governance, or activism.

Helix Arts, in NE England, developed a five-point critical framework for what they call 'dialogic participatory art' that goes some way towards reconciling the above questions – proposing a model that incorporates both a participatory, co-productive approach and an attention to the (positive) disruptive potential of art operating at multiple concurrent registers:

> "Dialogic participatory art:
>
> 1 enables people to explore what is meaningful to them
> 2 is creative, challenging and potentially disruptive
> 3 understands that our identities are the stories we tell ourselves about ourselves
> 4 is situated within, and has a deep understanding of, particular contexts
> 5 is a shared process of creative enquiry and learning between artists and participants"
>
> (Lowe, 2012, pp. 6–7)

New ways of working: intersections of art and resilience in practice

As indicated above, two major shifts have driven social enquiry in the arts: first, the move from dedicated spaces such as museums and galleries to a wider social context, and second, the emergence of dialogic and participatory responses to issues of power and visibility made visible by that move. This demands also a shift in the role of the artist, from creating artefacts to making interventions which open spaces of possibility and unfamiliar dynamics. This is a shift affected with varying degrees of success and commitment – perhaps expressed in its most ideal form in the concept of 'social sculpture': Beuys casts society in its entirety as a single, evolving, and collective artwork, in which all individuals participate as artists who can intervene at will in the process of creation. In *7,000 Oak Trees: City Forestation Instead of City Administration* (1982), for example, Beuys took advantage of a commission from the Dokumenta festival in Kassel to catalyse a large scale social project with a significant environmental legacy for the city (Körner and Bellin-Harder, 2009). Delivering a pile of granite stones to the site, he specified that each stone could be removed only to a new location within the city, where an oak was to be planted beside it. The work replaced traditional conceptions of sculpture with a direct intervention into everyday life. This blurring of the life/art boundary set the scene for a new emphasis in contemporary art practice: "Couldn't everyone's life become a work of art? Why should the lamp or house be an object, but not our life?" (Foucault, 1991, p. 350).

The rationale of art as intervention attempts to enact tangible, practical effects in ways that also articulate a cultural shift – to suggest new ways of seeing or doing and the possibility of engaging in transformative ways with the social sphere. In the work "*Palas por pistolas*" (2008), for example, Pedro Reyes coordinated a project in Culiacán, Mexico – a city with an extremely high rate of gun deaths. Voluntary donations of weapons were collected in exchange for domestic appliances. The 1,527 weapons were crushed in a symbolic public event, and the metal converted into an identical number of shovels, which were distributed through schools and art institutions, inviting people to plant 1,527 trees to combat deforestation in Mexico (Weintraub, 2012, pp. 259–264). Individual participation at different stages of the project built up incrementally to create a powerful, collectively enacted metaphor for the possibility of fundamental social change.

While projects such as these, at a grand scale, attempt to evoke a participatory transformative potential within the social realm, they also cast the artist in an orchestrating role. The enabling aspirations of socially-engaged art often exist in tension with an implicit hierarchy in which artists reproduce existing social stratification. One challenge for socially-engaged artists, then, is to find new ways of working which acknowledge and disrupt these dynamics.

Though these questions remain unresolved and ongoing challenges for any kind of practice that engages with the social world, participatory art differs substantially in aims and conceptual frameworks from social-scientific research. Furthermore, it offers a different array of methodological approaches – one that deserves further examination. One such characteristic is the ability of art to resonate simultaneously at different registers – combining immediately practical effect with other modes of cultural meaning and knowledge-making.

In the following section, we look at further examples from our own and other artists' work, and propose three characteristics of socially-engaged artistic process that speak to current concerns around resilience and community engagement: embracing uncertainty, expanded frames of reference, and creative language.

Embracing uncertainty

In the field of risk reduction and management, uncertainty may feature principally as an obstacle to effective analysis, and a complication in planning and mitigation (see for instance Apel et al., 2004). In contemporary art practice, however, uncertainty is not only integral to the working process, but a guiding principle, shaping the vectors of artistic enquiry. The artist working at the productive margin of their field does not usually work towards a predetermined result. Art practice is instead a process of devising strategies for working productively with uncertainty. This is particularly true of a concept-led or process-led art practice, such as socially-engaged art, in which the selection of media, technique, and methods respond to specific contexts where unfamiliar challenges give shape to the work. This is a process that often involves letting go of prior expectations and learning from accident, contingency, and unexpected encounter. Finding ways to relate to uncertainty as a generative field of possibility, and to operate comfortably and creatively within this field, is a form of resilient practice which has application at a practical level in situations such as extreme weather, where the destabilising effects of traumatic events present both challenges and opportunities for affected communities (Whittle et al., 2010).

Francis Alys' *When Faith Moves Mountains* (2002) was conceived in response to a climate of uncertainty in Peru following the collapse of the Fujimori government. Alys invited 500 students to work together to displace a sand dune by a few centimetres, in an epic choreographed shovelling event. Here the stated aim – to move the dune – was in fact a method used to bring about a transformative social encounter, and restore a sense of faith in the possibilities of collective action. In the words of one participant: "the people who took part felt totally involved and the fact that it took on such a huge dimension will generate one story after another which will be passed on like an oral tradition" (*When Faith Moves Mountains (the making of)*, 2002).

This approach can also work at more intimate scales to draw out and amplify existing currents within a community. In *Unconscious Power: the Act of Collective Creativity* (2014; see Figure 13.1) Seila Fernández Arconada worked with local residents and artists in Tongjianju – one of the last low-rise neighbourhoods in Chonqging, China, which originated as social housing and today faces rapid clearance and development. In this officially neglected public space, the abundant discarded material is reimagined and reused in different ways. The project explored the role of creativity, inspired by the creative practices of residents who generate artefacts and extravagant installations from found materials, incorporating them into the aesthetic and practical dimensions of their everyday lives.

Informal conversations and organised workshops with residents, alongside a collaborative public exhibition and event, avoided talking about art, and instead focussed on the transformative role of creative practice within daily lived experience. The project also brought a new attention to practices that otherwise went unremarked, and led to the establishment of *T1*, a creative platform working in Tongjianju to generate a longer-term legacy of the project within the local community.

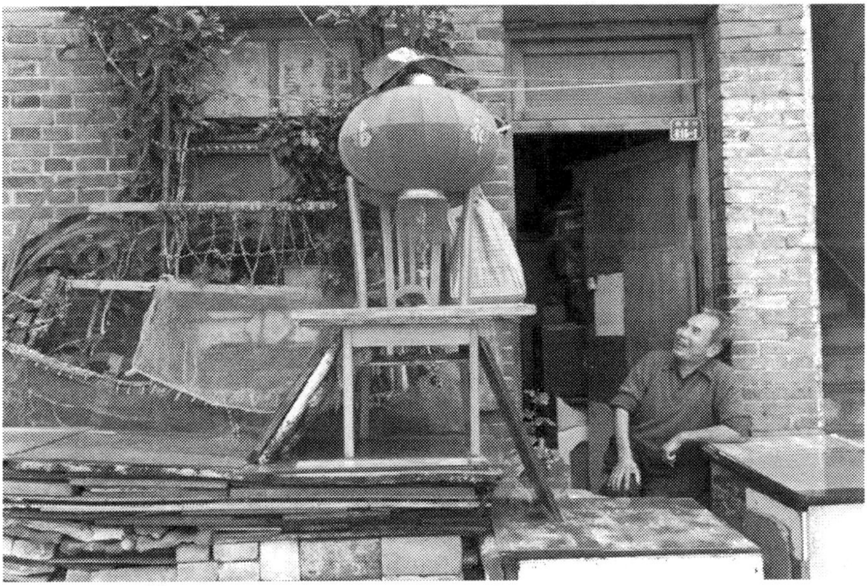

Figure 13.1 Unconscious power, the act of collective creativity.
Source: Seila Fernández Arconada in Tongjianju, China, 2014.

Expanded frames of reference

Creative practice encourages an appreciation of lateral, tangential and incidental processes that are often undervalued in rationalist frameworks. Although artistic experimentation may follow rigorously applied procedures, the intention is often to unsettle familiar conventions and to arrive at unexpected results. In a participatory art process, exploring the familiar from unfamiliar angles can offer participants an opportunity to understand themselves and the world in new ways (Lowe, 2012).

A related, though separate, dimension of socially-engaged practice is that artists frequently move between social contexts, and bring into contact worlds that would normally remain apart. Participatory art affords opportunities to encounter unfamiliar outlooks, and so offers expanded frames of reference through which to understand familiar experiences.

Finally, this aspect of creative practice can be a way of opening space for voices and narratives that are otherwise less heard. This goes some way to addressing issues of power and visibility, firstly by generating opportunities for those voices to become more audible, and secondly by opening spaces for communities to imagine themselves and the world differently. Clarissa Hayward, in '*De-Facing Power*' (2000, p. 39), writes that political freedom is 'the capacity to participate in shaping the limits that define what is socially possible.' Where that capacity is unequally distributed, socially-engaged art may be one way of beginning to redress the imbalance.

These possibilities are explored in Jeremy Deller's The Battle of Orgreave (2002) – the re-enactment of a historical confrontation between picketers and police that took place near the Orgreave coking plant in 1984 (The Battle of Orgreave, 2002). Deller worked with professional historic re-enactors, alongside non-professional participants who had been involved in the original conflict, from both sides of the picket lines. Here the role of the artist was not to produce an object or representation, but to frame a new kind of encounter (Thompson, 2012, p. 17). By bringing people together to revisit their past experiences and evolving sense of community identity through a creative encounter with others' stories, Deller offered an expanded frame of reference for understanding traumatic events and their ongoing effects in a divided community.

Creative language

Creative process operates as an expanded form of language, in that it enables us to process ideas and events, and to communicate about them, through embodied, material, and experiential registers alongside symbolic and cognitive dimensions. By providing multiple parallel lines of approach, art can help facilitate and enhance dialogue, rather than shutting it down. This has application not only regarding addressing traumatic events, but also to collaboration across disciplines and fields of experience or expertise, including between science and art.

Art and the sciences have a long shared history as research methodologies (Hesse-Honegger, 2001). Specialisation within the academies has increasingly separated them, but while disciplines clearly employ methodologies to support particular objectives, this chapter rejects traditional binaries of objectivity (attributed to science) and subjectivity (attributed to art). The challenges of thriving in an uncertain world are as much cultural as technical, and there is much to be said for cultivating approaches that reconcile these frames of response.

In *The Land of the Summer People* (2014 – ongoing; Figure 13.2) Seila Fernández Arconada works with Professor Thorsten Wagener at the University of Bristol, UK. The project explores the unstable relationships between human-beings, water and place by exploring flood impact in Somerset, England. Exploring methodologies of both art and scientific disciplines, the project aims to generate new ways of understanding research and disciplinary language, as each discipline generates its own terminology that can isolate and detach it from common discourse. Through a series of workshops, invited artists and student engineers have been gradually taken out of their respective comfort zones, combining their various skills and expertise to engage with each other and with flood-affected communities in Somerset. Creative process became a means of connecting and developing expanded frames of reference for researchers, artists, and residents engaging in different ways with the floods.

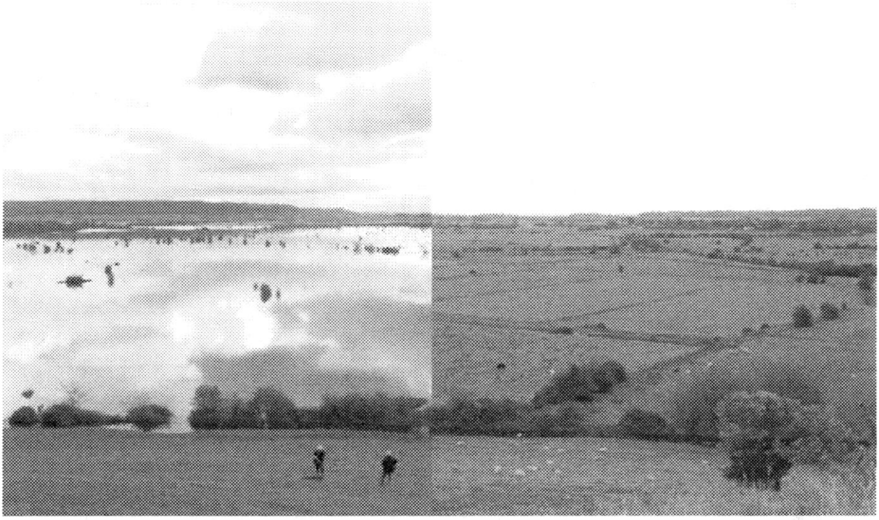

Figure 13.2 The land of the summer people.
Source: Seila Fernández Arconada in the Somerset Moors and Levels, 2014.

Artistic responses to social and environmental concerns can also take effect in practical ways. *HighWaterLine* began as a solo performance in which artist Eve Mosher walked the 200-year flood risk contours in her native New York with an ambulatory chalk marker (Nadir, 2015). After Hurricane Sandy faithfully replicated the artist's original chalk line, the work was reinvented as a community-based project that could be realised in different cities, in order to engage more meaningfully with communities at risk of flooding. The authors of this chapter became involved as community members when *HighWaterLine* was initiated in Bristol in 2014 (HighWaterLine, n.d.). The project avoided relying on 'obvious' partners and worked to build a broad and autonomous group – the process of planning and negotiating became a primary component of the work. The ensuing encounters and relationships have had multiple spin-off effects – for example an initiative to 'sunlight' a culverted stream in Greville Smyth Park and create a soft flood-management scheme, which – despite lack of funding and difficulties engaging local government support – has persisted thanks to the continuing efforts of residents inspired by the project.

Art practice can often have immediate practical and political effects – Beuys, for example, had an influential role in the emergence of environmental politics in Germany, establishing the Free International University for Creativity and Interdisciplinary Research (1973) and founding the German Green Party. Together, the three characteristics we have here outlined – *embracing uncertainty, expanded frames of reference* and *creative language* – offer a different way of thinking about both community and resilience when working in a socially-engaged setting. What is at stake in all the examples above is a redistribution in relations of power – situating the conditions of possibility for resilience in the different ways people can come together to understand both trauma and opportunity in new ways, and to imagine and demand a different world. In the following section, we look again at the role of these three concepts as expressed in a brief case study of our own joint work, and discuss some of the practical considerations we encountered, in attempting to enact them in practice.

Some: when – a brief case study

Many of the themes discussed in this chapter are illustrated in the authors' ongoing collaborative project *Some:when – celebrating cohesion through the watery heritage of the Somerset Moors and Levels*. Initiated by the artists in response to severe flooding in Somerset, England, in the winter of 2013–14, *Some:when* is based mainly in the vicinity of Langport, on the River Parrett. The process so far has involved a series of workshops (see Figure 13.3), encounters, journeys and public events centred around

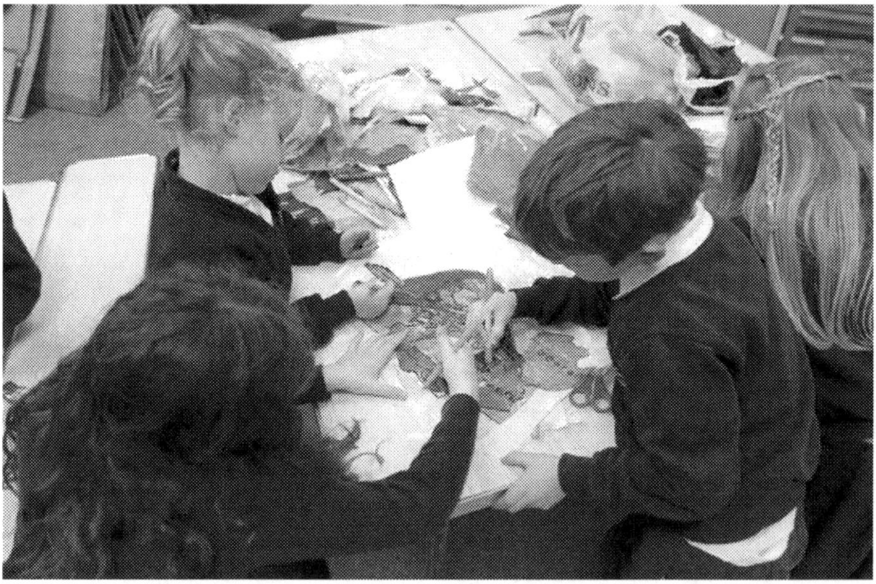

Figure 13.3 Some: when Project, 2014–5 Students at Curry Mallet CofE Primary School, Somerset, making collages from reclaimed plastic bags and wrappers as part of a workshop exploring Somerset's watery pasts and futures.

Source: Seila Fernández Arconada.

the construction of a Somerset 'flatner': a traditional flat-bottomed boat. This working craft was built for use on the region's numerous waterways, but also features conspicuously in the photographic record and community memory as a mode of transport in times of flood (Seaton, 2013; Smylie, 2012) – celebrated as a practical and affordable solution for navigating life in a changeable environment. The boat was chosen as a focal point for the project to highlight the centrality of both water and human ingenuity in shaping the history of life on the levels, and to evoke the past resilience of local communities in relation to present uncertainty.

Recent flooding has raised significant controversy around questions of how water can and should be managed in Somerset (Bates, 2014; British Broadcasting Corporation, 2014). The gestural and short-term political responses exacerbated controversy while doing little to resolve the questions. Flooding was framed as an exceptional traumatic event, with little attention to what flooding revealed about longer term problematic relationships. The *Some:when* project was conceived as a counter to this kind of reactive approach, which reinforces a particular model of resilience – based on resistance to crisis events rather than substantive change and adaptation to meet future challenges. We were struck by the discrepancy between public representation of the issues, and the kind of active discussion we saw taking place among community networks, both on the ground and through social media (see for example Flooding on the Levels Action Group, n.d.). Noting the inadequacy of top-down approaches to negotiating how we live in and with this changeable landscape, we began to draw connections to the longer history of flooding on the Moors and Levels, and ask how routes to resilience could be found in a deep and sustained relationship to landscape.

With *Some: when* we hoped to offer a new way of working with these questions, and an affirmative framework to counter the reductive presentation of public discourse. As a creative language, this framework offered a different way of bringing people together to address a potentially divisive theme. It was also chosen to suggest another frame of reference for thinking about flooding – embracing uncertainty as a generative force in the cultural history of the region, and in the development of the specific art project. Importantly, this way of working brought together a range of people to extend these ideas beyond our original concept as initiating artists. The flatner was built by hand in Langport using a mix of reclaimed and new materials (as well as skill and expertise) sourced variously from participants and local benefactors. The processes of negotiation, collaboration and celebration that accompanied the making of the boat were used to open space for conversations and encounters that approached difficult issues – flood management, land use, climate change and community politics – in a new way.

Our evocation of past resilience provided a starting point for participants to develop and share new frames of reference. At times this framing became simply an opportunity to engage with local heritage, while others seized the inspiration to imagine possible responses to current and future challenges. Providing a framework that people could relate to from different standpoints was also a playful way of bringing people together who might otherwise have been already divided along habitual lines determined by existing interests and agendas. Artistic practice was used as a different way in to looking at complex dynamics of power, access and privilege which shape responses to these issues, and to support a lively and constructive dynamic across habitual divisions. That this was realised to some degree was affirmed for us by participants, who noted as an achievement that *Some:when* events were attended by groups and individuals not normally seen together.

The project also connected with, and was shaped by, active currents within the local community. The creative space opened around the process of making the boat brought new energy and inspiration for groups such as the River Users' Group and Transition Town Movement. Dependence upon the good will and involvement of community members helped shape the project to suit participant's desires and interests. For example, a procession which carried the boat from the historic wharf to the town hall was intended partly to highlight issues of restricted access to the river, which is managed by the Environment Agency with minimal involvement of residents (see Figure 13.4). Without further research on the role of *Some: when* in contributing to broader social and political processes that took place at the time, we would avoid making claims for the direct effects of the project

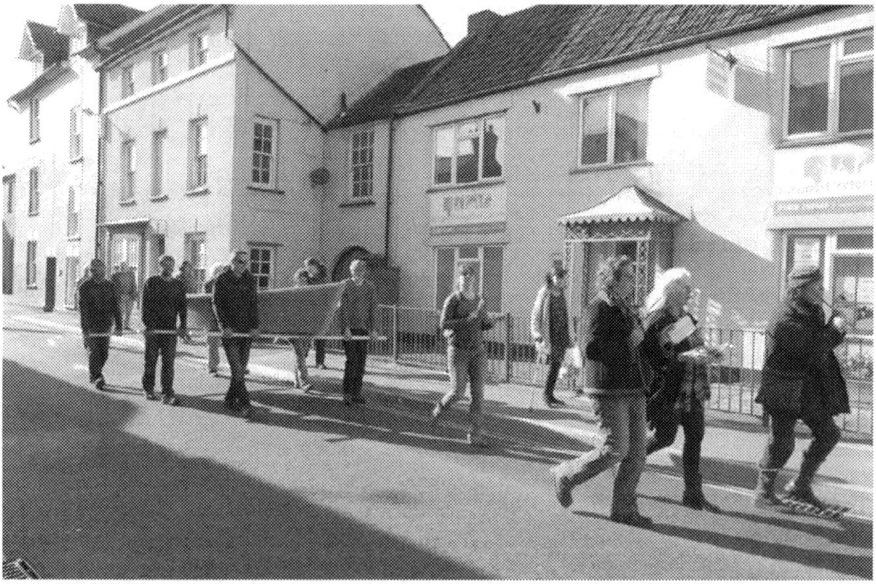

Figure 13.4 Some: when project – procession along Bow Street, Langport, 2015.
Source: Some: when project, anonymous workshop participant.

at this stage. One place we might start such an enquiry, however, is with participants of *Some: when* who, towards the end of the project, acted to diversify local government by collectively standing as candidates and so forcing an election. This could be a interesting study, but would require the kind of long-term, qualitative follow-up for which provision is lamentably rare in art funding, as in research.

Adopting uncertainty as a principle, and developing the project through dialogical process with participants, offered a different kind of imaginative space for political engagement which we saw people take up in their own lives. Importantly for the question of assessing resilience impacts, our way of working was embedded within existing contexts and was taken up by participants in relation to their own aspirations and concerns. We did not seek to maintain ownership of project outcomes, but attended instead to the integrity of our own authorial voices, as participants within a dynamic relationship.

The funding structure of the project became a factor in different ways, which both helped and hindered our attempts to contribute meaningfully to local communities. *Some:when* began in 2014 as an independent initiative rooted in our shared long-term interest in the area – not, as is usually the case, in response to a formalised artist opportunity. The project was funded initially by a small grant from the Somerset Community Foundation – later extended through crowdfunding and small business donations – and relied to a great extent on the active hospitality and participation of local residents.

Material concerns such as sourcing space, tools and materials for construction marked both the strengths and weaknesses of the project. The shared hunt for practical solutions became an immediate way for participants to take ownership from the start and facilitated the kind of dialogical relationship we have described above. At the same time, this framework raised the risk of placing a strain upon local resources which – though freely shared – we, as the artists, were not suitably placed to evaluate against any possible contribution or benefits of the project.

Finally, funding has been a significant constraint on the scope of the project – *Some: when* continues to have a gallery presence, but at the time of writing this is somewhat removed from the original community context, and it has been difficult to return to Langport to initiate a new stage for the work. Concerns that are briefly addressed in an art or research context often remain present and dynamic for the communities involved, after funding for artists or researchers has run out (Belfiore, 2002, p. 97). This is well articulated in the informal feedback we have received from participants, for example Annie Shillabeer, a youth worker very actively involved in the project, who described: "the joy of seeing the finished boat on the river and everyone's happiness, and thinking: 'this is just the start'" (see Figure 13.5).

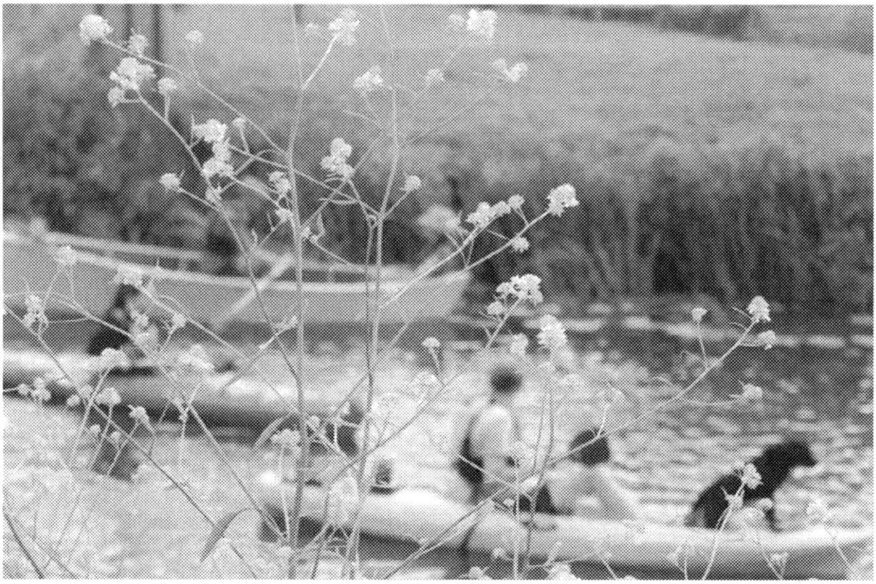

Figure 13.5 Some: when project – launching the flatner on the River Parrett.
Source: Simon Lee Dicker.

Conclusion

In this chapter, we have asked how insights from the theory and practice of socially engaged art can contribute to a wider understanding of resilience in the social sciences and beyond. We have looked at the frameworks that socially-engaged art offers, for thinking about the resilience of communities, and about how resilience might be supported through dialogic exchange and collaboration.

We have observed that resilience as a concept has multiple readings and applications, and suggested that a transformative approach is necessary, if resilience thinking is to avoid either replicating or obscuring the influence of structural disadvantage on the relative vulnerability of particular communities. Drawing on our own work and that of other socially-engaged artists, we have shown that transformative approaches can be entwined with immediate and practical outcomes through the capacity of art to work simultaneously at multiple registers.

We have discussed some of the ways in which artistic practice, in particular, offers new skills for engaging productively with uncertainty, generating expanded frames of reference, and building meaningful relations across perceived boundaries. We have shown that artistic practice offers routes to both greater cohesion and critical engagement when working with communities to promote greater resilience.

Finally, we have discussed some of the barriers to working productively in community settings, noting that the limitations of current funding schemes may restrict both the long-term meaningful contribution of socially-engaged art projects to the resilience of communities, and the capacity to evaluate and assess their impact to inform future policy. If we are to develop models of practice which meaningfully support community resilience, then, we suggest two things are important. On the one hand, supporting longer term involvement and follow-up evaluation on the part of artists and researchers, and on the other, finding ways of ensuring that short-term involvement facilitates and enables autonomous longer-term initiatives or sustainable afterlives within local community contexts.

While we find little value in uncritical treatments of socially-engaged art as a panacea for social problems or a tool for effecting community 'improvement', we conclude that that socially-engaged art does offer significant methodological and theoretical insights to the project of supporting community resilience, not least because of a long history of critical engagement with the challenges of working meaningfully in community settings.

Notes

1 A version of this chapter was first presented at the conference 'Resilience – Just Do It?', at the University of Groningen, 9 and 10 October 2014.

2 When discussing co-production and socially-engaged practice, it is difficult to avoid using the word 'community', despite its shortcomings. We have therefore tried instead to avoid the definite article and the unqualified singular form of the word; the implication being that we see community as always porous, fluid and contradictory rather than fixed and discrete.

References

Adger, W. N. (2000) 'Social and ecological resilience: Are they related?', *Progress in Human Geography*, 24(3), 347–364.

Apel, H., Thieken, A. H., Merz, B. & Blöschl, G. (2004) 'Flood risk assessment and associated uncertainty', *Natural Hazards and Earth System Science*, 4(2), 295–308.

Askins, K. & Pain, R. (2011) 'Contact zones: Participation, materiality, and the messiness of interaction', *Environment and Planning D: Society and Space*, 29(5), 803–821.

Bates, P. (2014) '*Flood Crisis: Dredging is a Simplistic Response to a Complex Problem*', The Guardian, 12th February [Online]. Available at: www.theguardian.com/environment/2014/feb/12/flood-crisis-dredging-climate-change [Accessed: 29/03/2016].

The Battle of Orgreave (2002) Directed by Mike Figgis, Jeremy Deller [Film]. Cornerhouse.

Belfiore, E. (2002) 'Art as a means of alleviating social exclusion: Does it really work? A critique of instrumental cultural policies and social impact studies in the UK', *International Journal of Cultural Policy*, 8(1), 91–106.

Bishop, C. (2005) 'The social turn: Collaboration and its discontents', *Artforum International*, 44(6), 178.
Bishop, C. (2006) 'Another turn (The "Social Turn: Collaboration and Its Discontents" by Claire Bishop) – Claire Bishop responds', *Artforum International*, 44(9), 24.
Bishop, C. (2012) *Artificial Hells: Participatory Art and the Politics of Spectatorship*, London, Verso Books.
Brint, S. (2001) 'Gemeinschaft revisited: A critique and reconstruction of the community concept', *Sociological Theory*, 199(1), 1–23.
British Broadcasting Corporation (2014) *'Somerset Floods Crisis: How the Story Unfolded'*, BBC News, 19 March [Online]. Available at: www.bbc.com/news/uk-england-somerset-26157538 [Accessed: 29/03/2016].
Brose, D. A. (2015) *Developing a Framework for Measuring Community Resilience, Washington (DC)*, National Academies Press (US) [Online]. Available at: www.ncbi.nlm.nih.gov/books/NBK285734/ [Accessed: 31/03/2016].
Bruguera, T. (2011) *'Introduction on Useful Art'*, New York, Corona, Queens, United States, 23 April [Online]. Available at: www.youtube.com/user/immigrantmove?blend=22&ob=5#p/u/4/MKPPmmNVuAs [Accessed: 1/11/2014].
Elms, D. (2015) 'Improving community resilience to natural events', *Civil Engineering and Environmental Systems*, 32(1–2), 77–89.
Evans, B. & Reid, J. (2014) *Resilient Life: The Art of Living Dangerously*, Cambridge, Polity.
Flooding on the Levels Action Group (n.d.) 'FLAG Flooding on the Levels Action Group – Facebook Group', Facebook [Online]. Available at: www.facebook.com/groups/FLAGSomerset/?fref=ts [Accessed: 29/03/2016].
Flowerdew, R. & Martin, D. (2005) *Methods in Human Geography*, 2nd ed., Harlow, Prentice Hall.
Foucault, M. (1991) '[1984] Interviewed by Rabinow, P. & Dreyfus, H. L.', New edition. In Rabinow, P. (Ed.), *The Foucault Reader: An Introduction to Foucault's Thought*, London: Penguin Books.
Gaventa, J. & Cornwall, A. (2006) 'Challenging the boundaries of the possible: Participation, knowledge and power', *IDS Bulletin*, 37(6), 122–128.
Hayward, C. R. (2000) *De-Facing Power*, Cambridge, Cambridge University Press.
Hesse-Honegger, C. (2001) *Heteroptera: The Beautiful and the Other, or Images of a Mutating World*, Zurich: Scalo Publishers.
HighWaterLine (n.d.) 'Bristol HighWaterLine', [Online]. Available at: http://bristol.highwaterline.org/ [Accessed: 18/07/2016].
Kester, G. (2000) 'Dialogical aesthetics: A critical framework for littoral art', *Variant*, 2(9).
Kester, G. (2006) 'Another turn (The "Social Turn – Collaboration and Its Discontents" by Claire Bishop)', *Artforum International*, 44(9), 22.
Körner, S. & Bellin-Harder, F. (2009) 'The 7000 Eichen of Joseph Beuys – experiences after twenty-five years', *Journal of Landscape Architecture*, 4(2), 6–19.
Lowe, T. (2012) *'A Quality Framework For Helix Arts' Participatory Practice'*, Helix Arts.
Macpherson, H., Hart, A. & Heaver, B. (2012) *Building Resilience through Collaborative Community Arts Practice: A Scoping Study with Disabled Young People and those Facing Mental Health Complexity*, Connected Communities.

Macpherson, H., Hart, A. & Heaver, B. (2014) 'Impacts between academic researchers and community partners: Some critical reflections on impact agendas in a "visual arts for resilience" research project', *ACME*, 13(1), 27–32.

Massumi, B. (2009) 'National enterprise emergency: Steps toward an ecology of powers', *Theory, Culture & Society*, 26(6), 153–185.

Matarasso, F. (2013) 'Creative progression reflections on quality in participatory arts', *UESCO Observatory Multi-Disciplinary Journal in the ARts*, 3(3), 1–15.

McEwen, L. & Jones, O. (2012) 'Building local/lay flood knowledges into community flood resilience planning after the July 2007 floods, Gloucestershire, UK', *Hydrology Research*, 43(5), 675–688.

McEwen, L., Reeves, D., Brice, J., Kam Meadley, F., Lewis, K. & MacDonald, N. (2012) 'Archiving memories of changing flood risk: Interdisciplinary explorations around knowledge for resilience', *Journal of Arts and Communities*, 4(1) 46–74.

Nadir, L. C. (2015) 'Walking the edge of the earth', *American Scientist*, 103(2), 110.

Rasmussen, M. B. (2009) 'The politics of interventionist art: The situationist international, artist placement group, and art workers' coalition', *Rethinking Marxism*, 21(1), 34–49.

Reyes, J. D. (2014) '*What Are We Trying to Get Ahead of?: Leaving the Idea of the Avant-Garde Behind*', A Blade of Grass [Online]. Available at: www.abladeofgrass.org/growing-dialogue/growing-dialogue-the-latest-thing-3/ [Accessed: 1/04/2016].

Seaton, J. (2013) *Langport & Huish Episcopi Through Time*, Stroud, Gloucestershire, Amberley Publishing.

Smith, N. (2006) '*There's No Such Thing as a Natural Disaster*', Understanding Katrina [Online]. Available at: http://understandingkatrina.ssrc.org/Smith [Accessed: 9/01/2011].

Smylie, M. (2012) *The Boats of the Somerset Levels*, Chalford, Amberley Publishing.

Tate (n.d.) '*APG: Artist Placement Group | Tate*', Tate Learn Online Resources [Online]. Available at: www2.tate.org.uk/artistplacementgroup/default.htm [Accessed: 18/07/2016].

Thompson, N. (2012) *Living as Form: Socially Engaged Art from 1991–2011*, Cambridge, MA, MIT Press.

Weintraub, L. (2012) *To Life! Eco Art in Pursuit of a Sustainable Planet*, Oakland, University of California Press.

When Faith Moves Mountains (the making of) (2002) Directed by F. Alys, C. Medina, & R. Ortega [Film]. Public Domain, 13:21.

Whittle, R., Medd, W., Deeming, H., Kashefi, E., Mort, M., Twigger Ross, C., Walker, G. & Watson, N. (2010) *After the Rain – Learning The Lessons From Flood Recovery in Hull, Final Project Report for 'Flood, Vulnerability and Urban Resilience: A Real-time Study of Local Recovery Following the Floods of June 2007 in Hull'*, Lancaster, UK, Lancaster University [Online]. Available at: www.lancaster.ac.uk/lec/sites/cswm/Hull%20Floods%20Project/AFTER%20THE%20RAIN%20FINAL%20REPORT.pdf [Accessed: 30/03/2016].

14 Resilience in practice – a transformative approach?

A conversation with Henk Ovink, first Dutch special envoy for international water affairs

Melanie M. Bakema and Britta Restemeyer

In 2015 Henk Ovink was appointed as the first Special Envoy for International Water Affairs in the Netherlands. It was an entirely new position with global outreach in the Dutch policy landscape. Ovink, who is also called 'the ambassador for the Dutch water sector' describes his role as a 'connector'. He travels to vulnerable places around the globe to connect foreign stakeholders to Dutch governments, businesses and research organizations, helping with Dutch expertise on water management where needed and desired. Among others, the governments of the United States, South Africa, Myanmar, Vietnam, and India have asked for Henk Ovink's advice in organizing policy processes, usually in relation to a recent water-related crisis. Prior to his position as a Water Envoy, Ovink was part of President Obama's Rebuilding Task Force in the United States of America after hurricane Sandy had severely damaged the New York region.

Henk Ovink works with governments, knowledge institutions, organizations such as the World Bank and the UN, the global business community as well as the civil society representatives. 'Building' resilience in vulnerable places especially in relation to water-related hazards are key aspects of his daily work. As, in addition to the above, his job offers Ovink the chance to see different policy contexts and cultures, the editors of this volume considered it valuable to gain an insight into Ovink's expertise of 'building' resilience on the international level. Melanie Bakema and Britta Restemeyer talked to Henk Ovink about his understanding of resilience, his vision on how to 'build' resilience in vulnerable places – something that Ovink terms 'the transformative approach' – and the lessons to learn from Ovink's experiences in the Netherlands as well as his projects around the world.

A special envoy for international water affairs – Why have the Netherlands created such a position?

Since the Netherlands is the only country with a position of 'a special water envoy', before enquiring further about resilience, we wanted to know a bit more about the position and the perception of Henk Ovink on this special role. It may appear logical for the Netherlands to be pioneers in the field of water management, with many parts of the country lying below sea level and Dutch water managers being renowned as 'conquerors of the sea'. But what specifically is the Netherlands' ambition with a Special Envoy for International Water Affairs? Is it philanthropy or ideology-driven, bringing Dutch expertise to vulnerable countries, or is it rather economy-driven with the underlying goal of bringing new projects to Dutch companies?

According to Ovink, it is a bit of both. Ovink explains:

> "Our Dutch Delta Approach is acknowledged worldwide and is attractive for nations, institutions, cities, NGO's and others around the globe. Our leadership emerged by distinctively managing our risks and uncertainties. Together with our global partners, we are now striving for comprehensive water security approaches worldwide: better policies, better governance, increased investments and innovations to face future risks and uncertainties, of course in partnership with Dutch governments, businesses and research organizations."

Henk Ovink's mission

Ovink's personal ambition and goals for his position are far from modest: "My water envoy's ambition? A new narrative, better partnerships and a whole new range of projects to inspire the world." For Ovink, the new narrative starts with acknowledging the complexity of what he calls the global water crisis and its impacts on society, referring to problems with both water quantity, as in floods and droughts and water quality, referring to hygiene of water to people and ecosystems. Ovink emphasizes that "water is at the heart of our uncertain future; it is through water that we feel the impact of climate change the most." According to Ovink, water is essential for our economy, our social and cultural well-being, since it is key to our food and energy production. However, Ovink also stresses the downsides of water: "The World Water Development Report of 2012 shows that of all worldwide disasters, 90% are water-related." Ovink, therefore, emphasizes that water can be an asset if managed right, but a severe risk if not.

By working on a better understanding of the complexity of the water crisis, Ovink hopes to find answers to questions like how to intervene, what actions can work, and where to start? To do this, Ovink is working on building partnerships "with institutional and non-institutional partners across the world, where different governments, businesses and research organizations circulate their knowledge, expertise and experience to help enforce water resilience approaches across the globe." Furthermore, he is striving for a 'global water innovation portfolio' which he is setting up with programmatic funding by the World Bank, other International Financial Institutions (IFI's), the Green Climate Fund and public and private investors. According to Henk Ovink, this global innovation portfolio aims at "finding the water-hotspots of the world, where all forces intertwine and subsequently define interventions that are catalytic, transformative and that can become inspirations to be scaled up and replicated for the globe."

Henk Ovink's understanding of resilience and his vision: the 'transformative approach'

In the light of the global water crisis, Ovink sees many reasons to seek for a new governance approach. According to Ovink, people are actively provoking a manmade ecological disaster without a true understanding of this ecological downfall and its impact on the economy (among other things). As an example, Ovink points out that 50% of the world's aquifers – our natural groundwater storage capacity – are beyond their tipping point, meaning that a natural recovery has become impossible. He, therefore, calls for a transition in the way risks and vulnerabilities are managed worldwide. According to Ovink, moving from response to preparedness – a shift from a rather reactive to a more proactive approach – should be central in every governance approach which focuses on management of (water) risks and disasters. Ovink disagrees with the so-called 'bounce-back' understanding of resilience, where the goal for the system would be to return to the state prior to the disaster as quickly as possible. Instead, Ovink argues that resilience is "about bouncing back differently and smarter, through collaboration, innovation and the best of science." This sounds beautiful in theory but how can this be achieved in practice?

Over the years, the Dutchman has developed what he terms 'the transformative approach,' "an approach with impact and transformative capacity, to help create an enabling environment where better science, research and data will find solid ground." In this context, Ovink stresses that "innovation and implementation should go hand in hand with inclusive collaborations across all sectors, all layers of government, all stakeholders from activists and vulnerable communities to private and public institutions." Based on his own visions and beliefs about how to stimulate change as well as experiences from the Netherlands and abroad, Ovink argues that 'building' resilience in practice requires five main ingredients:

1 *long-term planning coupled with short-term projects* in order to create a comprehensive approach and at the same time stimulate innovation;
2 *an inclusive and collaborative process*, in which partners of different backgrounds, experts as well as local inhabitants, would work towards a regional and comprehensive understanding of the problem and ideally create tailor-made responses;
3 *institutional capacity*, as the state needs to be capable of enabling an inclusive and collaborative approach coupled with *capacity building* among all stakeholders,

4 *funding and public-private partnerships*, which should ideally be built on trust and mutual gains to find new ways of financing;
5 and *monitoring and better cost-benefit-analyses* to evaluate the processes.

With respect to the latter point, Ovink addresses scientists, in particular, to develop new approaches since according to him, current cost-benefit-analyses lack the capacity to capture long-term, integrated approaches.

Ovink's 'transformative approach' sounds very promising, but also as a rather utopian policy process rarely encountered in practice. When asked whether his approach is not rather difficult to realize, Ovink enthusiastically declares: "No, it can be done! Currently, the rather slow pace of climate change causes a slow approach and a focus on reactive response, not a pro-active approach to preparedness. But we have a choice to make!" Clearly, Henk Ovink takes an optimistic stance, believing in the capacity of humans to bring about a global change. Nevertheless, Ovink adds: "I am not saying that change is easy, it is extremely hard to escape from existing conditions."

According to Henk Ovink,

> "change, unfortunately, often comes from situations that are very disruptive. Or, you need to organize a process that is taking place outside of existing frameworks. In that way, you create enough latitude for the transformative approach without it being fully detached. I like to call this a 'sabbatical detour', a step aside."

A 'sabbatical detour' is, according to Ovink, necessary to make room for change. However, such a detour must go in parallel and in interaction with the existing processes and conditions. The lessons from a detour need to be connected to the existing governance structures and processes.

> "It should not be the case that two separate governments are created; you need to bring the lessons back [to existing structures – eds.], you need to dare to test, learn and improve. Transparency, accountability, monitoring and evaluation are therefore highly relevant, otherwise we do not learn anything, or if we do there is no impact."

In addition, Ovink describes a set of principles that such a sabbatical detour within our governance processes needs to meet. First, it is important to not aim for solutions, but to focus on a collaborative process for getting a better understanding of the problem(s), since the complexity of present-day societal conditions is mostly determined by a myriad of issues, interdependent challenges and their impacts, a complex context, multiple partners and a variety of consequences. Second, through this process of enhancing our understanding, we must build capacity among all stakeholders to not only deal with these issues in one single project but to keep on dealing with them in a continuous and progressive way.

His emphasis on the necessity of inclusive and context-sensitive governance processes indicates that Ovink does not believe the transformative approach to be a blueprint for the world; instead, a regional (or eventually even local) interpretation is essential for success. In addition to the idea of sabbatical detour, during our conversation, Ovink drew out three main lessons based on his experiences with water governance processes in New York, Bangladesh, India, South Africa and the Netherlands. The three lessons, which are discussed below, are according to Henk Ovink essential for stimulating change and thereby making vulnerable places more resilient.

Lesson one: resilience – the importance of context and culture

Being sensitive to contextual and cultural factors is, according to Henk Ovink, a first very important lesson to take into consideration in the implementation of resilience strategies. Ovink passionately introduces the Dutch tradition of consensus building and working collaboratively in planning processes. Ovink points out the relevance of the so-called Dutch 'polder model' – a tradition of collaboratively searching for the best solutions to gain new land from water, which is strongly interwoven in the Dutch (planning) culture. Often, the Dutch experts tend to think that such model can be simply copied to other contexts. But a successful approach in one context is not a guarantee for success in another – the context and culture should not be overlooked to determine likeliness for success.

Ovink exemplifies this statement with the case of Bangladesh. The Dutch team of experts that was asked to give advice to Bangladesh initiated a coalition of different (local) stakeholders and various Dutch organizations which developed a 'Delta Plan for Bangladesh'. The plan is developed and enacted in 2016 and is aimed at making Bangladesh a more 'socially and technically' resilient delta. The delta of Bangladesh is the largest delta in the world and very complex, because of the large system of connected rivers and river basins. "One could say that this delta plan assures Bangladesh of a long-term approach for increasing its resilience. However, without institutional and human capacity, in the long run, this comprehensive strategy does not have ownership, meaning or added value." Henk Ovink is afraid that in the case of Bangladesh too much focus is on technological innovations, without paying any attention to the cultural innovation that is needed for a Delta Plan to succeed. In the Dutch context, the 'polder model' has been developed over centuries, which makes a Delta Plan in the Netherlands an appropriate and indeed successful instrument. Without such long-term experiences and decision-making culture, there is a risk that in Bangladesh projects aiming to copy the Dutch approach become standalone short-term interventions, without the necessary regional linkage and long-term perspective, Ovink argues. In his opinion, the plan with an integral resilience vision should go beyond technical innovations in order to trigger cultural innovation. Ovink explains:

> "I am not saying that the whole world needs to become like the Netherlands, not at all! I am saying the contrary; we do not have to think that what we do in the Netherlands is automatically appropriate for Bangladesh."

An important lesson that we can draw from this case is, therefore, to indeed obtain inspiration from the best practices of the Dutch case and spread it in a case-specific way to Bangladesh, taking into close account the cultural and contextual characteristics of Bangladesh.

However, Ovink also points out that it is too simplistic to see culture only as barrier for resilience strategies. He illustrates his argument with an example from Chennai in India where he was working after the floods of December 2015. Ovink was invited to Chennai directly after the floods to discuss and explore potential courses of action with international and local stakeholders. During the visit, Ovink noticed a big 'drive' and willingness among people to work collaboratively and learn together for the rebuilding challenge. Ovink was particularly impressed by the process; everyone was invited to meet with the international experts, including the most vocal community leader and the former alderman of the city who had to step down right after the disaster had occurred. "Where do you experience this? The former alderman sitting there, without a sense of personal revenge, trying to work on the problems and solutions as much as everyone else," Ovink exclaims. When he asked the local people and authorities in India where such willingness to collaborate comes from, he was told that part of the reason lies in the Tamil culture. It appeared to be a relevant part of the religion and culture of the local people to collaborate, to have all people together in one room regardless of their 'status' – the high officials together with the 'lay' people –, to discuss the shared issues, be transparent and by doing that, develop trust in each other. Ovink was positively surprised that during such meetings, there was no finger-pointing and that the people appeared to be completely honest about the vulnerabilities of their area towards the international visitors. As Ovink explains: "people were still proud [despite the disaster – eds.] and wanted to show their city, but they also did not hide anything." Although the recovery process is still ongoing, the culture in Chennai makes Henk Ovink optimistic about the future of this extremely vulnerable area.

Lesson two: the importance of political leadership in promoting 'movements for resilience'

The second lesson Henk Ovink draws out based on his experiences is the importance of leadership, which Ovink illustrates with examples from the US and South Africa.

When Barack Obama had just been inaugurated as the president of the United States in 2009, he spoke the famous words: "No Katrina on my watch". Soon after he was installed, Obama implemented a strategy to be prepared for a hazard such as a hurricane and by doing this, he distanced himself from his predecessor George W. Bush who did not take immediate action after Hurricane Katrina hit New Orleans. To develop a disaster preparedness strategy, Obama asked the ministers of Housing and Homeland Security at the beginning of his presidency to develop a new framework for disaster management, which would be operationalized in the case another disaster like Katrina would take place. And a disaster did indeed happen.

In 2012 hurricane Sandy hit the North East coast of the US, including the city of New York. This disaster revealed the vulnerability, tensions and disconnection between politics and people in the region. However, according to Ovink, New York and the federal government were ready to respond. In the turbulent period after the storm, Barack Obama installed the Hurricane Sandy Rebuilding Task Force, consisting of the heads of more than twenty federal departments, agencies or offices and headed by the (at the time) Secretary of Housing and Urban Development (HUD) Shaun Donovan.

During our conversation, Ovink explained that "as a signal and gesture [of solidarity – eds.], Obama went immediately to the region to show his commitment and dedication to provide first-aid quickly and start the rebuilding as soon as possible". Obama had declared: "Cut bureaucracy! We need help on the ground, now! Rebuilding and relief efforts that are struck because of default processes are not allowed." With his dedication, Barack Obama had, according to Ovink, implicitly made room for innovation and rethinking existing policies.

Building on the immediate action after Sandy, successes and preparedness that were possible because of already existing disaster management strategies, Obama also aimed to ensure a good recovery after Sandy, to "rebuild better". This ultimately resulted in the 'Rebuild by Design' program developed and led by Henk Ovink. Rebuild by Design brought together stakeholders from regional and local governments, private businesses and people from the communities and connected them to international experts in architecture, engineering, planning, ecology and design. Together these teams researched the interdependencies, vulnerabilities and opportunities of the region. Figure 14.1 represents one of the meetings in this collaborative designing process. The teams identified 42-proposals, each one of them aimed at increasing the resilience of the region. Ten project-plans across the region were developed with local coalitions of which six – the "winners" – are currently being realized in practice. Among these six are plans for Manhattan (the 'Big U', a comprehensive system in which the land is divided into compartments using landscaping and engineering measures to improve flood protection as well as social, economic and ecological services of the area) and Staten Island ('Living Breakwaters', using artificial oyster reefs as a protection shield).

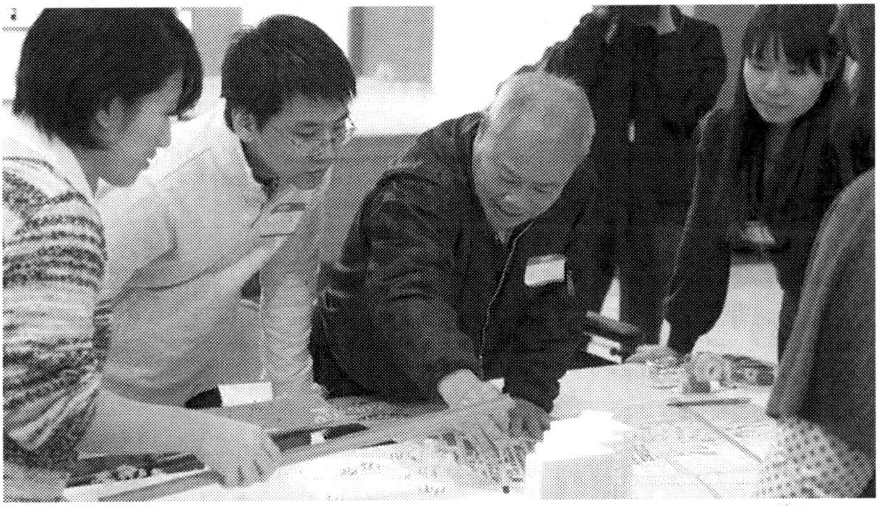

Figure 14.1 Collaborative design process in Rebuild by Design.
Source: Rebuild by Design/The BIG Team.

Recently, the OECD embraced Rebuild by Design as an inspiration for public-private partnerships and the UN presented it as an example for 'Institutional arrangements for national adaptation planning and implementation in the context of climate change'.

> "With Rebuild by Design a large and inspired coalition of stakeholders joined forces with the ambition to set a new standard for resilient development. Teams of engineers, scientists, architects and activists from all over the world came together with different levels of government, federal, state and local."

Henk Ovink proudly states. Supported by funding agencies such as the Rockefeller Foundation, Rebuild by Design evolved into a "movement for resilience" as Henk Ovink puts it.

According to Ovink, "Rebuild by Design would not have been possible without the political support of President Obama and the leadership of Secretary Shaun Donovan." The special Task Force that was set to work as a result enabled an inclusive process and facilitated the collaboration between people and policy-makers, which was highly important in getting political support for the eventual rebuilding efforts. Ovink praises the politicians who in the case of Hurricane Sandy did not get stuck at the borders defined by jurisdiction but followed what they believed to be the right response. "The issues at stake and the ecological and economic interdependencies cut across nations, states and cities. Understanding this complexity, perceiving the issues on this larger scale is where good politics started in the case of Hurricane Sandy," Ovink concludes.

In the case of South Africa, the political context was very different, but political leadership again played a crucial role in promoting a resilience strategy. Henk Ovink elaborates on his experiences there: "In South Africa, the problem is that there is at the same time too much, too little and too dirty water, and all three problems will even be exacerbated by climate change and economic, demographic and political challenges." Ovink explains that the problems are especially acute in the context of a lack of institutional capacity to deal with the above water issues on a regional level. Therefore, a water program called 'King Fisher', promoting an integral and long-term governance approach to deal with the problems at hand was established. Whereas in the case of Rebuild by Design the institutional context was largely shaped by the Task Force, and the leadership of President Obama and Secretary of Housing and Urban Development, in the case of King Fisher and South-Africa this political leadership was exercised by one woman, the Minister of Water Affairs and Sanitation, Nomvula Mokonyane. Mokonyane implemented a very strict strategy to get the water problems on the political agenda. "Since Mokonyane was convinced that implementing a strict water policy strategy was the only way to move things forward, she decided to be not three, but ten steps ahead of her political organization," Ovink explains. The strategy that Minister Mokonyane was pursuing was to set up a national water governance framework, including thirteen water catchment management agencies, through collaborations with Dutch organizations, regional partners and local initiatives. The Minister managed to get funding for her ambitious plan from international donor organizations such as the World Bank and the World Economic Forum.

> "This coalition has been able to implement innovative pilots and although it might be too early to judge whether all these initiatives add up to robust approach and long term success in water management, we can say that due to the political ambition of one minister and her taking the lead, we can see things moving on all levels, and moreover, in cooperation."

The experiences of Henk Ovink in both, US and South Africa, thus highlight the relevance of political leadership for stimulating change: strong leadership helps to set the problem on the political agenda, to form coalitions and to acquire adequate funding. Political leadership alone, however, does not provide guidelines about *how* to set up a collaborative process and *how* to create linkages between policy-makers and the (local) community. Confronted with the question of 'how' to set up a successful collaborative process and stimulate interaction, based on his experiences, Henk Ovink stresses the potential role of design. Ovink considers design to be both, a process and an instrument for collaborative policy making which is also the last important lesson he draws from his experiences.

Lesson three: the potential of design as an instrument to stimulate change towards greater resilience

Ovink's affection towards design comes from a long personal and professional history. In 2007, he initiated the Design and Politics research program in the Netherlands and to date operates as the chief editor of the 'Design and Politics' book series with NAI010 Publishers (2007 – ongoing, The Netherlands). As a curator of the International Architecture Biennale in 2012 in Rotterdam, The Netherlands, and in his role as Director of National Spatial Planning in The Netherlands, he explored the importance of design in policy-making and the connection of design and the 'sabbatical detour' discussed above. For Ovink, the Rebuild by Design program was the ultimate opportunity to test, explore and exploit the value of design in resilience building processes. As explained above, Rebuild by Design focused on 'rebuilding better' after Hurricane Sandy. As principal of the Rebuild by Design program, Henk Ovink set up a design competition and invited teams from all over the world to participate. However, it was not a 'regular' design competition.

> "Usually you launch a request for *proposals*, which means that teams suggest ideas to solve the identified problems. In Rebuild by Design, however, we launched a request for *qualifications*. We did not want to have experts with fixed ideas [as would be the case when asking for proposals – eds.], but we wanted them to ask questions first, explore the region together and then develop ideas in collaboration with regional and local stakeholders from government, businesses and civil society. We needed the best teams with different qualifications [characteristics, expertise and backgrounds – eds.] to join us in the US, so that we would have interdisciplinary teams working on proposals together with local stakeholders," Ovink explains.

According to Ovink, using design in plan-making processes has several strengths: it helps to unravel the past, analyse the present and envision the future. But above all, "design is essential for the collaborative and inclusive process, for building the alliances that are needed for realizing change." And collaboration was necessary for solving the complex problems which had been brought to light by hurricane Sandy.

> "We [the Rebuild by Design leading team – eds.] needed the talent from the region and from the world together. You cannot do it with your neighbour only, and neither only with a professor from Japan. If you do not try to involve everybody and everything, there is no point to start."

However, despite the good intentions, practice shows that participation processes often tend to be dominated by specific groups, and it is nearly impossible to include everybody equally. The groups with the dominant presence, in general, refer to 'the white, male, elderly and highly educated', whereas the groups with the least presence include the migrants, female, young and less well-educated people. When asked about the issues of inclusion and exclusion, Henk Ovink says:

> "I know about this problem [of exclusion – eds.], but in Rebuild by Design we really involved everyone. We contacted schools and we went to community centres. We had to invest a lot of time in people, in building trust and partnerships, but it was so rewarding to see the results and impacts on the community. We built partnerships that will last a lifetime. Capacity was built up along the way, thereby creating a real environment of opportunities."

Specifically, Ovink points out the value of the *competitive element* of design.

> "I believe the competitive nature of Rebuild by Design strengthened all aspects of the plan-making process. Joining forces to win, to overcome the disaster and to lift oneself up is a cultural thing. Pride, ambition and ownership are essential and were embedded in this design approach."

According to Ovink, the research phase of the Rebuild by Design program, which was organized by New York University's Institute for Public Knowledge and its Research Advisory Group, eventually turned into a comprehensive scientific and practical exploration of the region. Through design, people got acquainted with data and research. Visualization helped to make the research and the potential strategies more tangible, where texts would have left every person with their own interpretation of the words. However, Ovink also makes clear that just like the Dutch Delta Plan, Rebuild by Design cannot be simply approached as a blueprint and simply copied to a different context. Again, a regional, tailor-made approach and the support of strong leaders would have the potential for the best resilience outcomes.

Henk Ovink's recommendation for scientists in triggering resilience

At the end of our conversation, we asked Henk Ovink whether he had some specific recommendations to scientists regarding stimulating resilience. In response, Ovink refers to his experiences with Rebuild by Design pointing out that this project was not only successful in convincing the residents and designers to start a collaborative process; it also inspired and involved scientists. "When do things go wrong in the world? When everyone sticks to their own ivory tower. When do good things start to evolve? In the moment, you bring different parties together," Ovink explains. With this book, the editors aimed to come closer to an understanding of resilience in both scientific terms, but also in developing strategies and collective actions to implement resilience in practice. The different chapters contribute to, either one or both, of these aims, and a common element in studying resilience in all cases throughout this book is the emphasis on collaborative processes to understand and create more resilient places. When viewed from the perspective of practice, that especially Henk Ovink is devoted to, openness and willingness to collaboration are not only helpful in clarifying and working with a specific concept as resilience, it is also extremely relevant in 'building' a more resilient world together.

Ovink's main recommendation to scientists is: "Dare to share, dare to collaborate. You are often afraid that you put your own credibility at risk when you do so, but in fact, you will only strengthen it." Ovink encourages scientists to be more vocal and express their opinions more strongly, especially in relation to politics and policy-making processes. In the first chapter of this edited collection prof. Simin Davoudi emphasized the need for scientists and decision-makers to be critical about using resilience in practice and the potential influence of neoliberal agendas when 'operationalizing' resilience. From a practitioner's perspective, Henk Ovink encourages scientists to take a more active role in facilitating practitioners' work with resilience. Ovink argues that scientists should position themselves in relation to politics, policy and society instead of being afraid of them: "Organize yourself within instead of outside of it [politics, policy and society – eds.]" According to Henk Ovink, academics have an important societal role and an obligation to share not only their research findings but also opinions and reflections on what's happening in the world. Ovink illustrates his point with an example:

> "In the climate change debate, we all pinpoint to politicians and policymakers [for either starting or ignoring the need for a debate – eds.], which is legitimate and logical, but what efforts have the scientists made? They have been very careful and silent for a long time. Luckily that is changing, and that is needed."

Ovink's final advice therefore is:

> "I know that if the problems and the complexity are so extensive, scientists do not have an unambiguous answer. It is challenging and exciting, but have the courage to speak up and dare to form a coalition outside of your own world, and it will help and inspire us all!"

Index

Printed in the United States
By Bookmasters